CW00621171

Formulae for calculation of drug doses and drip

Solid drugs

$$\text{amount of stock} = \frac{\text{strength required}}{\text{stock strength}}$$

Liquid drugs

$$\text{amount of stock} = \frac{\text{strength required}}{\text{stock strength}} \times \text{volume containing stock strength}$$

Drugs measured in units

$$\text{amount of stock} = \frac{\text{no. units required}}{\text{no. units in stock solution}} \times \text{volume containing stock strength}$$

Preparation of solutions

$$\text{amount of stock} = \frac{\text{strength required}}{\text{stock strength}} \times \text{final total volume}$$

Children's dose (Clarke's Body Weight Rule)

$$\text{child's dose} = \text{adult dose} \times \frac{\text{weight of child (kg)}}{\text{average adult weight (70 kg)}}$$

Children's dose (Clarke's Body Surface Area Rule)

$$\text{child's dose} = \text{adult dose} \times \frac{\text{surface area of child}}{\text{surface area of adult (1.7 m}^2\text{)}}$$

Drip flow rate

$$\text{rate (drops/min)} = \frac{\text{volume of solution (ml)} \times \text{no. drops/ml}}{\text{time (minutes)}}$$

Note
- macrodrip delivers 15 drops/ml
- microdrip delivers 60 drops/ml
- see opposite for calculation nomogram

Concentrations

1 in 1000 means 1 g in 1000 ml of solution, therefore 1 g in 1000 ml is equivalent to 1 mg in 1 ml
1% solution contains 1 g of solute in 100 ml of solution

A Nursing Guide to Drugs

Margaret Havard BSc(Melb) RN DipNEd FCNA

THIRD EDITION

CHURCHILL LIVINGSTONE
MELBOURNE EDINBURGH LONDON AND NEW YORK 1990

CHURCHILL LIVINGSTONE
Medical Division of Longman Group UK Limited

Distributed in Australia by Longman Cheshire Pty Limited,
Longman House, Kings Gardens, 95 Coventry Street,
South Melbourne 3205, and by associated companies,
branches and representatives throughout the world.

First edition 1983
Second edition 1986
Third edition 1990

ISBN 0-443-04142-3

British Library Cataloguing in Publication Data
Havard, Margaret
  A nursing guide to drugs. – 3rd ed.
  1. Drugs
  I. Title
  615'..1

Library of Congress Cataloging in Publication Data
Havard, Margaret.
    A nursing guide to drugs/Margaret Havard. — 3rd ed.
      p. cm.
    Includes bibliographical references.
    1. Pharmacology. 2. Drugs. 3. Nursing. I. Title
    [DNLM: 1. Drug Therapy – nurses' instruction. 2. Drugs — nurses'
instruction. QV 55 H383n]
    RM300.H38 1990
    615'.1 — dc20
    DNLM/DLC
    for Library of Congress   89–22299

Produced by Longman Singapore Publishers (Pte) Ltd.
Printed in Singapore

Preface to the Third Edition

Each drug has been revised, new drugs have been added, and drugs which are used rarely have been omitted. Some drugs have been moved to a group to which they are more pharmacologically allied. A new section on Drugs in Lactation has been included in Appendix 1.

I especially wish to thank Allan Manser, Deputy Chief Pharmacist at the Royal Melbourne Hospital for the resource material, advice and interest in the preparation of this edition. I am greatly indebted to Allan Manser and Roslyn Hosking, who spent considerable time in proof reading and made the resources of the Pharmacy Department so freely available to me.

Also, I wish to thank Margaret Strang whose advice and typing was invaluable in the preparation of the manuscript.

I extend my gratitude to Jean for her patience and understanding, and to my constant companion and kneewarmer, Ambrose.

Melbourne 1990   M. E. H.

Preface to the First Edition

This book has been written to assist the student nurse and the qualified nurse, both in current practice or returning after a considerable interval, to learn about drugs and administer them safely, ultimately leading to improved nursing care.

As therapeutics occupies a major place in the prevention and management of disease, there is a need for each nurse to have access to an information source both in the classroom and the clinical situation. Nurses are expected to satisfy themselves as to the route, dosage, action and adverse effects of any drug they administer, but how often has a nurse been heard to say, 'What drug is that?' This need has resulted in a collection of facts about drugs as named and used most commonly in Australasia which will provide on-the-spot information.

The drugs have been arranged in systems where practicable, depending on the main pharmacological action or use, which allows their study in conjunction with other nursing subjects. In some cases the prototype drug has been dealt with in detail followed by lighter treatment of drugs similar in origin or effect; whilst in other areas drugs with similar effects are treated as a group.

In line with the trend toward ordering drugs by the generic name, drugs are given in the text by the generic name, the proprietary names being provided in the index.

Although doses are highly individualized, they are provided as a guide, any paediatric doses being clearly distinguished from adult doses. Interactions which increase or decrease the effects of a drug have been included where significant and only the common and important adverse effects have been listed. Nursing points, collected from many sources, have been highlighted especially where care is needed to avoid toxicity. Additional points of importance are noted at the end of the section on the presented drug or group of drugs.

For quick reference, a list of common abbreviations is on the outside back cover and a nomogram for calculating surface area on the inside back cover. Inside the front cover are a nomogram for calculating intravenous infusion rates and a series of formulae for calculating stock amounts of drugs, solutions, and children's doses and intravenous infusion rates.

So this book is to be used as a guide only and does not presume to take the place of product information, compatibility charts, the pharmacist or any other recognized information source. Where doubt exists, it must be dispelled by consultation with a hospital or local pharmacist, or a major publication of drug information listed in the bibliography.

Melbourne 1983   M. E. H

ACKNOWLEDGEMENTS

I am grateful for the tremendous encouragement and support from many friends and colleagues and I would like to express my thanks especially to pharmacists Elizabeth Creber, Ken Lawrie and David Taylor for the many hours spent in the early stages of preparation, and to the pharmacists, especially Jenny Johnstone and Bronwen Smith, who checked portions of the manuscript and provided so many helpful suggestions.

M. E. H.

Contents

1 The nurse's role in drug therapy

Importance of a history

The aim is to administer medication safely and efficiently and to observe the patient for both desirable and undesirable effects. Therefore the nurse will need to know the reason the drug or preparation is being given, its main pharmacological action, the usual dose range, dose interval, route, desired effect and potential adverse effects. Any allergies or idiosyncrasies will be noted by taking a careful history. Check the patient for an *Identicare* pendant or bracelet. This will include medical information if the patient is a diabetic, epileptic, haemophiliac, on anticoagulants or cortisone, or has a drug allergy.

Legal schedules

The supply, storage and use of drugs and preparations are under the control of governments. Substances are listed under certain schedules which dictate restrictions on usage and their management. Hospitals may also enforce further limitations.

Storage

All medications in a ward or department are kept in a locked cupboard, medication trolley or some other type of locked container, the key of which is kept by a nurse at all times. Drugs or preparations for external use are stored apart from those intended for internal use. Drugs of addiction are kept in a separate locked cupboard and are recorded in a special Register. It is usually necessary or preferable to refrigerate suppositories, pessaries, insulins, antisera, vaccines, some blood products, some intravenous solutions and some antibiotics (particularly if reconstituted). The trend toward single dose units being dispensed contributes to accuracy in dosage, better economy and less risk of product contamination.

Labelling

Only a pharmacist, medical officer or dentist may label or change the label on any pharmaceutical product.

Drug orders

A drug or preparation may be given only on a written or verbal order from a medical officer which must be clearly written and/or understood verbally. To conform with State law, a legal drug order must be legibly written in ink, dated and signed by the prescriber and must include the patient's name and identification number, the name and strength of the drug, the dose, route of administration, frequency of administration and duration of administration (if applicable). Any alteration to a drug order should be initialled. An unusual dose, drug strength or quantity should be underlined and initialled by the prescriber. If there is any doubt about the meaning of the order, contact the medical officer immediately for clarification *before* administration. Check the policy of the institution before taking telephone orders for drugs. Many errors may be eliminated if the nurse ensures that the intended drug has been ordered for the right patient, writes it on the correct patient's chart, then asks a second nurse, if available, to read the drug order silently while it is read back over the telephone to the medical officer. The order is signed by the prescriber as soon as possible, within 24 hours. A list of abbreviations in common use appears on the back cover of this book. Following a medical officer's order is thought by many to absolve the nurse from all responsibility; however legal judgements have shown that this is not always the case. The nurse is required to know the route and dosage, cause and effect of any drug ordered to be given and to possess the necessary skills to carry out the order. Information on any drug or preparation may be obtained from a pharmacist. Once in possession of this knowledge, the nurse is in a position to question an unclear order, to assess if he or she has the required skills to carry out the order, and to observe the effectiveness or otherwise of the drug.

Drug dosage

The dose will depend on the age, weight, sex, renal and hepatic function and general condition of the patient, and can be based on age, body weight or body surface area. As children usually require smaller doses than adults, various rules can be used to estimate the fraction of the adult dose (see inside front cover). However, despite very careful calculation of drug doses based on these rules, a dosage calculation supported by experience sometimes allows for individual variations, especially in children and the elderly.

Dose interval is also important. Anti-infective agents are given at regular intervals, 4-, 6- or 8-hourly to maintain adequate blood levels, and hormones are given at the same time each day for uniform effect.

The time of day must be suitable; e.g. diuretics are usually given after rising and hypnotics shortly before retiring.

Drug half-life

The half-life of a drug is a function of both elimination and distribution; in general terms it is the time required for one half of the amount of drug in the body to be eliminated. It is of practical use in calculating the frequency with which multiple doses of a drug can be administered to keep the blood level between the minimum effective concentration and the threshold for toxicity.

Therapeutic drug monitoring

Serum drug concentrations are measured to determine that therapeutic levels are being achieved and to exclude toxicity. Information which must accompany a request form should include the time the blood sample was taken, the time the last dose of the drug was given and its route of administration.

Drug route

The effectiveness of a drug often depends on the route of administration. Drugs are formulated to meet the requirements for rapid or slow absorption, metabolism or excretion so as to obtain the required blood levels. An oral preparation is given on an empty stomach, but if it causes gastric irritation it is given with or immediately after food. It is recommended that a capsule be preceded by a small volume of water and then taken with half a glass of water to prevent it being held in the oesophagus.

Check the policy of the institution as to whether the buttocks or lateral aspect of the thigh is to be used for IM injections.

Refer to the latest Nurses' Board (registering body) directive and the policy of the institution as to who is authorized to give IV injections or add any agent to IV infusions. A drug may be given by direct IV injection as a bolus in a volume of 20 ml or less in under 1 minute, or by slow IV injection over 5–15 minutes. This method is used when an immediate effect is required, or the drug becomes unstable on reconstitution or dilution. The intermittent infusion method is used when a drug is diluted, when interval dosing is desired and slow administration is required. The drug is diluted in 50–250 ml and infused over 15 minutes to 2 hours. This minimizes stability and incompatibility problems and gives the 'peak' and 'trough' effect in antibiotic therapy. When a drug must be highly diluted and a steady state blood level is to be maintained, the continuous infusion method is used in which the drug is diluted in 500–1000 ml and infused over 4–24 hours, e.g. potassium chloride requires high dilution and constant blood levels to prevent depression of cardiac function.

Control of IV flow rate may be by infusion pump, microdrip set or burette. When a drug is added to the burette during intermittent infusion, details of the additive are indicated on a label which is stuck onto the burette.

Drugs are not mixed with blood or blood products. Any IV drug admixture must be prepared aseptically, mixed thoroughly and labelled with the name and amount of the additive, name of person adding the agent, name of person checking the addition and the time of starting the infusion.

An IV admixture is not administered if there are signs of physical incompatibility such as a colour change, loss of clarity or precipitate formation. Chemical and physical compatibility and stability of admixtures should be checked *before* administration. If in any doubt, consult a pharmacist or a drug information centre.

Forms of presentation

A drug may have a systemic or local effect depending on whether it is taken orally, injected or applied topically.

Oral preparations

tablet: dried powdered drug mixed with a binding base and compressed into a variety of shapes; may be swallowed whole or crushed if required.

enteric coated tablet: coating applied to a tablet containing a drug which is a gastric irritant or is broken down by gastric acid; the tablet is swallowed whole.

slow release tablet: the tablet, swallowed whole, contains a drug which is released over a prolonged period.

capsule: a gelatin container, swallowed whole, containing a drug which is to be released or has an unpleasant taste; allows liberation of the drug when the capsule is dissolved in the stomach or intestine.

granule: a small pellet which is often the active substance.

mixture: contains several drugs dissolved or suspended in an aqueous vehicle.

linctus: a drug prepared as a sweet syrup, given in doses of small volume to be swallowed slowly without the addition of water, usually for the relief of cough.

lozenge: a solid drug form which acts by slow disintegration in the mouth and is used when a local drug action in the mouth or throat is required.

emulsion: a mixture of oil and water, the oil remaining dispersed by an emulsifying agent, the container being shaken before use.

suspension: solid insoluble particles of a drug are dispersed in a liquid; must be shaken well before use.

elixir: a flavoured sweetened alcoholic solution of a potent or unpleasant-tasting drug in a small dose-volume.

syrup: a drug contained in a concentrated sugar solution.

tincture: a drug contained in an alcoholic solution.

extract: a concentrated preparation of a drug which may remain in fluid form or be evaporated and the solid sediment incorporated into a tablet or capsule.

powder: usually mixture of 2 or more powdered medicaments intended for internal use.

Injections

Sterile aqueous or oily solutions and suspensions are given by a route other than the oral route, i.e. parenterally.

intramuscular: oily solutions, suspensions, potentially irritant substances or if rapid absorption is required; the site is not massaged if the Z-track technique used.

intravenous: if a very rapid effect is required or if the preparation is too irritant to the tissues.

subcutaneous: used if relatively slower absorption is required.

intradermal: given into the superficial skin layers, mainly in skin testing.

intrathecal: if a drug does not penetrate the blood-brain barrier, it is delivered to the cerebro-spinal fluid in the subarachnoid space, usually following lumbar puncture.

intra-arterial: drugs, mainly cytotoxic (anti-neoplastic) agents, are delivered directly to an organ or tissue.

intracardiac: a drug is delivered directly into the ventricle or myocardium for an immediate cardiac response.

intra-articular: a drug is injected into a joint cavity.

intraperitoneal: drugs such as antibiotics have direct contact with intraperitoneal organs during peritoneal dialysis.

Topical applications

drops: for the eye, ear and nose; avoid touching ear or nose with dropper and return dropper to bottle without washing (eye drops are sterile).

lotion: an agent contained in an aqueous, alcoholic or emulsified vehicle, applied to the skin without friction, having an astringent, emollient or other therapeutic action.

gel: aqueous preparation used to apply water soluble medicament to body surfaces for longer period than aqueous solution.

cream: a semi-solid emulsion which may be aqueous or oily.

ointment: a semi-solid preparation in a greasy base.

paste: a semi-solid preparation containing a high proportion of medicament which is not intended to be absorbed.

liniment: a thin cream or oily preparation applied to the intact skin by rubbing; may contain substances possessing analgesic, rubefacient,

soothing or stimulating properties.

paint: liquid preparation for application in limited amounts to the skin or mucous membranes.

pessary: solid preparation shaped suitably for vaginal administration containing an agent intended to act locally.

suppository: solid preparation shaped suitably for rectal administration and usually containing an agent intended for local or systemic medication.

inhalation: liquid preparation containing volatile substances which on vaporization are inhaled to produce a local or systemic effect via the respiratory tract by steam inhalation, nebulizer, atomizer or aerosol spray.

dusting powder: usually mixture of 2 or more substances in fine powder and should not be applied to open wounds or large areas of raw surface.

insufflation: powder intended for introduction into the ear, nose, throat, body cavities or wounds.

irrigation: washing of a body cavity or wound by a stream of water or other solution.

Guide for safe administration

Check

— check medical officer's order and when drug last given
— check container label with order when selecting the preparation, before measuring out, and when replacing the preparation.
— check drug calculation with a registered nurse, pharmacist or medical officer (ask the second person to do the calculation independently then compare answers, remembering that it is rare to give more than two tablets or one ampoule at a time)
— check patient's identity carefully
— check that the patient knows the reason for the medication and discuss any query with the medical officer before giving it
— check that the medication trolley is always under surveillance while unlocked.

Observe drug

— mix liquid contents thoroughly but rotate protein preparations gently to prevent denaturation and frothing
— note discolouration, precipitate or foreign bodies
— note expiry date

Administration of drug

— give only medications which you or a pharmacist has prepared
— give correct drug and dose
— give to correct patient
— give at the correct time
— give by the prescribed route, never handling tablets and waiting until oral medications are swallowed.

Chart

— chart on patient's drug administration sheet
— enter drugs of addiction in register.

Observe patient and chart

— note beneficial effects
— note, report and chart any adverse effects.

Adverse drug reactions

A suspected adverse drug reaction is any unintended or undesired effect thought to be due to a drug administered in a therapeutic situation, and is reported by the perescriber to The Adverse Drug Reactions Advisory Committee which is a sub-committee of The Australian Drug Evaluation Committee in Canberra. The Committee particularly requests reports of all suspected reactions to new drugs, all suspected drug interactions and reactions to other drugs which are suspected of significantly affecting the course of a patient's management. Therefore the nurse should be aware of the adverse effects of main drug groups and should observe the patient carefully for signs of any changes from normal each time a new drug is added to the regimen.

Adverse drug reactions include:

Overdose

— a characteristic but excessive pharmacological effect of the drug caused by an absolute or relatively larger than usual amount of drug in the body.

Intolerance

— a low threshold to the normal pharmacological action of a drug

Secondary effects

— indirect consequences of a primary drug action, e.g., superinfection from antibacterial agents, or postural hypotension from antihypertensive agents

Idiosyncracy

— inherent qualitatively abnormal reaction to a drug usually due to a genetic abnormality, e.g., haemolytic anaemia caused by primaquine in patients with glucose-6-phosphate dehydrogenase deficiency in red blood cells

Allergy (hypersensitivity)

— a reaction not explained by the pharmacological effects of the drug, caused by altered reactivity of the patient and generally considered to be an allergic manifestation due to the suspected drug and includes anaphylactic shock, bronchospasm, urticaria, angioneurotic oedema (immediate or delayed), serum sickness syndrome (arthralgia, lymphadenopathy, fever, urticaria, angioneurotic oedema), blood dyscrasias (thrombocytopenia, granulocytopenia, agranulocytosis, aplastic anaemia, haemolysis), rashes (non-urticarial), fever, syndromes resembling collagen diseases (polyarteritis nodosa, disseminated lupus erythematosis), hepatitis, cholestatic jaundice, severe haematemesis, peripheral neuritis and nephritis.

Side effects

— therapeutically undesired but unavoidable effects because they are normal physiological actions of the drug within normal dose ranges, e.g., drowsiness from antihistamines. It may be a desired effect, e.g., use of atropine in premedication to reduce salivary and bronchial secretions.

Drug interactions

When two or more drugs are given together, an interaction may occur which could reduce or enhance the therapeutic response or result in an adverse reaction. The interaction is usually characterized by potentiation or antagonism of the effect of one of the drugs. The drug interaction may be desired or undesired. Both drugs may act on the target site or may interact remotely from the target site. Interactions can occur during formulation, or mixing by the giver, before or at the point of absorption resulting in enzyme induction, competition for plasma protein binding sites, or during metabolism or excretion. Drugs which may be potentiated include digoxin, oral hypoglycaemics and oral anticoagulants because of their low therapeutic index, whereas bacteriostatics such as tetracycline antagonize the bactericidal effects of penicillins and cephalosporins.

Drug administration errors

A drug dose may be missed, occasionally doubling the next dose to compensate. The correct drug may be given at the wrong time or by the wrong route. The correct drug may be given but the dose is incorrect. A patient may receive the wrong drug. Any administration error could have an adverse effect on the patient and a mistake could have legal consequences. If a drug administration error does occur, the nurse involved must observe the effects on the patient and contact relevant medical and nursing personnel immediately the error is discovered.

Discharge planning

The patient is advised of the reason for the medication and how and when to take it at home. If the person is unsure of a metric dose, the gradation on the measure is indicated. Injection technique should be practised for several days prior to discharge. A responsible household member will have to be taught how to give the medication if the patient is unable to manage. Explain what effects to expect and what adverse effects to report.

Point out the need to keep taking the medication even if feeling well, as patient compliance is poor when prophylactic drugs are being taken such as antihypertensive agents, beta-adrenoceptor blocking agents and anti-infective agents.

Patient medication counselling

Medication counselling results in improved patient compliance and more effective therapy. Surveys have shown that patients often retain little of the information provided by the medical officer during a consultation.

Pharmacists who dispense the medication advise the patient about the directions for use, and mention expected effects which could cause inconvenience or worry to the patient such as drowsiness, or colour changes in urine or faeces, and also will stress the need to avoid certain foods, alcohol or self-medication where applicable. Compliance can be promoted by memory aids including a calendar, Dosett box, education booklets or guides. Despite this, nurses are often asked to explain certain aspects of a medication regimen. Therefore keep the information short, simple and practical. Use everyday language and relate it to the labelled instructions. Pay particular attention to elderly people who are frequently confused by a variety of medication being taken at different times. Rather than indicating that a certain side effect may occur, ask the patient to report any unusual effects to the pharmacist or medical officer. Avoid any apparent contradiction in advice by checking with the relevant pharmacist or prescriber.

Summary

The right patient receives the right dose of the right medication in the right form at the right time by the right route for the right duration of therapy. All medications should be checked by two people, one being a registered nurse. In some institutions, oral medications (except narcotics) may be checked and given by two student nurses who have completed pharmacology theory. Extra care must be taken in situations where the nurse is working alone. Any error is reported immediately and the patient is observed closely for any adverse effects. If any manufacturer's literature accompanies the drug, it will provide detailed and specific information for safe preparation and use.

WHEN IN DOUBT, CHECK.

2 · Drugs acting on the alimentary tract

ANTACIDS

Action

— compounds which relieve the pain of peptic ulcer, reflux oesophagitis and hyperacidity by neutralizing gastric acidity and reducing pepsin activity

Use

— gastritis
— peptic ulcer
— hiatus hernia
— reflux oesophagitis
— taken with medication known to cause gastrointestinal irritation

Preparations

Several compounds form the basis of most antacids: aluminium hydroxide, magnesium hydroxide, magnesium carbonate and magnesium trisilicate. Aluminium hydroxide is often used alone, but is combined with magnesium hydroxide to offset the side effect of constipation. The potent local anaesthetic oxethazaine is added for rapid pain relief. An antifoam agent, simethicone, is added to some preparations to relieve flatulence. The addition of alginic acid forms a frothy raft which suppresses oesophageal reflux, so protecting the mucosa of the lower oesophagus. Bismuth subnitrate, an insoluble salt, has a protective and antacid action but is of doubtful value.

Dose

i) 5–20 ml liquid (30 ml Mylanta II® for duodenal ulcer); OR

ii) 1–4 tablets sucked or chewed (Mucaine® swallowed whole with water); OR
iii) 1 sachet (4 g) granules chewed and followed by a little water; OR
iv) ½–1 sachet (1–2 g) Infant Gaviscon® mixed with each milk feed or mixed with water and taken after each meal

Antacids are usually taken immediately after meals and at bedtime, or as required to remain symptom-free.

Adverse effects

— constipation (aluminium salts)
— diarrhoea (magnesium salts)
— rarely, intragastric mass formation when alginic acid preparation given with Prosobee® to infants
— the high sodium content of Infant Gaviscon® excludes its use in premature infants or if water loss is excessive

Interactions

— the absorption of many drugs is reduced, particularly of oral iron, cimetidine, ranitidine, chlorpromazine, digoxin and the tetracyclines, if taken with antacids, so preferably taken 2 hours apart if possible

Nursing points

— select the correct preparation (Mylanta II® is double the concentration of Mylanta®)
— shake liquids well before pouring
— leave preparation at bedside for self-medication, if required
— tablets to be chewed thoroughly (except Mucaine®)

— medication may be followed by a small amount of water or milk
— may be given in continuous intragastric drip as 1 part antacid to 2 or 3 parts water and run at 5 to 20 drops/min
— note persisting pain, constipation or diarrhoea

Note

— antacids do not appear to hasten ulcer healing
— liquid preparations are faster acting than tablets but tablets may be sucked to produce a continuous effect
— see anticholinergics

ACTIVATED CHARCOAL

Action

— gastrointestinal adsorbent

Use

— flatulence
— poisoning (see p. 298)

Dose

2 or 3 tablets t.d.s.

Interactions

— regular ingestion may affect normal gastrointestinal absorption pattern including some orally administered drugs

Nursing point

— warn patient that charcoal colours the faeces black

Note

— may be used locally as deodorant in ostomy pouches, wounds and ulcers
— NEVER GIVEN WITH AN EMETIC

ANTIULCERANTS

CARBENOXOLONE

Action and use

— accelerates healing rate of gastric and duodenal ulcers

Dose

Gastric ulcer

50–100 mg t.d.s. with or immediately after food (Biogastrone®)

Duodenal ulcer

50 mg capsule swallowed whole with liquid 15 to 30 minutes a.c. (Duogastrone®)

Adverse effects

— sodium and water retention, oedema, hypertension
— hypokalaemia, alkalosis
— impaired glucose tolerance
— rarely, headache, nausea

Interactions

— therapeutic properties of carbenoxolone inhibited by spironolactone
— carbenoxolone therapy increases the risk of cardiac glycoside toxicity

Nursing points

— no added salt diet
— encourage the eating of potassium-rich bananas, tomatoes, apricots, cantaloupe, dates, grapefruit, prunes, raisins, strawberries, watermelon and oranges
— check weekly for oedema, weight gain and raised blood pressure

CIMETIDINE

Action

— histamine H_2 receptor antagonist which reduces gastric acid secretion

Use

— benign gastric and duodenal ulcer
— reflux oesophagitis
— gastrinoma (Zollinger-Ellison syndrome)
— scleroderma oesophagitis
— prophylactically where 'stress ulcers' are common in cases of extensive burns and severe trauma

Dose

i) 200–400 mg orally t.d.s. with meals and 400 mg nocte, OR
ii) 400 mg orally with breakfast and 400 mg at bedtime; OR
iii) 200 mg diluted in 100 ml 5% glucose or other compatible IV solution and infused over 15–20 minutes and repeated every 4–6 hours up to a maximum of 2 g/24 hours; OR
iv) 200 mg diluted in isotonic saline or other compatible solution up to 20 ml and given as bolus over 2 minutes 4–6 hourly; OR
v) continuous IV infusion not exceeding 75 mg/hr/24 hours

Adverse effects

— headache, tiredness, dizziness
— diarrhoea, constipation
— muscular pain
— rash
— confusion, bradycardia, tachycardia, hypotension (IV)
— gynaecomastia

Interactions

— absorption reduced by antacids
— enhances effects of phenytoin, propranolol, labetolol, metoprolol, chlordiazepoxide, diazepam, lignocaine, procainamide, theophylline and oral anticoagulants

Nursing points

— when taken at mealtimes should be ingested *with* the meal
— patient encouraged to continue treatment for 4 to 6 weeks after which a maintenance dose may be prescribed
— monitor heart rate and blood pressure during IV administration

Note

— antacids may be required for symptomatic relief but taken 1 hour apart
— adverse effects more likely if the patient is elderly or has renal dysfunction

RANITIDINE

Action and use

— as for cimetidine (see p. 9) but less antiandrogenic

Dose

i) 300 mg orally nocte or 150 mg orally b.d. initially for 4–6 weeks then 150 mg orally nocte; OR
ii) 150 mg orally nocte (maintenance); OR
iii) 150 mg orally t.d.s. initially and increased as necessary to 600–900 mg/day (Zollinger-Ellison syndrome); OR
iv) 50 mg diluted in 20 ml isotonic saline and given slowly over 5 minutes which may be repeated 6–8 hourly; OR
v) continuous IV infusion at 25 mg/hr for 2 hours which may be repeated 6–8 hourly

Adverse effects

— nausea, vomiting, diarrhoea, constipation
— tiredness
— rash

Interactions

— antacids significantly reduce absorption of ranitidine

— increases blood level of metoprolol significantly
— enhances effect of warfarin

Nursing points

— not taken with antacid preparations
— patient encouraged to continue treatment for 4– 6 weeks after which a maintenance dose may be prescribed

Note

— as for cimetidine
— all unused admixtures of ranitidine injection with infusion fluids should be discarded 24 hours after preparation

MISOPROSTOL

Action

— synthetic prostaglandin E_1 analoque
— reduces gastric acid secretion so protects mucosa when exposed to ulcerogenic agents (mucosal cytoprotective)

Use

— acute gastric and duodenal ulcers for up to 4 weeks

Dose

200 micrograms t.d.s. and nocte

Adverse effects

— diarrhoea
— nausea, abdominal discomfort
— headache, dizziness

Note

— contraindicated in pregnancy

FAMOTIDINE

Action

— histamine H_2 receptor antagonist which reduces gastric acid secretion

Use

— duodenal ulcer
— benign gastric ulcer
— Zollinger-Ellison syndrome
— prevention of recurrence of duodenal ulceration

Dose

i) 40 mg orally nocte (treatment duodenal ulcer, benign gastric ulcer) OR
ii) 20 mg orally nocte (maintenance duodenal ulcer); OR
iii) 20 mg orally 6-hourly (Zollinger-Ellison syndrome)

Adverse effects

— headache, dizziness
— constipation, diarrhoea

Note

— treatment continued for 4–8 weeks, but duration may be shortened if endoscopy reveals that ulcer has healed

SUCRALFATE

Action

— selectively adheres to ulcer base which protects ulcer site from potential ulcerogenic properties of acid, pepsin and bile
— complexes with pepsin and bile directly

Use

— acute non-malignant gastric and duodenal ulcers for up to 8 weeks

Dose

1 g t.d.s. 1 hour a.c. and nocte

Adverse effects

— constipation, gastric discomfort
— headache
— urticaria

Interactions

— antacids decrease mucosal binding of sucralfate if taken less than ½ hour before or after sucralfate
— impairs absorption of phenytoin, warfarin

Nursing points

— antacid taken at least ½ hour before or after sucralfate

Note

— not recommended if severely impaired renal function (contains 190 mg aluminium)
— not recommended if actively bleeding ulcer

TRI-POTASSIUM DI-CITRATO BISMUTHATE (TDB)

Action and use

— gives symptomatic relief presumably by providing a protective barrier at the peptic ulcer site

Dose

1 tablet chewed ½ hour a.c. t.d.s. and 2 hours after the last main meal

Adverse effects

— darkening of the faeces and tongue
— nausea, vomiting

Interactions

— inactivated if taken at the same time as milk and antacids, so if an antacid is necessary, it is taken at least 1 hour before or after TDB
— absorption of the tetracyclines reduced

Nursing points

— no liquids for at least ½ hour before or after taking medication
— milk is taken only with meals or in tea
— warn patient that stool may become darker

— patient encouraged to complete the full 4-week course
— the usual dose is taken even if meals are missed
— no eating between meals

ANTICHOLINERGIC AGENTS

ATROPINE SULPHATE

Action

— reduces production of sweat, saliva, lachrymal, nasal, bronchial, gastric and intestinal secretions
— reduces gastrointestinal mobility
— increases heart rate by blocking vagal stimulus
— mydriatic, cycloplegic
— raises intraocular pressure
— stimulates respiration, inhibits micturition (high doses)

Use

— pylorospasm, pyloric stenosis
— renal and biliary colic
— premedication before induction of general anaesthesia to diminish risk of vagal inhibition of the heart and to reduce salivary and bronchial secretions
— given with prostigmine which reverses the effects of non-depolarizing muscle relaxants
— bradycardia in early myocardial infarction
— enuresis
— antidote to parasympathetic stimulants such as pilocarpine, carbachol and bethanecol and also to irreversible anticholinesterases

Adult dose

i) 0.3–0.6 mg SC or IM usually with morphine 10–15 mg 1 hour before anaesthesia; OR
ii) 0.3–0.6 mg IV immediately before induction of anaesthesia; OR
iii) 0.6–1.2 mg slowly IV plus neostigmine to reverse the effects of skeletal muscle relaxants; OR
iv) 0.4–0.6 mg slowly IV at 3–5 minute intervals to a total dose of 2 mg to achieve the desired heart rate
v) 0.6 mg IM t.d.s. to relieve biliary or renal colic;OR
vi) 1–2 mg IV initially, then 2 mg IM or IV every 5–60 mins if necessary for poisoning due to irreversible

anticholinesterases (severe cases 2–6 mg up to a total dose of 50 mg/24 hours

Paediatric dose

Premedication

i) premature infants 65 micrograms IM; OR
ii) full term infants 100–200 micrograms IM; OR
iii) older children 20 micrograms/kg IM

Other

0.03–0.06 mg in a mixture preparation may be given 5–15 minutes before each feed up to 4 times a day.
Phenobarbitone may be added to the mixture.

Note

— dose reduced in hot weather or if child febrile

Adverse effects

— dry mouth, dysphagia, constipation
— urinary hesitancy and retention
— flushing and dryness of skin
— tachycardia, palpitations, arrhythmias
— mydriasis, photophobia, cycloplegia
— raised intraocular pressure
— toxic doses cause tachycardia, hyperpyrexia, restlessness, confusion, excitement, hallucinations, delirium, and may progress to circulatory failure and respiratory depression

Interactions

— additive anticholinergic effects with quinidine, antidepressants and some antihistamines

Nursing points

— ensure written informed consent has been obtained from patient before premedication given
— patient allowed to rest following premedication to avoid postural hypotension

— note tachycardia, raised intraocular pressure and urinary retention, especially in the elderly
— advise patient to avoid risky activities if has blurred vision, dizziness or drowsiness
— dark glasses worn if continuous mydriasis and cycloplegia
— infants and young children are especially susceptible to atropine toxicity, even from the absorption of eye preparations, so note irritability, dry mouth, tachycardia, mydriasis, fever and rash

HYOSCINE HYDROBROMIDE
(known as scopolamine hydrobromide in USA)

Chemically related to atropine sulphate, but causes more CNS depression.

Use

— premedication
— combined with morphine or pethidine to produce 'twilight' sleep during first stage of labour
— prevention and treatment of motion sickness
— intractable hiccups
— cycloplegic and mydriatic

Adult dose

Premedication

0.4 to 0.6 mg SC or IM as premedication 1 hour before induction of anaesthesia together with morphine OR papaveretum OR pethidine

Travel sickness

Based on 0.3 mg tablet which is taken ½ hour before travelling and the dose repeated in 4–6 hours if necessary 1–2 tablets up to a maximum of 4 tablets/24 hours

Paediatric dose

Premedication

0.008 mg/kg IM usually with papaveretum 0.4 mg/kg

Travel sickness

Based on 0.3 mg tablet which is taken ½ hour before travelling and the dose repeated in 4–6 hours if necessary
2–7 years: ¼ tablet up to a maximum of 1 tablet/24 hours
over 7 years: ½–1 tablet up to a maximum of 2 tablets/24 hours

Adverse effects

— as for atropine sulphate, together with
— confusion in the elderly
— bradycardia

Interactions

— as for atropine sulphate

HYOSCINE METHOBROMIDE (known as methscopolamine bromide in USA)

Action

— inhibits gastric secretion
— decreases volume and acidity of gastric secretion
— delays gastric emptying
— reduces peristalsis

Use

— adjunct in management of peptic ulcer and gastric disorders associated with hyperacidity and hypermotility
— post-gastrectomy dumping syndrome
— controls obstinate, longstanding functional diarrhoea
— diarrhoea associated with irritable colon, ulcerative colitis, intestinal resection, ileostomy
— reduces sweating and therefore aggravation of certain dermatoses
— excessive salivation

Dose

2.5–5 mg orally ½ hour a.c. and nocte

Adverse effects

— dry mouth, dysphagia, heartburn, nausea, constipation

— flushing and dryness of skin
— palpitations
— blurred vision, drowsiness, dizziness
— inability to micturate

Interactions

— additive anticholinergic effects with antidepressants and some antihistamines

Nursing points

— warn patient against driving a vehicle or operating machinery if drowsy or ·vision blurred
— thirst may be relieved by water, chewing gum or mints or sucking hard sweets

Note

— contraindicated in glaucoma
— anticholinergic effects may decrease with continued therapy

ATROPINE METHONITRATE

Use

— gastrointestinal spasm
— alleviation of paroxysms of whooping cough (pertussis)

Adult dose

1–3 mg orally t.d.s. (tablets)

Paediatric dose

Drops of alcoholic solution 0.6% 4-hourly

up to 6 months: 2–4 drops
6 months–2 years: 3–6 drops
2–6 years: 4–6 drops
6–10 years: 6–12 drops

Adverse effects and interactions

— similar to atropine sulphate

Note

— **discontinued in Australia**

— store in cool place in airtight container to prevent evaporation
— drops may be given in water or fruit juice

DICYCLOMINE HYDROCHLORIDE

Use

— gastrointestinal spasm
— relieves infant colic

Adult dose

10–40 mg t.d.s. a.c. or p.c. (tablets or syrup)

Paediatric dose

Infants

Not given to infants under 6 months old

6 months–2 years

5–10 mg (syrup) diluted with an equal volume of water 15 minutes a.c. up to 4 times in 24 hours

2–12 years

10 mg t.d.s. or q.i.d. a.c. or p.c. (tablets or syrup)

Adverse effects and interactions

— similar to atropine sulphate

DICYCLOMINE WITH SIMETHICONE

Use

— relieves flatulence and abdominal discomfort due to entrapped gas
— relieves infant colic

Adult dose

10 ml syrup 3–4 times daily and nocte

Paediatric dose

Infants under 3 months: 1 ml diluted with an equal volume of water before feeds up to 4 times daily for 2–3 days to establish that the infant can tolerate the medication. If tolerated, 2.5 ml before feeds up to 6 times daily

3 months–4 years: starting dosage as for infant under 3 months then if tolerated, 5 ml before feeds up to 4 times daily

Adverse effects and interactions

— similar to atropine sulphate

SIMETHICONE

Action and use

— safe, inert antifoaming agent which relieves flatulence and abdominal discomfort due to entrapped gas, also relieves infant colic

Adult dose

40 mg (drops 40 mg/0.6 ml) q.i.d. between meals and nocte

Paediatric dose

i) 40 mg (drops 40 mg/0.6 ml) a.c. 4- to 6-hourly (Mylicon®); OR
ii) 50 mg a.c. (Infacol Wind drops)

HYOSCINE BUTYLBROMIDE (known as scopolamine butylbromide in USA)

Use

— gastrointestinal spasm
— renal and biliary colic
— delayed first stage of labour
— diagnostic aid in radiology
— spasmodic dysmenorrhoea

Dose

i)   20 mg orally q.i.d.; OR
ii) 1–2 rectal suppositories (10–20 mg) q.i.d.; OR
iii) 20–40 mg IM or slowly IV

Adverse effects and interactions

— if high doses, similar to atropine sulphate

MEBEVERINE

Use

— irritable colon syndrome, primary or associated with gastrointestinal inflammation

Dose

135 mg orally t.d.s. before or with food

Adverse effects

— occasionally, dizziness, headache

Interactions

— similar to atropine sulphate

PROPANTHELINE BROMIDE

Action

— similar peripheral effects but less of the central effects of atropine sulphate

Use

— irritable colon syndrome
— renal colic
— pancreatitis
— diagnostic aid in radiology

Dose

i)   15 mg orally t.d.s. 30 mins before meals and 30 mg nocte; OR
ii) 15–30 mg orally q.i.d.; OR
iii) 30 mg orally 45 mins before radiology

Interactions

— similar to atropine sulphate

EMETIC

IPECACUANHA SYRUP (APF)

Action and use

— induces vomiting by acting locally on the gastric mucosa and centrally on the chemoreceptor trigger zone
— has expectorant action in smaller doses

Adult dose

30 ml

Paediatric dose

1 year: 15 ml
2 years: 20 ml
3 years: 25 ml
over 4 years: 30 ml

Adverse effects

— persistent vomiting
— bloody diarrhoea
— cardiac arrhythmias

Nursing points

— action enhanced if dose followed by 200–300 ml of water or clear liquid (100–200 ml for children)
— expect emesis within 30 minutes
— dose repeated if required
— if vomiting has not occurred following repeat dose, seek medical advice
— contra-indicated if patient unconscious or if caustic, corrosive or petroleum products or anti-emetic drugs have been ingested

Note

— in the event of acute poisoning, a regional Poisons Information Centre is available to provide advice on the telephone (see Appendix).

ANTI-EMETICS AND ANTINAUSEANTS

METOCLOPRAMIDE

Action

— reduces intensity of impulses to the vomiting centre caused by local emetics in the pylorus and duodenum
— raises threshold of chemoreceptor trigger zone preventing vomiting caused by central emetics
— increases rate of gastric emptying by enhancing peristalsis
— reduces gastro-oesophageal reflux
— raises prolactin levels

Use

Diagnostic

— increases transit time of barium in radiological examination
— facilitates and accelerates introduction of tubes or biopsy capsules into small intestine

Therapeutic

— controls nausea and vomiting which may be drug- or disease-induced, post-operative or associated with labour or irradiation
— enhances absorption of aspirin in a migraine attack (given 10 minutes before aspirin)
— persistent hiccups
— adjunct to other methods of emptying stomach prior to induction of general anaesthesia in an emergency
— controls nausea and vomiting associated with intolerance to cytotoxic drugs

Adult dose

i) 10 mg orally or IM 1–3 times daily; OR
ii) 10–20 mg IV; OR
iii) up to 2 mg/kg added to at least 50 ml of compatible diluent and infused IV over at least 15 mins prior to commencement of cytotoxic therapy and repeated 2-hourly up to

a maximum of 10 mg/kg/24 hours
(high dose formulation)

Paediatric dose

under 5 years: 1–2 mg IM 2–3 times
daily according to age; OR
under 1 year: 1 mg orally b.d.
1–3 years: 1 mg orally 2–3 times daily
3–5 years: 2 mg orally 2–3 times daily
5–14 years: 2.5–5 mg orally, IM or IV
1–3 times daily

Note

— paediatric dose should not exceed
  0.5 mg/kg/day

Adverse effects

— constipation or diarrhoea
— drowsiness, lassitude
— extrapyramidal reactions (Parkinson
  type) especially if used in
  combination with phenothiazines e.g.
  promethazine
— hypertensive crisis if patient has
  phaeochromocytoma

Interactions

— reduces absorption of oral digoxin
  (solid dose form)
— increases absorption of aspirin,
  paracetamol and oral diazepam
— effects of metoclopramide on
  gastrointestinal motility antagonized
  by anticholinergic agents and
  narcotic analgesics

Nursing points

— compatible with morphine or
  pethidine when mixed in the same
  syringe as long as the resultant
  solution is used within 15 minutes
  and there is no precipitation
— warn patient against driving a vehicle
  or operating machinery if drowsy
— protect from light
— discard any ampoules showing
  yellow discolouration
— benztropine or diphenhydramine
  reverses extrapyramidal reactions

DOMPERIDONE
Action and use

— a dopamine antagonist used similarly
  to metoclopramide

Dose

10–20 mg orally, 3–4 times daily before
meals.

Adverse effects, Interactions, Nursing points

— see metoclopramide

PROCHLORPERAZINE
Action and use

— a centrally acting phenothiazine used
  as an anti-emetic and antivertigo
  agent
— used as an antipsychotic in larger
  doses

Adult dose

i) 5–10 mg orally 2–3 times daily; OR
ii) 12.5 mg deep IM stat; OR
iii) 25 mg rectal suppository stat

Paediatric dose

i) 0.25–0.35 mg/kg/day orally; OR
ii) 0.2 mg/kg/day IM

Adverse effects

— drowsiness
— extrapyramidal reactions (Parkinson
  type)
— restlessness and excitement in
  children
— hypotension if given IV

Interactions

— reduces efficacy of levodopa
— enhances the CNS depressant
  effects of alcohol and some
  analgesics, sedatives and
  tranquillizers

Nursing points

— protect from light
— not normally mixed in the same syringe with other drugs but is compatible with morphine, pethidine or papaveretum when mixed in the same syringe as long as the resultant solution is used within 15 minutes and there is no precipitation
— warn patient against driving a vehicle or operating machinery if drowsy

THIETHYLPERAZINE

Action and use

— a centrally-acting phenothiazine used as an anti-emetic and antivertigo agent

Dose

i) 10 mg orally 1–3 times daily; OR
ii) 10 mg IM or slowly IV; OR
iii) 10 mg rectal suppository 1–3 times daily

Note

— see prochlorperazine

HYOSCINE

Action

— antiemetic

Use

— protects against nausea, vomiting and dizziness due to motion sickness

Adult and paediatric dose (over 10 years)

1.5 mg in a transdermal therapeutic system or patch (releasing 1 mg/72 hours) delivers a primary dose initially from an adhesive layer then a controlled release of a maintenance dose from a reservoir layer.
    Patch applied to dry, hairless, unbroken skin behind ear. (If journey of shorter duration than 72 hours, patch should be removed earlier.) For more prolonged protection, remove first patch after 72 hours and apply a fresh system.

Adverse effects

— dry mouth
— drowsiness, impaired concentration
— slight hypotension, bradycardia
— mydriasis, blurred near vision
— serious confusion, visual hallucinations (remove patch immediately, wash site of application and, if necessary, reverse by physostigmine adults 1–2 mg, children 0.5–1 mg slowly IV or IM and repeat as required)
— occasionally disorientation, memory disturbance, dizziness, restlessness, hallucinations, confusion, difficulty with micturition, rash and erythema, acute narrow-angle glaucoma, dry itchy or red eyes
— rarely, dizziness, nausea and delayed hypersensitivity at site of application 3 days or more after removal

Interaction

anticholinergic activity of hysoscine increased by antidepressants and some antihistamines

Instructions for use

— remove patch from sachet
— peel off clear hexagonal foil protective liner
— press patch (silvery side against skin) firmly on to a dry, hairless, cleaned area of unbroken skin behind the ear
— wash hands thoroughly after applying or removing patch
— wash site of application after removing patch
— if patch becomes detached, replace with a fresh one behind other ear

Nursing points

— caution against driving a vehicle or operating machinery if drowsy
— caution against taking alcohol during the use of hyoscine

— wash hands after handling patch to avoid mydriasis and blurred vision if direct contact with eyes
— cutting patch in halves or quarters reduces adverse effects

Note

— use with caution in people over 65 years
— only one system (patch) should be in use at any one time

OTHER ANTIEMETICS AND ANTINAUSEANTS

See meclozine, perphenazine and promethazine

PANCREATIC ENZYMES

Action

— oral preparations containing the pancreatic enzymes protease, lipase and amylase which catalyse the hydrolysis of protein, fat and starch respectively

Use

— pancreatitis
— pancreatic enzyme replacement therapy
— mucoviscidosis (cystic fibrosis of the pancreas)

Preparations and dose

PANCRELIPASE

Dose

1–2 capsules taken with each meal, or capsule contents sprinkled on soft food that does not require chewing

PANCREATIN

Dose

i) 0.75 g powder (small children) with each meal (Viokase®); OR
ii) 0.5–2 g powder q.i.d. a.c. (Pancrex V®); OR
iii) 1–3 tablets or capsules swallowed whole with meals (Viokase®); OR
iv) 1–2 tablets swallowed whole during or after meals (Combizym®); OR
v) 5–15 tablets q.i.d. a.c. (Pancrex V®); OR
vi) 2–6 Forte tablets q.i.d. a.c. (Pancrex V®)
vii) contents of 1–2 capsules (neonates) mixed with feeds (Pancrex V 125®); OR
viii) contents of 1–2 capsules (infants) mixed with feeds (Pancrex V®); OR
ix) contents of 2–6 capsules (older children) q.i.d. with meals (or capsules may be swallowed whole) (Pancrex V®)

Adverse effects of pancreatic enzymes
— buccal and perianal soreness (pancreatin)
— occasionally, hypersensitivity reactions to preparations of porcine origin such as sneezing, lachrymation and rash

Nursing points for pancreatic enzymes
— store preparations in airtight containers in a cool place and note expiry date
— protect the enteric coating on the beads by avoiding crushing, chewing and contact with alkalis
— if pancreatin powder is mixed with liquids or feeds, the resulting mixture should not be allowed to stand for more than 1 hour prior to use
— barrier cream will prevent irritation of skin around the mouth and anus

Note
— pancrelipase (Cotazym®) and pancreatin (Viokase®) are of porcine origin and should be avoided in patients hypersensitive to pork products
— pancrelipase has more enzyme activity than pancreatin

BULK LAXATIVES
Action
— increases the volume of the faeces by absorbing water so stimulates peristalsis
— effective in 12–24 hours

Use
— constipation
— pre-operative bowel emptying
— colostomy and ileostomy control
— diverticular disease

Preparations and dose
ISPAGHULA
Dose
1 sachet (3.5 g) b.d. p.c. stirred into a glass of water

PSYLLIUM
Dose
1 rounded teaspoon (5 ml) or 1 sachet 1–3 times daily stirred into a glass of water, milk or fruit juice

Note
— also may be used as an appetite suppressant

STERCULIA
Dose
1–2 heaped 5 ml teaspoons of granules once or twice daily, the granules being placed dry on the tongue and swallowed whole with plenty of water

Note
— select the correct formulation of Normacol®, i.e. standard, special or antispasmodic

Adverse effects of bulk forming laxatives

— flatulence, discomfort
— if the recommended method of administration is not adhered to, oesophageal and intestinal obstruction and faecal impaction may occur

Nursing points for bulk forming laxatives

— generous amounts of water should be given with all bulk forming laxatives
— no bulk forming laxatives given if nausea, vomiting, undiagnosed abdominal pain or faecal impaction
— advise the patient to avoid the 'laxative habit' and encourage normal bowel function by increased fibre and fluid intake and regular exercise

Note

— see methylcellulose (p. 145)

SALINE LAXATIVES

Action and use

— retain water in the intestinal lumen by osmosis which results in increased bulk so stimulates peristalsis
— effective in 1–2 hours
— may be taken following an anthelmintic

Preparations and dose

MAGNESIUM SULPHATE

Dose

5–15 g in 250 ml water orally before breakfast

SODIUM PHOSPHATE

Dose

Contents of 1 disposable enema unit (130 ml)

SODIUM CITRATE WITH SODIUM LAURYL SULPHOACETATE

Adult and paediatric dose

contents of 1 disposable enema unit (5 ml)

ELECTROLYTE GASTROINTESTINAL LAVAGE

Action

— cleanses bowel by inducing diarrhoea and causing little change in water and electrolyte balance

Use

— colon preparation for radiological procedures
— before gastrointestinal examination, proctoscopy, sigmoidoscopy, colonoscopy
— before colonic surgery

Dose

Dissolve and mix the powder provided in 4 litres of water.

i) 1 litre orally each hour for 4 hours the evening prior to examination or surgery; OR
ii) 20–30 ml/min via nasogastric tube

Adverse effects

— nausea, vomiting
— bloating
— rectal irritation

Nursing points

— patient to fast 3–4 hours prior to administration
— only clear liquids
— cordial or clear fruit juice may be added to improve flavour
— keep mixture refrigerated
— preparation considered to be complete when patient passing clear fluid from bowel
— observe patient closely if impaired gag reflex or unconscious (nasogastric intubation)

Note

— contains polyethylene glycol, potassium chloride, sodium bicarbonate and sodium sulphate

Adverse effects of saline laxatives

— excessive use may cause dehydration, electrolyte imbalance

Interactions of saline laxatives

— most oral magnesium salts reduce absorption of oral iron, digoxin, tetracycline and chlorpromazine

Nursing points for saline laxatives

— advise the patient to avoid the 'laxative habit' and encourage normal bowel function by increased fibre and fluid intake and regular exercise
— no oral saline laxatives given if nausea, vomiting, undiagnosed abdominal pain or faecal impaction

STIMULANT OR IRRITANT LAXATIVES

Action

— increase peristalsis through irritation of intestinal sensory nerve endings
— effective in 4–8 hours

Use

— chronic constipation
— before proctoscopy, sigmoidoscopy
— colon preparation for radiological procedures

Preparations and dose
BISACODYL
Adult dose

i) 10–20 mg nocte (tablets or rectal suppositories); OR
ii) 10 mg nocte (micro-enema); OR
iii) 10 mg orally on 2 nights preceding radiological examination and 1 rectal suppository 90 minutes prior to examination

Paediatric dose

1–2 years: 5 mg (tablets or rectal suppositories)
over 2 years: 5–10 mg (tablets or rectal suppositories)

Note

— tablets are enteric coated, so swallowed whole
— no antacids within $\frac{1}{2}$ hour of taking tablets
— insert suppository high in rectum against rectal wall
— sufficient lubrication will be produced by warming the suppository in the hand before removing it from the foil wrapper
— suppository effective within 20–60 minutes of insertion
— micro-enema usually effective within 15–60 minutes.
— available as pack containing 3 × 5 mg tablets, a 10 mg suppository and a mild saline laxative, which can

be used for complete bowel preparation before abdominal X-ray examinations such as barium meal and barium enema

CASTOR OIL

Dose

5–20 ml in milk or fruit juice before breakfast

Note

— effective in 2–6 hours
— used as purgative in treatment of food poisoning

SENNA

Adult dose

i) 2–4 tablets nocte, OR
ii) 1–2 teaspoons granules nocte eaten plain or mixed with hot or cold milk

Paediatric dose

i) 1–2 tablets once or twice daily; OR
ii) ½–1 teaspoon granules once or twice daily

Note

— urine may become red or yellow

Nursing points for stimulant or irritant laxatives

— advise the patient to avoid the 'laxative habit' and encourage normal bowel function by increased fibre and fluid intake and regular exercise
— no oral stimulant or irritant laxatives given if nausea, vomiting, undiagnosed abdominal pain or faecal impaction

LUBRICANT LAXATIVES

Action

— soften faeces

Use

— allow defaecation without straining
— painful anorectal disorders

Preparations and dose

DOCUSATE SODIUM (dioctyl sodium sulphosuccinate)

Adult dose

i) 50–240 ml orally daily after evening meal; OR
ii) retenion enema (100–150 ml diluted solution); OR
iii) evacuant enema (300–500 ml diluted solution); OR
iv) flushing enema (500–1500 ml diluted solution); OR
v) 1 rectal suppsitory

Paediatric dose

2–10 years: 50 mg orally daily or b.d.
over 10 years: 120 mg orally daily

under 12 months: ½ rectal suppository or 30–60 ml diluted enema solution.
over 12 months: 1 rectal suppository or 60–120 ml diluted enema solution.

Note

— the diluted solution is obtained by adding 1 part of enema concentrate to 23 parts of sterile water
— oral formulation also prepared in combination with the stimulant laxative, senna

GLYCERINE SUPPOSITORIES

Adult and paediatric dose

1–2 of the appropriate size for adults, children or infants

Note

— store below 25 °C, preferably in a refrigerator

LIQUID PARAFFIN

Dose

15–45 ml nocte or 2–4 evenly-spaced doses daily

Note

— prolonged use may interfere with the absorption of fat-soluble vitamins
— possibility of aspiration pneumonia or anal seepage and irritation
— avoid taking within 2 hours of other medications
— more palatable if mixed with or followed by orange juice
— also prepared in combination with the stimulant laxative, phenolphthalein

Nursing points for lubricant laxatives

— advise the patient to avoid the 'laxative habit' and encourage normal bowel fuction by increased fibre and fluid intake and regular exercise
— no oral lubricant laxatives given if nausea, vomiting, undiagnosed abdominal pain or faecal impaction

SYNTHETIC DISACCHARIDE LAXATIVE

LACTULOSE

Action

— administered orally as 50% w/w syrup which is not much absorbed in the gastrointestinal tract
— broken down in colon by saccharolytic bacteria to acetic and lactic acids
— acids stimulate peristalsis and exert local osmotic effect in the colon
— reduces ammonia production in the gut
— both bulk forming and irritant laxative

Use

— chronic constipation
— hepatic encephalopathy

Adult dose

10–45 ml daily after breakfast mixed with water, milk or fruit juice

Paediatric dose

under 1 year: 3 ml
1–5 years: 5–10 ml daily
6–14 years: 8–15 ml daily

Adverse effects

— nausea, diarrhoea, flatulence (large doses)

Nursing points

— avoid other laxatives during lactulose therapy because loose stools resulting from their use may be mistaken for adequate lactulose dosage
— advise patient to avoid the 'laxative habit' and encourage normal bowel function by dietary means as soon as practicable

Note

— contra-indicated in patients on galactose and/or lactose-free diet
— begin on higher dose and reduce after 3 days depending on response

RETENTION ENEMA

PREDNISOLONE SODIUM PHOSPHATE

Use

— ulcerative colitis

Dose

100 ml introduced into the rectum each night on retiring

Nursing point

— advise patient to introduce the solution in the left lateral position, discard disposable plastic bag then lie prone for 3–5 minutes then go to sleep in any comfortable position

ANTIDIARRHOEAL AGENTS

ALUMINIUM HYDROXIDE GEL WITH KAOLIN

ALUMINIUM HYDROXIDE GEL WITH KAOLIN AND PECTIN

KAOLIN WITH PECTIN

Action

— reduce the amount of free water in the bowel

Use

— nonspecific diarrhoea

Dose

30 ml initially, then 15 ml after each unformed stool

Interactions

— reduces the absorption of many drugs, particularly oral iron and the tetracyclines, so taken 2 hours apart if possible

Note

— underlying cause of diarrhoea should be investigated
— other preparations available containing attapulgite, simethicone, codeine phosphate and anti-infective agents in various combinations

CODEINE PHOSPHATE

Action

— reduces peristalsis by suppressing intestinal motility

Use

— relief of acute nonspecific diarrhoea

Dose

30–60 mg orally 6-hourly

Adverse effects

— nausea, vomiting
— dizziness, drowsiness
— constipation

Nursing point

— if dose 30 mg or greater, warn patient about reduced tolerance to alcohol and warn against driving a vehicle or operating machinery if drowsy

Note

— underlying cause of diarrhoea should be investigated

DIPHENOXYLATE WITH ATROPINE

Action

— diphenoxylate reduces peristalsis and atropine discourages excessive self-medication of the pethidine-related diphenoxylate

Use

— symptomatic treatment of acute and chronic diarrhoea

Dose

5 mg (2 tablets) 3–4 times daily then reduced as required

Adverse effects

— drowsiness, headache, depression
— dizziness, restlessness, euphoria
— numbness of extremities
— anorexia, nausea, vomiting
— abdominal distension, paralytic ileus
— (from atropine) tachycardia, dry mouth

Note

— not for children
— underlying cause of diarrhoea should be investigated

LOPERIMIDE

Action

— reduces peristalsis by suppressing intestinal motility

Use

— relief of acute nonspecific diarrhoea

Dose

4 mg (2 capsules) then 2 mg after each unformed stool up to 16 mg/day

Adverse effects

— nausea, flatulence, abdominal pain
— constipation

Nursing point

— instruct patient to discontinue drug if no improvement within 48 hours

Note

— underlying cause of diarrhoea should be investigated
— nursing mothers taking loperimide should not breast-feed their infants

SULPHASALAZINE

Action

— a sulphonamide, thought to have an anti-inflammatory effect on the intestinal wall, but no antibacterial effect on intestinal flora

Use

— ulcerative colitis (maintenance therapy)
— Crohn's disease

Adult dose

i) 1–2 g orally q.i.d. initially, then 500 mg q.i.d.; OR
ii) 1–2 rectal suppositories mane and nocte after defaecation. Dose halved after 4–5 weeks

Paediatric dose

40–60 mg/kg/day in 4–6 divided doses initially either tablets or suppositories, then 20–40 /mg/kg/day for maintenance

Adverse effects and interactions

— as for sulphonamides
— reduces absorption of digoxin

Nursing points

— tablets taken preferably after meals
— night-time interval between doses should not exceed 8 hours

Note

— enteric-coated tablets available if gastrointestinal intolerance

ANTHELMINTICS

Other affected household members may require concurrent treatment, living quarters and clothing will need to be washed thoroughly and scrupulous attention paid to personal hygiene

Action

— some agents kill worms or inhibit development of eggs or larvae
— some agents paralyse the worms, dislodging them thereby allowing their removal (a saline laxative may also be indicated)

Preparations

DIETHYLCARBAMAZINE

Use

— filariasis (prophylaxis and treatment)
— onchocerciasis
— tropical eosinophilia
— loasis
— roundworm

Adult dose

Tropical eosinophilia

13 mg/kg orally as a single dose after breakfast daily for 4–7 days

Roundworm

13 mg/kg orally as a single dose after breakfast daily for 7 days

Others

2 mg/kg orally t.d.s. p.c. for 3–4 weeks

To reduce allergiç and other unwanted reactions

2 mg/kg orally daily p.c. first day,
2 mg/kg orally b.d. p.c. second day,
then 2 mg/kg orally t.d.s. p.c. third day and thereafter for 30 days

Paediatric dose

Roundworm

6–10 mg/kg t.d.s. p.c. for 7–10 days

Adverse effects

— (filariasis) headache, weakness, malaise, nausea, vomiting, rash
— (onchocerciasis) facial oedema, itchy eyes
— allergic reaction

Note

— administer with care to avoid or control allergic or other untoward reactions
— severe reactions may develop after a single dose when heavy infestations are treated

MEBENDAZOLE

Use

— whipworm, hookworm, roundworm and pinworm

Dose (Adults and children over 2 years)

i) 100 mg orally as single dose, repeated after 2–4 weeks (pinworm); OR
ii) 100 mg orally mane and nocte for 3 consecutive days (others). Second course may be necessary after 3 weeks.

NICLOSAMIDE

Use

— tapeworm

Adult dose

2 g orally as a single dose after breakfast

Paediatric dose

2–8 years: 1 g orally as a single dose after breakfast
under 2 years: 0.5 g orally as a single dose after breakfast

Nursing points

— tablet chewed thoroughly and taken with a little water after a light breakfast
— if treating pork tapeworm infestation, drastic saline purgation is necessary 2 hours after medication

Note

— if dwarf tapeworm, half the initial single dose is taken daily for the next 6 days

PYRANTEL

Use

— thread-, round- and hookworm

Dose

Based on 10 mg pyrantel base/kg for adults and children given as a single oral dose

Adverse effects

— nausea, vomiting, abdominal cramps, diarrhoea
— dizziness, drowsiness, insomnia, rash

Note

— granules can be either sprinkled on food or taken as a drink by reconstituting with water or milk (10 ml/sachet)

THIABENDAZOLE

Use

— roundworm, pinworm, threadworm, hookworm, and whipworm

Dose

Based on 25 mg/kg for adults and children given orally after breakfast and the evening meal for 2 successive days up to a maximum of 1.5 g per dose
May be repeated in 7 days

Adverse effects

— anorexia, nausea, vomiting, dizziness
— allergic reaction

OTHER ANTHELMINTICS

See metronidazole and tinidazole

TOPICAL RECTAL MEDICATION

Actions and preparations

— adrenaline, ephedrine and phenylephrine are local decongestants
— benzocaine, lignocaine and cinchocaine relieve pain and spasm
— bismuth compounds and zinc oxide reduce inflammation
— clemizole has an antipruritic effect
— hydrocortisone, prednisolone and fluocortolone have an anti-inflammatory, antipruritic and local decongestant effect

Use

— painful anorectal conditions accompanied by swelling and inflammation

Dose

Insert suppository or ointment into rectum morning and evening and after each bowel action

3 Drugs affecting the cardiovascular system

CARDIAC GLYCOSIDE

DIGOXIN

Action

— preparation of digitalis which is excreted via the kidneys
— increases the force of contraction in the failing heart (positive inotropic action)
— slows heart rate (negative chronotropic action)
— increases myocardial excitability (high doses)
— IV digoxin takes effect in 5–10 minutes and has maximum effect in 2 hours
— oral digoxin takes effect in about an hour, has its maximum effect in 6 hours and may remain effective for up to 6 days

Use

— congestive cardiac failure
— atrial cardiac arrhythmias

Adult digitalizing (loading) dose

If no cardiac glycoside given in last 2 weeks:
  i) 0.75–1.5 mg (geriatric 0.5–0.75 mg) orally as single dose or 3 or 4 divided doses 4- to 6-hourly; OR
  ii) 0.5–1 mg (geriatric 0.25–0.5 mg) slowly IV over 5 minutes as single dose or in divided doses of 0.25–0.5 mg (geriatric 0.125–0.25 mg) 4- to 6-hourly

Adults and children over 10 years maintenance dose

62.5 micrograms–0.25 mg daily or b.d.

Paediatric digitalizing (loading) dose

If no cardiac glycoside given in last 2 weeks:
premature and full term neonates: 30–40 micrograms/kg IM
infants beyond neonatal period: 40–50 micrograms/kg IM
2–9 years: 30–40 micrograms/kg IM
Half total digitalizing dose usually given initially, a further quarter in 6 hours, the remaining quarter after a further 6–12 hours.

Paediatric maintenance dose

neonates: 4–5 micrograms/kg/dose IV or orally 12-hourly

over 2 years: 6 micrograms/kg/dose IV or orally 12-hourly

Adverse effects

— anorexia, nausea, vomiting, diarrhoea
— bradycardia, ectopic beats, coupled beats, ventricular tachycardia, ventricular fibrillation (late)
— headache, mental confusion, visual disturbances

Interactions

— risk of digoxin toxicity increased by hypokalaemia which may result from the associated administration of potassium-losing diuretics, laxatives, corticosteroids or amphotericin B
— digoxin blood levels increased by nifedipine, verapamil, spironolactone, quinidine and calcium salts
— effectiveness of digoxin reduced by phenytoin, neomycin, cholestyramine, cholestipol, sulphasalazine, kaolin-pectin and some antacids

— hyperkalaemia may antagonize cardiac effects of digoxin
— metoclopramide reduces absorption of solid dose form of digoxin

Nursing points

— note any improvement such as return of heart rate to within normal limits, less cyanosis, easier breathing, less oedema, reduced pulse deficit and increased urinary output
— select the correct digitalis preparation noting especially when the weaker product of digoxin Lanoxin PG® (paediatric-geriatric), paediatric elixir or paediatric injection is prescribed
— before giving the preparation, check the heart rate and rhythm. If heart rate less than 60 beats/min (adults), any arrhythmia, pulse deficit or any other adverse effects present (especially anorexia, nausea), withhold the drug and notify the medical officer.
— for a dose of 0.125 mg, give 2 tablets of 62.5 micrograms not half a 0.25 mg tablet
— digoxin causes prolonged intense pain if given IM and severe local irritation if given SC
— digoxin may be added to isotonic saline or glucose and given slowly IV over at least 5 minutes
— digoxin not given as IV infusion
— blood sample for serum digoxin level taken at least 6 hours after last dose
— advise the patient of the need for accurate and regular dosage and to report effects such as anorexia, nausea, vomiting, headache, fatigue and dyspnoea

Note

— anorexia, nausea and vomiting may occur in the absence of digoxin toxicity as a result of gastric irritation and stimulation of the vomiting centre by the drug itself or as a result of congestive cardiac failure

— digoxin withdrawn 3 days before patient undergoes cardiac surgery or cardioversion
— non-urgent treatment may be started with maintenance doses to achieve a steady state gradually
— optimum serum digoxin levels are 0.5–2 nanogram/ml and values of 3 nanogram/ml suggest toxicity
— the therapeutic digoxin blood level is close to the toxic level leaving only a narrow margin of safety
— it may be several days before a reduction in digoxin dose is reflected in a new blood level
— there are 1000 micrograms (μg) in 1 milligram (mg)
— dosage highly individualized

ANTI-ARRHYTHMIC AGENTS

Anti-arrhythmic agents are classified according to properties (Vaughan Williams)

Class I — interfere with depolarization of cardiac membrane (membrane-stabilizing agents)
Class II — beta-adrenoceptor blocking drugs
Class III — prolong duration of cardiac action potential
Class IV — interfere with calcium conductance (slow channel calcium blockers)

QUINIDINE SULPHATE

Action

— Class I agent
— prolongs refractory period
— decreases myocardial excitability
— slight anticholinergic action

Use

— prophylaxis and treatment of paroxysmal atrial and ventricular arrhythmias

Dose

i) 200 mg orally t.d.s. or q.i.d. (prophylaxis); OR
ii) 200–400 mg orally 2- to 4-hourly to a maximum of 3 g daily (therapeutic); OR
iii) 600 mg orally 8- to 12-hourly (SR, therapeutic)

Adverse effects

— allergy including rash, angioneurotic oedema, severe hypotension, respiratory depression or arrest, thrombocytopenic purpura (rare)
— ventricular arrhythmias or heart block
— anorexia, nausea, diarrhoea, colic
— cinchonism including tinnitus, deafness, vertigo, visual impairment

Interactions

— increased effectiveness of digoxin, coumarin anticoagulants, some beta-adrenoceptor blocking drugs and some skeletal muscle relaxants
— effect reduced by phenobarbitone, phenytoin and rifampicin

Nursing points

— not to be confused with the antimalarial quinine
— idiosyncrasy detected by noting the effect of a test dose of 200 mg
— gastrointestinal irritation may be reduced by taking drug with food
— count apical heart rate for a full minute
— note and report changes in heart rate, rhythm and character, blood pressure or cardiac monitor pattern especially if one or more ventricular extrasystoles every six normal beats
— sustained release tablets must be swallowed whole

QUINIDINE BISULPHATE

— as for quinidine sulphate

Dose

0.5–1.25 g orally b.d. sustained release tablet with food, then 0.75 g orally b.d. after conversion of atrial fibrillation

Note

— possible hypersensitivity to quinidine ascertained by test dose of 0.25 g

AMIODARONE

Action

— Class III agent
— prolongs refractory period of atrial, nodal and ventricular tissues
— increases coronary blood flow
— reduces cardiac oxygen requirements

Use

— atrial fibrillation

— supraventricular and ventricular tachycardia refractory to other anti-arrhythmic drugs
— angina pectoris
— Wolff-Parkinson-White syndrome

Loading dose

200 mg orally t.d.s. for 1 week, then reduce to 200 mg orally b.d. for 1 week

Maintenance dose

i) 200–400 mg orally daily; OR
ii) 200 mg orally 5 out of 7 days; OR
iii) 200 mg orally alternate days

Adverse effects

— reversible benign yellowish-brown corneal microdeposits
— skin photosensitivity and discolouration
— peripheral neuropathy
— insomnia
— thyroid dysfunction
— nausea
— alveolitis (rare but fatal)

Interactions

— increases plasma levels of digoxin, quinidine and procainamide
— activity of warfarin increased significantly
— potentiates bradycardic effect of verapamil and beta-adrenoceptor blocking agents

Nursing points

— advise patient to avoid skin exposure to direct sunlight

Note

— the onset of action is 5–10 days and the half-life is 20–60 days
— during long-term therapy, the patient should have a neurological assessment, thyroid and liver function monitored and regular ophthalmological examination

BRETYLIUM

Action

— Class II and III agent
— potent adrenergic neurone blocking agent
— increases myocardial contractility

Use

— control ventricular arrhythmias resistant to standard treatment

Dose

i) 5 mg/kg IM 6- to 8-hourly; OR
ii) 10 mg/kg/24 hours by slow IV infusion

Adverse effects

— nausea, vomiting (necessitating reducing dose or stopping drug)
— tissue necrosis at injection site

Interactions

— enhanced by levodopa and some beta-adrenoceptor blocking drugs
— increased risk of serious arrhythmias when large doses of tricyclic antidepressants added to bretylium therapy
— effects reduced by previous treatment with the antihypertensive guanethidine

Nursing points

— used only in coronary or intensive care units where facilities for monitoring and treating serious arrhythmias are available
— patient remains recumbent during therapy because of the risk of severe hypotension
— blood pressure monitored frequently during therapy

DISOPYRAMIDE

Action and use

— Class I agent
— as for quinidine

Dose

i) 200–300 mg orally (loading dose) then 100–200 mg 6-hourly; OR

ii) 2 mg/kg (maximum 150 mg) IV bolus over 10–15 minutes followed by slow IV infusion of 0.4 mg/kg/hr up to maximum of 800 mg/24 hours

— see recent pharmacology text for paediatric dose

Adverse effects

— difficulty in micturition, dry mouth, blurred vision
— nausea, vomiting, diarrhoea, colic
— hypotension following rapid IV injection

Interactions

— enhances the effect of some beta-adrenoceptor blocking drugs

Nursing points

— disopyramide should not be premixed with any other drugs
— anticholinergic action may aggravate any urinary difficulty

Note

— nursing mothers taking disopyramide should not breast-feed their infants

FLECAINIDE

Action

— Class 1 agent
— analogue of procainamide
— increases PR interval and QRS duration

Use

— suppression and prevention of ventricular tachycardia and ventricular extrasystoles
— some supraventricular tachycardias

Dose

i) 100 mg orally 12-hourly initially, increasing gradually to 300 mg 12-hourly or 200 mg 8-hourly; OR

ii) 2 mg/kg slowly IV over 10 minutes or diluted with 5% glucose and given as a mini-infusion

Adverse effects

— dizziness, headache, fatigue
— visual disturbances
— gastrointestinal disturbance
— palpitation, chest pain
— dyspnoea
— rash
— tinnitus

Interactions

— cimetidine increases absorption of flecainide

Nursing points

— have available isoprenaline, dopamine or dobutamine, mechanical ventilator and facilities for cardiac monitoring and defibrillation
— dilute for IV infusion only with 5% glucose
— infusion admixture stable only for 24 hours at 25°C

LIGNOCAINE

(known as lidocaine in USA)

Action

— Class I agent
— reduces cardiac irritability

Use

— control of ventricular arrhythmias especially premature ventricular contractions
— local anaesthetic

Dose

i) 1 mg/kg slowly IV over 1–2 minutes initially followed by 2–4 mg/min IV infusion; OR

ii) 321 mg of IM preparation (whole ampoule) slowly IM into deltoid muscle for rapid absorption

Adverse effects

— dizziness, drowsiness, muscle twitching, convulsions
— bradycardia, hypotension, respiratory and/or cardiac arrest

Nursing points

— check that drug solutions to be given IV are for IV use
— monitor IV infusion rate closely by using a microdrip set or burette
— aspirate before giving IM injection to ensure drug not being given IV
— constant heart rate, blood pressure and cardiac monitoring
— have diazepam, isoprenaline and atropine available

Note

— see local anaesthetics

MEXILETINE

Action and use

— Class I agent
— similar to lignocaine but has a longer duration of action and can be given orally

Loading dose

i) 200–250 mg IV bolus over 10 minutes followed by IV infusion of 250 mg added to 500 ml of compatible solution at the rate of 120 ml/hr for first hour; OR
ii) 400 mg orally

Maintenance dose

i) continue IV infusion as prepared at 30 mg/hr depending on response; OR
ii) 200–250 mg orally t.d.s. 2 hours after oral loading dose or after IV infusion stopped

Adverse effects

— nausea, vomiting, unpleasant taste
— drowsiness, dizziness, visual disturbances,

— nystagmus, convulsions, ataxia
— hypotension, bradycardia

Interactions

— ammonium chloride and phenytoin increase drug excretion rate
— sodium bicarbonate reduces drug excretion rate

Nursing points

— mexiletine for injection is compatible with isotonic saline, isotonic glucose and isotonic sodium bicarbonate
— prepared infusion solutions discarded 24 hours after preparation
— monitor IV infusion rate closely by using a microdrip set or burette
— constant heart rate, blood pressure and cardiac monitoring
— check urinary pH as renal excretion increases with low pH
— have atropine available to reverse bradycardia or hypotension
— drug withdrawn gradually over 1 or 2 weeks

PHENYTOIN

Action

— Class I agent
— has positive inotropic effect and enhances conduction
— properties similar to procainamide and quinidine
— anticonvulsant (see p. 132)

Use

— arrhythmias due to digitalis
— ventricular arrhythmias not controlled by lignocaine or procainamide
— grand mal and psychomotor epilepsy (see p. 132)

Dose

i) a loading dose of 1 g orally over 12–24 hours, followed by 100 mg 6-hourly; OR
ii) 3.5–5 mg/kg IV initially, repeated if necessary at a rate not exceeding 50 mg/min

Adverse effects (associated with rapid IV injection)

— bradycardia, hypotension, respiratory depression
— thrombophlebitis

Interactions

— multiple drug interactions (too numerous to list)

Nursing points

— not added to IV infusion solutions
— not mixed with other drugs
— avoid perivascular or SC injection of this highly alkaline solution
— supplied as 'Ready-Mix' solution
— constant heart rate, blood pressure and cardiac monitoring
— IV administration must not exceed 50 mg/min
— have diazepam, atropine, metaraminol and sodium bicarbonate available

PROCAINAMIDE

Action and use

— Class I agent
— similar in action to quinidine and procaine, but used mainly for ventricular arrhythmias
— peripheral vasodilator

Dose

i) 1 g orally initially followed by 50 mg/kg daily given in divided doses at 3-hour intervals or 0.5–1 g 4- to 6-hourly; OR
ii) 0.5–1 g IM 6-hourly until oral therapy commenced; OR
iii) in extreme emergency, 0.2–1 g diluted and given by IV infusion at 25–50 mg/min monitored by ECG and blood pressure recordings

Adverse effects

— nausea, vomiting, urticaria, rash
— fever, chills, agranulocytosis
— severe hypotension and ventricular arrhythmias especially if given IV

— psychosis with hallucinations (rare)
— syndrome resembling lupus erythematosus (rare)

Interactions

— enhances the effect of some beta-adrenoceptor blocking drugs
— cimetidine increases procainamide blood levels

Nursing points

— capsules should be swallowed with water and should not be broken or chewed
— patient remains recumbent during infusion
— frequent heart rate, blood pressure and ECG monitoring during infusion
— if fall in blood pressure exceeds 15 mm Hg, infusion is discontinued temporarily
— advise patient to report sore mouth or throat, fever or respiratory tract infection
— solutions darker than light amber must be discarded

VERAPAMIL

Action

— Class IV agent
— calcium antagonist which impedes the transport of calcium ions across the cell membrane
— increases the refractory period
— reduces myocardial oxygen requirements

Use

— prophylaxis and treatment of angina pectoris
— cardiac arrhythmias
— essential hypertension, hypertensive crises

Dose

i) 40–120 mg orally t.d.s. or q.i.d.; OR
ii) 5 mg slowly IV repeated in 5–10 minutes if required or followed by IV infusion at 5–10 mg/hr
— see recent pharmacology text for paediatric dose

Adverse effects

— nausea, dizziness
— hypotension, transient heart block after rapid IV injection
— ventricular fibrillation

Interactions

— not given with or immediately after beta-adrenoceptor blocking agents
— digoxin blood levels increased by verapamil, even higher when quinidine added to therapy
— quinidine reduces verapamil levels

Nursing points

— constant heart rate, blood pressure and cardiac monitoring
— have adrenaline or orciprenaline available

ANTIHYPERTENSIVE AGENTS

One or more antihypertensive agents may be used in conjunction with diuretics and/or beta-adrenoceptor blocking agents allowing smoother control of hypertension using smaller drug doses

CAPTOPRIL

Action

— prevents conversion of angiotensin I to angiotensin II by inhibition of the angiotensin converting enzyme, kininase II, resulting in decreased aldosterone production

Use

— severe hypertension where other therapy has failed

Dose

25 mg orally t.d.s. 1 hour a.c. gradually increased up to a maximum of 150 mg t.d.s.

Adverse effects

— taste disturbance, gastric irritation, aphthous mouth ulcers
— rash, pruritus
— leucopenia, agranulocytosis
— proteinuria, nephrotic syndrome, renal failure
— hyperkalaemia

Interactions

— patients, newly commenced on diuretic therapy, may have a severe hypotensive response within 3 hours of initial dose
— increases serum potassium levels especially if concurrent use of potassium-sparing diuretics or potassium supplements
— antihypertensives which cause increased renin activity enhance effect of captopril

Nursing points

— check for urinary protein prior to treatment then monthly for first 8 months and periodically thereafter
— blood pressure recorded frequently for 1 hour after initial dose
— medical supervision should be maintained for at least 1 hour after initial dose
— report immediately any rash, fever or sore throat, as these are early signs of leucopenia
— advise patient to keep appointments during initial therapy and report any rash, fever or sore throat immediately

ENALAPRIL

Action

— a prodrug which is rapidly hydrolysed to enalaprilat, a potent angiotensin converting enzyme inhibitor
— enalaprilat prevents conversion of angiotensin I to angiotensin II by inhibition of the angiotensin converting enzyme, kininase II, resulting in decreased aldosterone production

Use

— essential hypertension
— renovascular hypertension

Dose

i) 10–20 mg orally daily (essential hypertension)
ii) 2.5–5 mg orally daily initially increasing gradually to 20 mg daily (renovascular hypertension)

Adverse effects

— dizziness, headache, fatigue
— nausea, diarrhoea
— persistent cough
— postural hypotension
— rash
— hyperkalaemia
— occasionally, loss of taste

Interactions

— observe closely for hypotensive response if enalapril therapy initiated in patients on diuretics
— increases lithium blood level

Note

— patient advised that if fluid loss from any cause, e.g., vomiting, diarrhoea, blood loss, stop drug and take added salt
— mothers taking enalapril should not breast-feed their infants
— plasma creatinine monitored 2–4 weeks after starting drug

CLONIDINE

Action

— inhibits central sympathetic outflow resulting in reduced sympathetic tone

Use

— moderately severe hypertension
— in smaller doses for migraine prophylaxis, vascular headaches and menopausal flushes

Dose (hypertension)

i) 75 micrograms orally b.d. or t.d.s. initially then 150–300 micrograms t.d.s.; or
ii) 150–300 micrograms IM; or
iii) 150–300 micrograms diluted in 10 ml isotonic saline given slowly IV over 5 minutes

Adverse effects

— drowsiness, depression
— dry mouth, constipation, nausea, vomiting
— bradycardia, postural hypotension
— weight gain

Interactions

— clonidine may enhance the effects of central nervous system depressants such as alcohol, sedatives etc.
— tricyclic antidepressants reduce effect of clonidine
— beta-adrenoceptor blocking agents reduce effect of clonidine
— thiazide diuretics enhance effect of clonidine

Nursing points

— may be a transient hypertensive response of 5–10 mm Hg lasting for about 5 minutes after IV injection (reduced by slower IV administration)
— monitor supine and standing systolic and diastolic blood pressure
— note oliguria, oedema and weight gain
— warn patient against driving a vehicle or operating machinery if drowsy
— warn patient to sit or lie down at the onset of faintness (postural hypotension)
— advise patient to avoid postural hypotension by moving gradually to a sitting or standing position especially after sleep
— advise patient that postural hypotension is aggravated by prolonged standing, hot baths or showers, hot weather, physical exertion, large meals and alcohol ingestion
— warn patient against ceasing therapy suddenly or missing a dose (prevents rebound hypertension)
— note instability in previously controlled diabetic

Note

— oral therapy terminated gradually over 7 days
— mothers taking clonidine should not breast-feed their infants

DEBRISOQUINE

Action

— blocks transmission of sympathetic nerve impulses at nerve terminals by preventing release of noradrenaline so reduces peripheral vascular resistance

Use

— mild, moderate and severe hypertension

Dose

5–20 mg orally b.d. increasing by 10–20 mg every 3–4 days depending on response up to 150 mg b.d.

Adverse effects

— postural and exercise hypotension
— nausea, headache, malaise, sweating
— impotence
— occasionally, fluid retention, depression, nocturia, frequency of micturition

Interactions

— antihypertensive effect reduced by chlorpromazine, tricyclic and monoamine oxidase inhibitor antidepressants, amphetamines and other sympathomimetic agents
— enhances effects of phenylephrine
— less debrisoquine required if patient taking levodopa

Nursing points

— monitor supine and standing systolic and diastolic blood pressure
— see clonidine for ways of avoiding postural hypotension (this page)
— advise patient to discuss taking any OTC preparations with the medical officer or pharmacist

DIAZOXIDE

Action

— IV diazoxide causes a fall in blood pressure by dilatation of the arterioles
— increases blood glucose levels

Use

— hypertensive crises
— intractable hypoglycaemia
— to reduce the danger of haemorrhage
  in hypertensive patients undergoing
  renal biopsy or arteriography

Adult dose

i) 1–3 mg/kg up to a maximum of
   150 mg as minibolus IV over 30
   seconds for hypertensive crisis,
   avoiding extravasation. May be
   repeated at 5–15 minute-intervals as
   required; OR
ii) 300 mg as bolus IV over 30 seconds
    for hypertensive crisis, avoiding
    extravasation. May be repeated in $\frac{1}{2}$
    hour, giving up to 4 doses in 24
    hours if required

Paediatric dose

1–3 mg/kg given as for adults

Adverse effects

— hypotension, reversible shock
— transient nausea, vomiting, abdominal
  discomfort
— transient hyperglycaemia, sodium and
  water retention

Interactions

— less diazoxide required if patient
  taking beta-adrenoceptor blocking
  agents
— thiazide diuretics enhance the
  hyperglycaemic and hypotensive
  effects of diazoxide

Nursing points

— must be given undiluted IV within 30
  seconds
— not given SC or IM
— patient remains recumbent during
  and for $\frac{1}{2}$ hour after the injection
— the blood pressure is recorded
  before the injection and at 1 minute
  intervals after injection for the first 5
  minutes, then at 5 minute intervals
  until blood pressure begins to rise
  then hourly as required

— check for glycosuria if treatment
  prolonged
— store in a cool dark place

Note

— have noradrenaline available to
  reverse severe hypotension
— should be used in eclampsia with
  discretion

FELODIPINE

Action

— calcium antagonist which impedes
  the transport of calcium ions across
  the cell membrane.
— decreases peripheral vascular
  resistance
— mild naturetic and diuretic effect

Use

— hypertension

Dose

2.5 mg orally b.d. in fixed relation to
food for consistent absorption for first
week, then 5–10 mg orally b.d.

Adverse effects

— flushing, peripheral oedema
— nausea
— headache, dizziness, fatigue, muscle
  weakness

GUANETHIDINE

Action

— causes depletion of noradrenaline
  stores in peripheral sympathetic
  (adrenergic) nerve terminals
— effective in 2–3 days and continues
  for 7–10 days after withdrawal
— sensitizes effector cells to
  catecholamines

Use

— mild, moderate and severe essential
  hypertension

— hypertension secondary to renal disease
— malignant hypertension

Dose

Hospitalized patients

5–50 mg orally daily increased by 25 or 50 mg daily or alternate days according to response up to 150 mg daily

Outside hospital

10 mg orally daily increased by 10 mg at weekly intervals according to response up to 150 mg daily

Adverse effects

— postural and exertional hypotension
— bradycardia
— diarrhoea
— failure of ejaculation
— fluid retention
— nasal congestion
— severe hypertensive reaction in patient with phaeochromocytoma

Interactions

— antihypertensive effects enhanced by levodopa and beta-adrenoceptor blocking agents
— effects of guanethidine may be reduced by tricyclic antidepressants, monoamine oxidase inhibitors and phenothiazines
— patients taking guanethidine are sensitive to adrenaline, amphetamine and other sympathomimetic agents
— patients taking large doses of tricyclic antidepressants are subject to serious cardiac arrhythmias if given guanethidine

Nursing points

— taken as single daily dose preferably in morning
— monitor supine and standing systolic and diastolic blood pressure
— note oedema and weight gain
— see clonidine for ways of avoiding postural hypotension (p. 40)

— have oxygen, atropine, phentolamine, vasopressors and solutions for volume replacement available

Note

— **discontinued in Australia**
— contra-indicated if patient has phaeochromocytoma
— monoamine oxidase inhibitors should be discontinued for 1 week before starting guanethidine
— guanethidine withdrawn 2 weeks prior to surgery but in emergencies, high doses of atropine are given to prevent excessive bradycardia

HYDRALAZINE

Action

— causes peripheral vasodilatation
— may have partial alpha-adrenoceptor blocking effect
— increases plasma renin activity

Use

— moderate to severe hypertension
— hypertensive crises especially in pre-eclampsia and renal disease

Adult dose

i) 25 mg orally b.d. increasing over several weeks to 100 mg b.d. as required (rarely 150 mg b.d.); or
ii) 20–40 mg IM repeated as required; or
iii) 10–20 mg diluted in isotonic saline and given slowly IV or infused IV at 1 mg/min

Paediatric dose

0.3–1 mg/kg/day orally initially, gradually increasing to 4 mg/kg/day in 2 divided doses (maximum 200 mg/day)

Adverse effects

— postural hypotension, tachycardia, palpitations, angina pectoris
— flushing, sweating, headache
— anorexia, nausea, vomiting

— localized oedema
— syndrome resembling lupus erythematosus (rare)

Interactions

— antihypertensive effect enhanced by MAO inhibitors, tricyclic antidepressants and thiazide diuretics
— beta-adrenoceptor blocking agents given in combination to counteract reflex tachycardia

Nursing points

— absorption enhanced when taken with food
— hydralazine injection should not be added to other drugs in a multiple infusion solution
— hydralazine should not be added to glucose solutions or biological fluids
— discard any unused solution
— hydralazine injection is diluted in isotonic saline
— warn patient against ceasing therapy suddenly (prevents rebound hypertension)
— have noradrenaline and angiotensin available
— see clonidine for ways of avoiding postural hypotension (p. 40)

Note

— mothers taking hydralazine should not breast-feed their infants

METHYLDOPA

Action

— although mechanism is still uncertain, is believed to act mainly through an inhibition of central sympathetic outflow

Use

— mild, moderate or severe hypertension
— acute hypertensive crises

Dose

i) 250 mg orally b.d. or t.d.s. initially, then increased gradually as required to 2 g/day in 2–4 divided doses; OR
ii) 250–500 mg added to 100 ml 5% glucose and given by slow IV infusion over 30–60 min

Adverse effects

— transient drowsiness, headache and weakness
— oedema, weight gain
— postural hypotension, bradycardia
— nasal stuffiness
— haemolytic anaemia
— positive direct Coombs' test

Interactions

— methyldopa dose may need to be reduced when beta-adrenoceptor blocking agents added to regime
— pressor response to noradrenaline and phenylpropanolamine increased

Nursing points

— monitor supine and standing systolic and diastolic blood pressure
— note oliguria, oedema and weight gain
— warn patient against driving a vehicle or operating machinery if drowsy
— see clonidine for ways of avoiding postural hypotension (p. 40)

MINOXIDIL

Action

— reduces peripheral vascular resistance
— reflex-mediated increase in cardiac output
— increases plasma renin activity

Use

— as adjunctive therapy with beta-adrenoceptor blocking drugs and diuretics in adults with severe refractory hypertension

Dose

5 mg orally as single daily dose, increasing gradually to 50 mg b.d.

Adverse effects

— peripheral oedema and possible weight gain
— tachycardia
— hypertrichosis (excessive hairiness)
— reduced haemoglobin (temporary)

Interactions

— effects enhanced by concurrent antihypertensive and beta-adrenoceptor blocking agents
— increased sympathetic nervous activity caused by minoxidil is counteracted by beta-adrenoceptor blocking agents

Nursing points

— monitor supine and standing systolic and diastolic blood pressure
— note oedema, weight gain

Note

— patient warned of hypertrichosis, a reversible elongation, thickening and enhanced pigmentation of fine body hair

PRAZOSIN

Action

— causes peripheral vasodilatation but seldom produces tachycardia

Use

— mild, moderate or severe hypertension
— congestive cardiac failure not caused by mechanical obstruction

Dose

0.5 mg orally nocte initially, increasing gradually to 2 mg b.d. or t.d.s. then after 4 to 6 weeks, 3–20 mg daily in divided doses

Adverse effects

— postural hypotension, palpitations
— headache, lassitude, drowsiness

Interactions

— antihypertensive effect enhanced when given with a diuretic and other antihypertensive agents especially beta-adrenoceptor blocking agents allowing smaller doses to be given to reduce the incidence of adverse effects

Nursing points

— advise patient to take the first dose and any increase in dosage on retiring to reduce the 'first dose' effect of dizziness, weakness, sweating and sudden loss of consciousness
— see clonidine for ways of avoiding postural hypotension (p. 40)

RESERPINE

Action

— central nervous system depressant and sedative
— causes depletion of noradrenaline stores in peripheral sympathetic nerve terminals
— causes depletion of catecholamines and serotonin stores mainly in the brain and heart
— effective in 4–5 days and continues for many days after withdrawal

Use

— hypertension
— hypertensive emergencies
— adjunct to treatment of thyrotoxic heart disease
— sedative in mild anxiety states and chronic psychoses

Dose

Hypertension

i) 0.25–0.5 mg orally daily initially gradually increasing to 1 mg daily as a single dose or 4 divided doses p.c;
   OR
ii) 2.5–5 mg IM (hypertensive crisis)

Psychiatry
2.5–5 mg IM initially then 0.25–2 mg orally daily in 2 or 3 divided doses

Adverse effects

— nasal congestion
— depression, drowsiness, lethargy
— diarrhoea, fluid retention
— severe depression with suicidal tendency (high doses)
— occasionally, extrapyramidal reaction

Interactions

— hypotensive effects enhanced by thiazide diuretics
— reserpine may enhance the effect of some beta-adrenoceptor blocking agents and increase the risk of cardiac glycoside toxicity
— antagonized by sympathomimetic amines and tricyclic antidepressants

Nursing points

— gastrointestinal irritation is reduced by taking drug after food
— monitor supine and standing systolic and diastolic blood pressure
— note weight gain
— report signs of mental depression as therapy must stop

Note

— **discontinued in Australia including compounds**
— should not be used while breast-feeding as it causes nasal stuffiness, respiratory difficulty, bradycardia and feeding problems in the infant
— reserpine withdrawn 2 weeks prior to surgery but in emergencies, high doses of atropine are given to prevent excessive bradycardia

RESERPINE WITH DIHYDRALAZINE

Calming effect of reserpine combined with an increase in renal and cerebral blood flow caused by dihydralazine produces a gradual and sustained reduction in hypertension using lower drug doses

Dose

1 tablet t.d.s. p.c. gradually increasing to 2 tablets t.d.s. if required

SODIUM NITROPRUSSIDE

Action

— potent short-acting IV agent which produces peripheral vasodilatation by a direct action on blood vessels

Use

— hypertensive crises
— elective hypotension to reduce surgical haemorrhage

Dose

— reconstitute contents of 50 mg vial with 2–3 ml 5% glucose in water
— no other diluent should be used
— the reconstituted stock should be diluted in 500 ml 5% glucose in water (100 micrograms/ml) or 1000 ml 5% glucose in water (50 micrograms/ml) depending on the desired concentration
— no other drugs to be added
— protect from light by wrapping immediately in aluminium foil, black plastic sheeting or some other opaque material
— a burette, infusion pump or micro-drip regulator should be used to deliver the solution IV at 0.5–10 micrograms/kg/min

Adverse effects

— postural hypotension, tachycardia, palpitations
— dizziness, drowsiness, headache
— nausea, vomiting, sweating, muscle twitching, agitation (if too rapid reduction in blood pressure)

Interactions

— enhanced by antihypertensive agents, volatile-liquid anaesthetics and most other circulatory depressants

Nursing points

— patient remains recumbent during infusion to avoid severe postural hypotensive effects
— if prepared IV solution highly coloured (blue, green or dark red) replace it
— monitor blood pressure frequently and vigilantly so that drip rate can be regulated very closely depending on response (systolic blood pressure should not be less than 60 mm Hg (7980Pa))
— any stock or prepared solutions should not be kept or used longer than 4 hours
— avoid extravasation

OTHER ANTIHYPERTENSIVE AGENTS

See verapamil, nifedipine

ANTI-ANGINA AGENTS

GLYCERYL TRINITRATE TABLETS

Action

— relaxes smooth muscle, including vascular muscle
— reduces myocardial oxygen demand by peripheral vasodilatation
— effective in 2–3 minutes with a duration of 30 minutes

Use

— prophylaxis and treatment of angina pectoris

Dose

600–1200 micrograms SL or in buccal cheek pouch and allowed to dissolve at the first sign of an attack, or if about to undertake an activity known to cause an attack

Adverse effects

— flushing of the face, throbbing headache
— tachycardia, dizziness

Interactions

— alcohol may enhance vascular effects and produce hypotension

Instructions to patient

— tablet taken as early in the attack as possible
— tablet not swallowed but allowed to dissolve under the tongue or in pouch of cheek
— ½ tablet (300 micrograms) may be adequate early in onset
— once pain is relieved or headache becomes severe, tablet may be removed or swallowed
— if 2 fresh tablets and rest in a chair do not relieve chest pain within 15 minutes, a medical officer should be consulted
— keep tablets airtight in manufacturer's bottle and do not put

other drugs or any materials apart from the manufacturer's packing into the bottle
— store in a cool place; should not be kept close to the body or in direct sunlight
— unopened bottle has shelf-life of 2 years if stored below 25°C
— tablets unused 3 months after first opening a bottle should be discarded and a fresh supply obtained
— tell 2 other household members where main supply kept

Nursing points

— patient to have access to tablets if accustomed to self-medication
— medication ineffective if swallowed
— patient may sit or lie down for 10 to 20 minutes after taking tablet to avoid dizziness
— once pain is relieved or headache becomes severe, tablet may be removed or swallowed
— ½ tablet (300 micrograms) may be adequate early in onset
— if 2 fresh tablets and a rest do not relieve the attack within 15 minutes, a medical officer should be notified or the patient taken to an emergency department
— keep tablets below 25°C in a glass, airtight container protected from light and replace after 3 months and do not put other drugs or any materials apart from the manufacturer's packing into the bottle
— tolerance disappears after withdrawal for one week
— ensure patient receives instructions leaflet

Note

— abrupt withdrawal following chronic use may precipitate angina
— use with caution if increased intraocular or intracranial pressure

GLYCERYL TRINITRATE OINTMENT

Action and use

— application to the hairless aspect of the forearm or occasionally the chest

or thigh results in a prolonged vasodilating effect from continuous absorption through the skin, so prevents or relieves anginal pain particularly at night (see glyceryl trinitrate tablets).
— effective within 30 minutes with a duration of 3–8 hours

Preparations and dose
NITRO-BID® OINTMENT 2%

— measure out the required amount of ointment on to the supplied Dose Measuring Applicator and smooth it over a 15 cm (6'') square on the chosen skin area
— the dose ranges from 5 cm applied every 8 hours to 12 cm every 4 hours, but begins with 1 cm (6 mg) every 4 to 8 hours, increasing the dose by 1 cm with each successive dose until optimal dosage reached

NITROLATE® OINTMENT 3%

i) capsule is cut open and the contents squeezed on to the chosen skin area and smoothed over a 7.5 cm (3'') square; OR
ii) the ointment may be spread over a similar area on a piece of paper or plastic wrap and applied to the skin. 7.5 mg (half a capsule) to 60 mg (four capsules) may be applied every 3 to 4 hours if necessary and before retiring

Adverse effects and interactions

— as for glyceryl trinitrate tablets

Nursing points for ointment

— patient to apply ointment where possible, then wash hands
— staff or patient may use a plastic glove or supplied applicator to apply ointment
— for improved absorption and less rubbing off, the area may be covered with plastic wrap and held by adhesive tape

— excess ointment may be removed with a gauze swab, soap and water and the patient placed in the recumbent position
— tell the patient that the Nitrolate® ointment capsules are NOT to be swallowed

GLYCERYL TRINITRATE PAD

Action and use

— as for glyceryl trinitrate tablets but applied topically to maintain a steady state concentration of glyceryl trinitrate for as long as pad in contact with the skin for at least 24 hours

Dose

Pad releasing 5 mg/24 hours applied once each day initially, or for greater response, apply a pad releasing 10 mg/24 hours

Adverse effects and interactions

— as for glyceryl trinitrate tablets

Nursing points

— separate protective foil cover and apply to a hairless skin site not subject to excessive movement, preferably the chest or inner aspect of arm
— pad applied once each day and if loosens or falls off, new pad applied

GLYCERYL TRINITRATE SOLUTION (IV USE)

Action

— relaxes vascular smooth muscle causing reduction in systolic, diastolic and mean arterial blood pressure
— reduces myocardial oxygen demand by peripheral vasodilatation

Use

— angina pectoris refractory to other treatment

— congestive cardiac failure associated with acute myocardial infarction
— control peri-operative hypertension
— produce controlled hypotension during neurosurgery and orthopaedic surgery

Dose

— dilute 50 mg in a 500 ml *glass* bottle of either 5% glucose or isotonic saline to make a concentration of 100 micrograms/ml
— no other drugs to be added
— both a micro-drip regulator and infusion pump used to deliver the solution IV at an initial rate of 5 micrograms/min then adjusted as required for pain relief while maintaining adequate systemic blood pressure

Adverse effects

— headache
— tachycardia, palpitations
— nausea, vomiting, abdominal pain, retrosternal discomfort
— apprehension, restlessness, dizziness
— muscle twitching
— overdose, severe hypotension, reflex tachycardia

Interactions

— IV glyceryl trinitrate may slow morphine metabolism
— tricyclic antidepressants and anticholinergic agents may potentiate hypotensive effect of IV glyceryl trinitrate

Nursing points

— depending on fluid requirements, 100 mg may be added to 500 ml of infusion fluid to make a concentration of 200 micrograms/ml or 200 mg may be added to give a maximum concentration of 400 micrograms/ml
as glyceryl trinitrate is absorbed strongly by plastics, glass solution bottles are used and 50 ml of preparation is discarded when

priming the general purpose PVC administration set
— invert prepared solution several times for uniform dilution
— unused portions of prepared solution discarded after 24 hours
— continuous monitoring of heart rate, blood pressure and chest pain, especially at commencement of infusion and after dose increase
— store stock in refrigerator but do not freeze

Note

— if Tridilset® administration set is used which has non-absorbing tubing, follow the manufacturers' instructions closely

DILTIAZEM
Action

— calcium antagonist which impedes the transport of calcium ions into cells during membrane deplorization of cardiac and vascular smooth muscle
— reduces myocardial oxygen requirements
— potent dilator of coronary arteries

Use

— moderate to severe angina pectoris

Dose

30 mg orally t.d.s. a.c. and nocte initially, increasing gradually to 60–90 mg t.d.s. a.c. and nocte

Adverse effects

— oedema, atrioventricular block, bradycardia, hypotension
— rash, urticaria
— gastrointestinal disturbances
— headache, dizziness
— flushing

Interactions

— effects of diltiazem enhanced by beta-adrenoceptor blocking drugs

— diltiazem increases blood digoxin levels, trough blood levels of cyclosporin and blood creatinine level
— diltiazem blood levels decreased by diazepam

Nursing points

— monitor closely for bradycardia, hypotension, atrioventricular block
— have available atropine, isoprenaline, dopamine or dobutamine, diuretics

Note

— blood digoxin levels should be monitored closely 6–8 days after commencing combination
— sudden withdrawal of diltiazem has been associated with severe angina

NIFEDIPINE
Action

— calcium antagonist which impedes the transport of calcium ions into cells during depolarization so causes improvement in the myocardial oxygen supply and reduction in myocardial work by reducing afterload

Use

— prophylaxis and treatment of angina pectoris
— hypertension

Dose

10 mg orally t.d.s. increasing to 20 mg q.i.d. (angina)
20–40 mg orally b.d. (hypertension)

Adverse effects

— peripheral oedema, hypotension, palpitations, tachycardia
— flushing, dizziness, light headedness
— headache, weakness

Interactions

— increases digoxin blood levels

— may cause cardiac failure if used concurrently with beta-adrenoceptor blocking agents

Nursing points

— capsules not to be substituted for tablets and vice versa
— protect stock from direct sunlight

PENTAERYTHRITOL
Action

— as for glyceryl trinitrate but more prolonged
— effective within 1 hour with a duration of 5 hours

Use

— prophylaxis of angina pectoris
— reduce severity of angina attack
— reduce glyceryl trinitrate requirements

Dose

i) 10–40 mg orally q.i.d. a.c.; OR
ii) 80 mg orally b.d. a.c. (SA)

Adverse effects

— rash (necessitating stopping drug)
— headache
— gastrointestinal disturbances

Nursing points

— select correct preparation
— SA means sustained action

PERHEXILINE
Action

— appears to have a depressant effect on all smooth muscle
— has cardiac membrane effect similar to that of quinidine and procainamide
— reduces exercise-induced tachycardia
— has mild diuretic effect

Use

— reduce the frequency of moderate to severe angina attacks resistant to other conventional treatment

Dose

100 mg orally daily initially, then 50–300 mg orally daily in 2 divided doses depending on response

Adverse effects

— anorexia, nausea, vomiting
— weight loss
— dizziness, headache, weakness, tremors, fatigue
— hepatotoxicity
— neuropathy, ataxia
— severe hypoglycaemia

Interactions

— hypoglycaemia provoked by concurrent use of hypoglycaemic agents and beta-adrenoceptor blocking agents

Nursing point

— warn patient against driving a vehicle or operating machinery because of the possibility of dizziness, weakness and ataxia

SORBIDE NITRATE
Action

— milder but more prolonged than glyceryl trinitrate
— effective SL within 5 minutes with a duration of 2 hours
— effective orally within 30 minutes with a duration of 5 hours

Use

— prophylaxis and treatment of angina pectoris
— acute and chronic congestive cardiac failure

Dose

i) 5–10 mg (sublingual tablet) prophylactically or 2- to 3-hourly for acute angina; OR
ii) 10–30 mg (oral tablet) q.i.d. for prophylaxis
iii) 2–5 sprays on chest from about 20 cm, then rub in (transdermal spray) in the morning after washing and nocte p.r.n.

Adverse effects

— headache
— flushing

Nursing points

— patient to have access to tablets if accustomed to self-medication
— once pain is relieved or headache becomes severe, tablet may be removed
— reduced dosage and analgesics may be required if headache severe
— if 2 fresh sublingual tablets and a rest do not relieve the acute anginal attack within 15 minutes, a medical officer is notified or the patient taken to an emergency department
— advise the patient to keep the tablets airtight in the manufacturer's bottle in a cool place
— remember that the 5 mg tablet is for sublingual administration and the 10 mg tablet is taken orally

Note

— use with caution if increased intraocular pressure

OTHER ANTIANGINAL AGENTS

See dipyridamole, verapamil and beta-adrenoceptor blocking agents

PERIPHERAL VASODILATORS

BETAHISTINE

Action

— histamine-like drug which increases blood flow in the microcirculation

Use

— vertebral basilar insufficiency
— Ménière's syndrome
— vertigo
— improvement in hearing acuity
— nausea and/or vomiting and tinnitus

Dose

8 mg orally t.d.s. or q.i.d. initially, then 4–8 mg b.d.

Adverse effects

— mild skin or gastrointestinal disturbances
— occasionally, headache, dizziness, insomnia

Nursing points

— observe for improvement in mental state in patients with vertebral basilar insufficiency
— note reduction of symptoms in Ménière's syndrome

Note

— should not be used in conjunction with antihistamines

CYCLANDELATE

Action

— produces vasodilatation by direct action on vascular smooth muscle

Use

— cerebrovascular disease
— peripheral vascular disease

Dose

200–400 mg orally q.i.d.

Adverse effects

— gastrointestinal disturbances
— high doses, nausea, flushing

DIHYDROERGOTOXINE

Action

— causes generalized peripheral vasodilatation

Use

— cerebrovascular disease
— peripheral vascular disease
— Ménière's syndrome
— cervical syndrome

Dose

Acute cerebrovascular disturbance

i) 0.3 mg diluted in 20 ml 5% glucose in water and given slowly IV; OR
ii) 0.3 mg IM daily to several times daily while monitoring blood pressure closely

Chronic cerebrovascular insufficiency

0.375 mg SL t.d.s.

Peripheral vascular disease

i) 0.3–0.6 mg IM or SC daily or alternate days together with 0.25 mg SL t.d.s.; OR
ii) 0.3–0.6 mg diluted in 10 ml isotonic saline and given IA daily in affected limb followed by 0.25–0.5 mg SL t.d.s.

Adverse effects

— nasal congestion
— headache
— gastrointestinal disturbances

ISOXSUPRINE

Action

— alpha-adrenoceptor blocking agent
— beta-adrenoceptor stimulating agent

(not blocked by propranolol)
— produces peripheral vasodilatation by a direct effect on vascular smooth muscle acting primarily on blood vessels within skeletal muscle
— produces cardiac stimulation
— produces uterine stimulation

Use

— cerebral and peripheral vascular disease

Dose

10–20 mg orally 3–4 times daily

Adverse effects

— nausea, vomiting
— postural hypotension, tachycardia, palpitations

NICOTINYL ALCOHOL

Action

— produces vasodilatation by direct action on vascular smooth muscle
— as for nicotinic acid but more prolonged

Use

— peripheral vascular disease
— Ménière's syndrome
— migraine

Dose

12.5–50 mg orally several times daily with fluid after food

Adverse effects

— mild transient flushing of face and neck

OXPENTIFYLLINE

Action

— a xanthine derivative thought to increase blood flow in the affected microcirculation

Use

— peripheral vascular disorders

Dose

400 mg orally 2–3 times daily with or after food

Adverse effects

— gastrointestinal disturbances
— dizziness, headache, tremor

Interactions

— combined use with other xanthine derivatives or with sympathomimetics may cause excessive CNS stimulation

Nursing point

— controlled release tablet swallowed whole

Note

— patients on warfarin need closer monitoring of prothrombin activity

PHENOXYBENZAMINE

Action

— a powerful long acting alpha-adrenoceptor blocking agent

Use

— hypertensive episodes caused by phaeochromocytoma
— urinary retention caused by neurogenic bladder or prostrate hypertrophy
— peripheral vascular disorders

Dose

10 mg nocte initially, increasing gradually to 10–30 mg b.d. as required

Adverse effects

— nasal congestion, miosis, dry mouth
— postural hypotension, tachycardia

Nursing points

— see end of section on peripheral vasodilators

Note

— 2 weeks required to reach optimal dosage level
— may be given in critical care unit by slow IV infusion in severe shock unresponsive to conventional treatment

PHENTOLAMINE

Action

— as for phenoxybenzamine

Use

— diagnostic agent for phaeochromocytoma
— relieve paroxysmal hypertension in cases of confirmed phaeochromocytoma, in conjunction with a beta-adrenoceptor blocking agent
— prophylactic measure before and during surgical removal of phaeochromocytoma
— peripheral vascular disorders

Dose

i) 5 mg IV (diagnostic); OR
ii) 5–10 mg IM or IV 2 hours prior to surgery for relief of paroxysmal hypertension or as prophylactic measure; OR
iii) 10 mg IM or IV daily or b.d. in severe cases of peripheral vascular disorder

Adverse effects

— tachycardia

Nursing points

— see end of section on peripheral vasodilators

Note

— superseded in diagnosis of phaeochromocytoma now that catecholamines in the blood and urine can be estimated

Nursing points for peripheral vasodilator agents

— pulse and blood pressure taken with patient both lying and standing
— note tachycardia and hypotension when standing
— see clonidine for ways of avoiding postural hypotension (p. 40)
— observe for improvement of skin colour, temperature and peripheral pulses
— note if less sensitivity to cold, also avoid undue exposure to cold
— prevent ulceration of affected lower extremities by advising careful skin care, close attention to toe nails, properly fitting shoes and hosiery and avoidance of garters, hot water bottles and any trauma
— note if patient can walk further without pain
— advise patient to avoid smoking and alcohol
— medical officer may suggest elevating the head of the bed on 15 cm blocks to improve circulation to legs

Note

— have noradrenaline available
— note and report sweating, falling heart rate and blood pressure in a patient being treated for phaeochromocytoma

OTHER PERIPHERAL VASODILATORS

See hydralazine, nicotinic acid and prazosin

BETA-ADRENOCEPTOR BLOCKING DRUGS

Action

Blocks the beta-adrenoceptors of the sympathethic nervous system, some drugs having more specificity for the receptors dominant in the heart (β_1), other drugs blocking the principal sympathetic receptors in the lungs (β_2) as well as β_1 receptors resulting in:
— reduced rate of impulses through the cardiac conducting system
— reduced cardiac rate and force of contraction
— reduced cardiac output
— reduced blood pressure
— reduced response to stress and exercise
— bronchospasm

Use

— prophylaxis in angina pectoris
— cardiac arrhythmias
— hypertension, usually in conjunction with thiazide diuretics
— migraine prophylaxis
— hypertrophic sub-aortic stenosis
— psychiatry
— thyrotoxicosis
— glaucoma (eye drops)

Preparations and dose

ALPRENOLOL

Dose

i) 50–200 mg orally q.i.d.; OR
ii) 200 mg orally b.d. (SR)

ATENOLOL

Dose

50–100 mg orally daily initially, increasing to 100 mg b.d. depending on response

Note

— cardioselective therefore less likely to cause bronchospasm

ATENOLOL WITH CHLORTHALIDONE

Dose

1–2 tablets daily

LABETALOL

Dose

100–200 mg orally b.d. p.c. initially, increasing to 2400 mg daily in 2–4 divided doses

Note

— alpha- and beta-adrenoceptor blocking agent therefore also likely to cause postural hypotension

METOPROLOL

Dose

i) 50–100 mg orally daily, b.d. or t.d.s.; OR
ii) 5 mg IV at 1–2 mg/min repeated at 5-minute intervals as required up to a total dose of 15 mg

Note

— cardioselective therefore less likely to cause bronchospasm

OXPRENOLOL

Dose

i) 20–40 mg orally b.d. or t.d.s. but may reach the maximum daily dose of 320 mg; OR
ii) 160–320 mg orally mane (SR); OR
iii) 1–2 mg IM (reconstituted in 1 ml isotonic saline); OR
iv) 1–2 mg slowly IV over 30 seconds and repeated in 10–20 minutes as required (reconstituted in 5 ml isotonic saline)

PINDOLOL

Dose

i) 7.5–15 mg orally daily in 1–3 divided doses preferably a.c. (hypertension); OR

ii) 10–30 mg orally daily in 3 divided doses (cardiac arrhythmias), OR
iii) 0.4 mg slowly IV in emergency with further doses of 0.2 mg as required by IV burette over 10 minutes; OR
iv) 2.5 mg orally b.d. increasing to q.i.d. (migraine prophylaxis)

PINDOLOL WITH CLOPAMIDE

Combining the thiazide-like diuretic clopamide with pindolol gives an antihypertensive effect

Dose

1 tablet daily or b.d.

PROPRANOLOL

Adult dose

i) 30–320 mg orally daily in 2–4 divided doses; OR
ii) 1 mg slowly IV over 1 minute repeated at 2-minute intervals as required up to a maximum of 10 mg (5 mg if under anaesthesia); OR
iii) 20 mg orally b.d. or t.d.s. increasing to 40–80 mg t.d.s. (migraine prophylaxis)

Note

— atropine 1–2 mg IV precedes IV propranolol to prevent excessive bradycardia

Paediatric dose

1 mg/kg/day orally increasing gradually to 5 mg/kg/day

SOTALOL

Dose

i) 80–240 mg orally b.d. a.c. (up to 640 mg/day); OR
ii) 0.5–1.5 mg/kg slowly IV over 10 minutes and repeated 6-hourly as necessary, prepared as a solution containing 2 mg/ml in isotonic saline or 5% glucose; OR
iii) 10 mg/hr IV infusion

Note

— possesses additional class III
   antiarrhythmic activity

TIMOLOL

i) 5–15 mg orally b.d. or t.d.s.
   (hypertension, angina pectoris); OR
ii) 1 drop 0.25% ophthalmic solution
   into affected eye b.d. (glaucoma);
   0.5% solution may be required if
   response inadequate

Adverse effects of beta-adrenoceptor blocking drugs

— bradycardia, heart block, postural
   hypotension
— acute congestive cardiac failure
— impairment of peripheral circulation,
   muscle cramps
— bronchospasm
— weakness, fatigue, headache, nasal
   stuffiness
— rash
— vivid dreams

Interactions

— activity of insulin and oral
   hypoglycaemic agents enhanced
   which may mask hypoglycaemic aura
   in diabetics
— enhances cardiac depressant effects
   of most antihypertensive and anti-
   arrhythmic agents and also some
   general anaesthetic agents
— enhances the effects of
   phenothiazines, ergot derivatives and
   levodopa
— hypotensive effects of clonidine
   reduced
— hypotensive effect increased by
   indomethacin

Nursing points for beta-adrenoceptor blocking drugs

— before giving drug, note bradycardia
   (especially if heart rate less than
   50/min), hypotension, dyspnoea,
   cyanosis and circulation in
   extremities

— labetolol, metoprolol and propranolol
   are taken in fixed relation to food for
   consistent absorption
— check weight and keep fluid chart to
   detect fluid retention
— if given IV, monitor ECG, blood
   pressure and central venous pressure
   and have available atropine,
   aminophylline, orciprenaline and
   isoprenaline
— see clonidine for ways of avoiding
   postural hypotension (p. 40)
— dosage is reduced gradually over
   7–10 days to decrease the risk of
   angina pectoris, acute myocardial
   infarction or cardiac arrhythmias

Note

— breast-fed infants of mothers taking
   beta-adrenoceptor blocking drugs
   (except propranolol) should be
   monitored closely for bradycardia and
   hypoglycaemia
— contraindicated in asthma, chronic
   obstructive airways disease, heart
   block and bradycardia.

SYMPATHOMIMETIC AGENTS

Sympathomimetic (adrenergic) agents mimic the effects of sympathetic nerves stimulation. Various agents cause different effects depending on whether the influence is on alpha- or beta-receptors.

Alpha receptor stimulation effects

— vasoconstriction (skin, skeletal muscle, abdominal viscera)
— uterine contraction
— mydriasis
— sphincter contraction (stomach, intestine, urinary bladder)

Beta-1 receptor stimulation effects

— increased heart rate and myocardial contractility
— increased atrio-ventricular conduction
— shortened refractory period
— lipolysis, glycogenolysis, promotion of insulin release

Beta-2 receptor stimulation effects

— vasodilatation (skeletal muscles, coronary vessels, abdominal viscera)
— bronchodilation
— uterine relaxation

ADRENALINE

(known as epinephrine in USA)

Action

— increases heart rate, output, myocardial contractility and blood pressure
— dilates skeletal muscle blood vessels
— constricts blood vessels in skin and mucous membranes
— causes bronchodilatation
— increases glycogenolysis
— inhibits insulin and histamine release
— inhibits uterine contraction
— reduces intraocular pressure
— causes CNS stimulation

Use

— relief of bronchospasm
— relief of mucosal and conjunctival congestion
— heart block and cardiac arrest
— anaphylaxis
— serum sickness
— hypersensitivity reactions
— prolongs action and delays systemic absorption of local anaesthetics
— applied topically to control superficial bleeding
— simple glaucoma

Adult dose

Bronchospasm

i) 0.2–0.5 ml 1 in 1000 solution SC, repeat in 15–30 minutes if required; OR
ii) 1 or 2 inhalations (0.35–0.7 mg) from metered dose aerosol allowing a 2-minute interval between inhalations

Status asthmaticus

i) 0.5 ml 1 in 1000 solution SC at 10-minute intervals for 3 doses; OR
ii) 0.05–0.1 ml 1 in 1000 solution SC initially repeated every 15–60 seconds until relief

Cardiac arrest

i) 0.25–1 ml 1 in 1000 solution diluted to 5 ml with isotonic saline given IV (rarely); OR
ii) 1–8 micrograms/min by IV infusion

Paediatric dose

i) 10 micrograms/kg IV; OR
ii) 0.05–1.0 micrograms/kg/min by IV infusion

Adverse effects

— anxiety, restlessness, tremor, dyspnoea
— tachycardia, palpitation
— sweating, vomiting
— weakness, dizziness, headache
— coldness of extremities
— tissue necrosis at injection site

— gas gangrene at IM site if microbial contamination
— tolerance after repeated use
— hyperglycaemia
— high doses, cardiac arrhythmias, cerebral haemorrhage, pulmonary oedema

Interactions

— adrenergic effects enhanced by reserpine, guanethidine, thyroid hormone, tricyclic antidepressants and other sympathomimetic agents
— IV adrenaline used concurrently with cardiac glycosides, quinidine, cyclopropane or halothane can result in cardiac arrhythmias
— IV adrenaline used with propranolol causes bradycardia

Nursing points

— select correct type of solution and note concentration, dose and route carefully
— use tuberculin syringe for accuracy
— protect stock from light
— discard any discoloured or precipitated solutions
— when giving SC, aspirate to ensure not in vein and inject very slowly
— if ordered IM *NOT* given into buttocks
— rotate injection sites
— if IV injection, monitor cardiac rate and blood pressure especially in first 5 minutes
— ensure adequate fluid intake as bronchial secretions are reduced with prolonged use
— inhalation may cause epigastric pain and the mouth and throat should be rinsed with water after inhaling
— adrenaline is incompatible with alkaline solutions such as sodium bicarbonate
— have phentolamine and propranolol available

ANGIOTENSIN
Action

— increases peripheral arterial

resistance leading to marked and rapid rise in blood pressure but of relatively short duration

Use

— shock not involving hypovolaemia and where other pressor agents have failed or ceased to be effective

Dose

— dissolve 2.5 mg in 5 ml sterile water then add to infusion solution immediately before use
— no other drugs to be added
— a burette, infusion pump or micro-drip regulator should be used to deliver the solution IV at 3–10 micrograms/min
— refer to a specialist text or manufacturer's literature

Adverse effects

— hypertension, bradycardia (both rare)

Nursing points

— monitor blood pressure
— check infusion rate regularly
— monitor fluid status closely
— rate reduced gradually once patient's condition stabilized
— not mixed with blood or serum
— have atropine available

Note

— **discontinued in Australia**
— should not be given to patients being treated with MAO inhibitor or within 14 days of stopping treatment

DOBUTAMINE

Action

— cardioselective beta-adrenoceptor stimulant effects of short duration

Use

— short term treatment of cardiac

failure secondary to acute myocardial infarction or cardiac surgery

Dose

— reconstitute contents of 250 mg vial with 10 ml sterile water (add another 10 ml if not completely dissolved) then add to recommended infusion solution
— a burette, infusion pump or drip regulator should be used to deliver the solution IV at 2.5–10 micrograms/kg/min
— refer to a specialist text or manufacturer's literature

Adverse effects

— marked increase in heart rate and blood pressure
— ventricular ectopic activity

Interactions

— myocardium may be sensitized to the effect of dobutamine by cyclopropane, halothane and related general anaesthetics

Nursing points

— not added to sodium bicarbonate or any other strongly alkaline solution
— monitor infusion for rate and free flow to avoid extravasation
— monitor cardiac rate and rhythm by ECG
— monitor blood pressure, CVP and urinary output frequently
— reconstituted dobutamine stable for 48 hours in refrigerator and for 6 hours at room temperature (below 25°C)

DOPAMINE

Action

— stimulates alpha, beta and dopamine receptors
— renal and mesenteric vasodilatation (low doses)
— effective within 5 minutes with a duration of 10 minutes

— physiological precursor of noradrenaline and adrenaline

Use

— correction of haemodynamic imbalance in acute hypotensive states

Dose

— contents of 1 or more ampoules added to recommended infusion solution
— a burette, infusion pump or micro-drip regulator should be used to deliver the solution IV commencing at 2.5–5 micrograms/kg/min and increasing up to 50 micrograms/kg/min as required
— refer to a specialist text or manufacturer's literature

Adverse effects

— tachycardia, palpitations, ectopic beats
— anginal pain, dyspnoea
— hypotension
— nausea, vomiting, headache
— peripheral vasoconstriction
— gangrene of feet if pre-existing peripheral vascular disease

Interactions

— myocardium is sensitized to the effect of dopamine by cyclopropane, halothane and related general anaesthetics
— effect of dopamine enhanced greatly by MAO inhibitors necessitating starting at 1/10 the usual dose of dopamine
— alpha- and beta-adrenoceptor blocking drugs exhibit complex interactions with dopamine

Nursing points

— not added to sodium bicarbonate or any other strongly alkaline solution
— monitor infusion for rate and free flow to avoid extravasation

— monitor cardiac rate and rhythm by ECG frequently, reporting tachycardia, new arrhythmias
— monitor blood pressure, CVP and urinary output frequently, reporting excessive increase in blood pressure, marked decrease in pulse pressure and reduction in urinary output
— check conscious state and nail bed capillary filling frequently
— note changes in temperature or colour of extremities if pre-existing peripheral vascular disease
— stable for 24 hours after dilution
— check with pharmacist before adding any drug to dopamine
— have phentolamine available as antidote for peripheral ischaemia following extravasation

ISOPRENALINE (known as isoproterenol in USA)

Action

Beta-adrenoceptor stimulant effects resulting in:
— increased cardiac output, excitability and heart rate
— peripheral vasodilatation (IV)
— bronchodilatation
— CNS stimulation

Use

— adjunct in management of shock
— prevention and treatment of heart block
— cardiac arrest
— bronchospasm

Adult dose

Metered aerosol

— 1 or 2 inhalations (0.1–0.2 mg) from metered dose aerosol for acute relief of bronchospasm up to 6 times daily
— if 2 inhalations required, allow a 2-minute interval
— a metered dose aerosol delivering 0.5 mg is also available.

Injection

i) 0.1–1 mg SC or IM (1:5000 solution contains 0.2 mg/ml); OR
ii) 0.01–0.2 mg IV (1 in 50 000 solution 0.02 mg/ml)

Infusion

— dilute 2 mg (10 ml of 1:5000 solution) in 500 ml 5% glucose to make a concentration of 4 micrograms/ml
— use a burette or micro-drip regulator to deliver the solution (1 in 250 000) IV at 0.5–5 micrograms/min

Paediatric dose

0.02–0.05 mg IV
(1 in 5000 solution contains 0.2 mg/ml).

Adverse effects

— tachycardia, palpitation
— nervousness, tremors
— flushing, sweating
— headache
— dry mouth (metered aerosol)

Interactions

— adrenergic effects enhanced by the concomitant use of most sympathomimetics but may be alternated if given 4 hours apart
— antagonized by beta-adrenergic receptor blocking agents
— cardiac arrhythmias may occur if used with cyclopropane or related general anaesthetic agents
— increases theophylline blood levels

Nursing points

— select correct preparation for correct route
— do not use discoloured or precipitated solutions
— see salbutamol for nursing points on metered aerosol (p. 71)
— warn patient to seek medical advice if not obtaining adequate relief
— the infusion rate is adjusted according to the heart rate, ECG,

CVP, systemic blood pressure and urine output (reduce if heart rate exceeds 110 beats/min).

Note

— sudden death can occur following excessive use of sympathomimetic aerosols.

METARAMINOL

Action

— mainly alpha-adrenergic stimulant effects with some beta effects resulting in increased blood pressure and peripheral vasoconstriction
— indirectly causes release of noradrenaline from storage sites
— overall effects similar to noradrenaline but less potent and more prolonged action
— effective within 1–2 minutes (IV) with a duration of 20 minutes
— effective within 5–15 minutes (SC or IM) with a duration of 1 hour

Use

— prevention and treatment of acute hypotension occurring with spinal anaesthesia
— as adjunct in treatment of hypotension

Dose

i)   2–10 mg IM or SC (occasionally) for prevention of hypotension, OR
ii) 15–100 mg diluted in 500 ml of isotonic saline or 5% glucose regulated by burette or micro-drip, the IV infusion rate adjusted to maintain the blood pressure at the desired level; OR
iii) in extreme emergency 0.5–5 mg IV bolus followed by IV infusion as above

Adverse effects

— tachycardia, palpitations, reflex bradycardia
— flushing, sweating, tremor
— nausea, vomiting
— decreased urinary output
— tissue necrosis at injection or infusion site

Interactions

— pressor response enhanced by guanethidine and MAO inhibitors
— pressor effect decreased by alpha-adrenergic blocking agents

Nursing points

— allow at least 10 minutes to elapse between IM doses and change IV infusion rate cautiously to prevent cumulative effect
— observe infusion site for extravasation
— monitor heart rate and systemic blood pressure every 5 minutes until stabilized then every 15 minutes during and for several hours after infusion completed
— reduce rate gradually prior to discontinuing IV infusion to avoid rebound hypotension
— note and report reduced urinary output
— have available phentolamine, propranolol and atropine

NORADRENALINE (known as norepinephrine and levarterenol in USA)

Action

Mainly alpha-adrenergic stimulant effects with some beta effects resulting in:
— increased systemic blood pressure
— increased coronary artery blood flow
— peripheral vasoconstriction

Use

— treatment of acute hypotensive states where blood volume is adequate

Dose

— dilute 2 ml of the 1 in 1000 solution in 500 ml of 5% glucose to make a concentration of 4 micrograms/ml

— no other drugs to be added
— noradrenaline should not be added to isotonic saline, whole blood or plasma
— administer via existing infusion line or into second separate IV site through well secured IV cannula
— a burette or micro-drip regulator should be used to deliver the solution IV at 8–12 micrograms/min initially then adjusted to maintain the blood pressure at the desired level, usually 2–4 micrograms/min

Adverse effects

— tachycardia, palpitations, reflex bradycardia
— anxiety, restlessness, tremor, sweating
— vomiting
— sudden rise in blood pressure which may cause cerebral haemorrhage
— tissue necrosis at infusion site

Interactions

— pressor response significantly increased by guanethidine and methyldopa
— tricyclic antidepressants and MAO inhibitors increase cardiovascular effects of noradrenaline ie. heart rate and blood pressure increase
— contraindicated with cyclopropane and halothane

Nursing points

— select correct solution
— coloured or precipitated solutions are not used
— monitor heart rate and blood pressure every 2 minutes until stabilized at desired level then every 5 minutes
— patient should never be left unattended
— monitor conscious state, temperature and colour of extremities, urinary output and infusion site for extravasation every 15 minutes
— reduce rate gradually prior to discontinuing infusion to avoid rebound hypotension

— have available phentolamine, propranolol and atropine.

OTHER SYMPATHOMIMETIC AGENTS

See drugs used in bronchial asthma, miotics, mydriatics, nasal decongestants

ANTIMIGRAINE PREPARATIONS

ERGOTAMINE

Action

— alpha-adrenoceptor blocking agent causing vasoconstriction
— serotonin antagonist

Use

— relief of acute attacks of migraine and other forms of vascular headache
— not for prophylaxis

Dose

i) 2 mg SL initially, repeated in ½–1 hour if required (restricted to 6 mg/day and 10 mg/week); OR
ii) 1 inhalation (0.45 mg) from metered aerosol initially, repeated in 5 minutes if required (restricted to 6 inhalations in 24 hours and 15/week)

Adverse effects

— muscle cramps, stiffness, tiredness
— numbness and tingling of extremities
— nausea, vomiting, diarrhoea
— rarely, ergotism consisting of severe peripheral vasoconstriction, hypertension and gangrene of extremities

Nursing points

— smallest dose given during prodrome of attack if possible
— encourage patient to lie in quiet, darkened room for about 2 hours
— ensure maximum doses not exceeded

Note

— avoid ergot preparations during pregnancy because of the oxytocic effect
— nursing mothers should avoid taking ergot preparations as it produces vomiting, diarrhoea, weak pulse and unstable blood pressure in the infant

— additional caffeine increases ergotamine absorption and also exerts a vasoconstricting effect
— antihistamines are added for anti-emetic and sedative effects
— belladonna group members are added for anti-emetic and anticholinergic effects
— phenobarbitone provides a sedative effect
— itobarbitone relieves nervous tension and reduces the stimulant effects of caffeine
— if preparation contains a sedative or antihistamine, warn patient against driving a vehicle or operating machinery if drowsy

Ergotamine preparations and dose

DIHYDROERGOTAMINE

Dose

i) 1–2 mg SC or IM initially, followed by 1 mg in 30–60 minutes if required; OR
ii) 0.5 mg slowly IV for cluster headache.

ERGOTAMINE WITH CAFFEINE

Dose

2 tablets or 1 rectal suppository initially, then 1 tablet or ½ suppository ½-hourly if required (restricted to 6 tablets or 3 suppositories in 24 hours or 10 tablets or 5 suppositories/week).

Note

— suppositories contain additional itobarbitone and belladonna

ERGOTAMINE WITH CAFFEINE AND DIPHENHYDRAMINE

Dose

1 capsule initially, repeated in ½ hour if required (restricted to 6 in 24 hours or 10/week)

ERGOTAMINE WITH CAFFEINE AND CYCLIZINE

Dose

1–2 tablets initially, then ½–1 tablet ½-hourly if required (restricted to 3 tablets in 24 hours or 6/week)

OTHER ANTIMIGRAINE PREPARATIONS

CLONIDINE

Use

— migraine prophylaxis
— menopausal flushing

Dose

25 micrograms orally b.d. initially increasing after 2 weeks as required to 50–75 micrograms b.d.

Adverse effects

— drowsiness, dry mouth
— gastrointestinal disturbances

Note

— see entry in antihypertensive section (p. 39)

CYPROHEPTADINE

Use

— migraine prophylaxis and treatment

Dose

4 mg orally initially, repeated in ½ hour if required (restricted to 8 mg in a 4 to 6 hour period)
Relief maintained with 4 mg 4- to 6-hourly

Note

— see entry in antihistamine section

METHYSERGIDE

Action

— serotonin antagonist
— vasoconstrictor

Use

— migraine prophylaxis
— cluster headaches
— control diarrhoea of carcinoid disease

Dose

1 mg orally nocte for 2 days then
1–2 mg b.d. or t.d.s. with meals

Adverse effects

— nausea, vomiting
— insomnia, vertigo
— rash, oedema
— numb, painful extremities
— retroperitoneal fibrosis

Note

— a 1 month drug-free interval after 6
  months reduces the risk of
  retroperitoneal fibrosis
— dose gradually reduced during last 2
  weeks of course to avoid rebound
  headache
— in case of idiosyncratic arterial spasm
  have available papaverine, heparin
  and phenindione or warfarin
— not used in pregnancy or if peripheral
  vascular disease present

PARACETAMOL WITH ATROPINE AND PAPAVERINE AND NICOTINIC ACID

Action

— analgesic, antipyretic

Use

— relief of acute attack of migraine and
  severe headache

Dose

1 or 2 tablets initially repeated in 1 hour
if required (restricted to 8 tablets in 24
hours)

PIZOTIFEN

Action

— serotonin antagonist
— antihistamine
— appetite stimulant

Use

— migraine prophylaxis
— cluster headache

Adult dose

0.5 mg orally mane and 1 mg nocte,
increasing to 1.5 mg t.d.s.

Paediatric dose

0.5 mg orally b.d. or t.d.s., increasing to
1 mg t.d.s. in older children

Adverse effects

— sedation, initially
— increased appetite, weight gain

OTHER AGENTS USED TO TREAT MIGRAINE

See aspirin, paracetamol, codeine,
doxylamine, metoclopramide, propranolol
and pindolol

SCLEROSING AGENTS

ETHANOLAMINE

Medical officer injects varicose veins with 2–5 ml

SODIUM TETRADECYL SULPHATE

Varicose veins are treated by 0.5–1 ml injected at each of 4 sites by the medical officer, then compression applied for about 6 weeks by firm bandaging with crepe bandages and an elastic stocking to cover the bandages, both reapplied as required

Note

— the possibility of anaphylaxis, though rare, necessitates the availability of adrenaline, aminophylline, hydrocortisone, an antihistamine and equipment for mucus extraction and endotracheal intubation

PHENOL 5% IN ALMOND OIL

Medical officer gives 3–5 ml by submucosal injection to treat internal haemorrhoids

PROSTAGLANDIN

ALPROSTADIL (PROSTAGLANDIN E₁)

Action

— relaxes the ductus arteriosus in early postnatal life

Use

— to temporarily maintain the patency of the ductus arteriosus until corrective or palliative surgery can be performed in neonates who have congenital heart defects and depend upon a patent ductus for survival

Dose

— 0.1 micrograms/kg/min by continuous IV infusion into a large vein or through an umbilical artery catheter placed at the ductal opening.
— refer to a specialist text or manufacturer's literature

Adverse effects

— flushing, bradycardia, hypotension, tachycardia, oedema
— apnoea
— fever, seizures
— diarrhoea
— disseminated intravascular coagulation
— hypokalaemia

Nursing points

— used only in paediatric intensive care units where facilities for monitoring and treating apnoea are available

4 Drugs acting on the respiratory system

COUGH SUPPRESSANTS

PHOLCODINE

Action

— morphine derivative with no analgesic properties
— depresses the cough centre in the medulla and so allows relief for the inflamed respiratory membranes

Use

— relief of unproductive cough (in many proprietary preparations)

Adult dose

5–15 mg t.d.s. and nocte

Paediatric dose

2 to 4 years: 2.5 mg 2–4 times daily
4 to 10 years: 5 mg 2–4 times daily
Not recommended for children under 2 years

Adverse effects

— nausea, drowsiness

Nursing points

— sip undiluted linctus slowly
— has enhanced effect if not followed immediately by liquid

DEXTROMETHORPHAN

Action

— non-narcotic derivative
— depresses the cough centre in the medulla

Adult dose

15–30 mg t.d.s. and nocte as linctus or lozenge allowing lozenge to dissolve slowly in the mouth

Paediatric dose

2–10 years: 7.5–15 mg q.i.d.
Not given to children under 2 years

Adverse effects

— nausea, drowsiness

Nursing points

— sip undiluted linctus slowly
— has enhanced effect if not followed immediately by liquid

Note

— no analgesic effect
— does not depress respiration
— may be purchased over the counter
— contained in many proprietary preparations

DIHYDROCODEINE

Action

— as for morphine but much less potent

Use

— relief of unproductive cough

Adult dose

10 mg orally 4- to 6-hourly

Paediatric dose

not given to children under 2 years
over 2 years: 0.2 mg/kg 4- to 6-hourly

Adverse effects

— constipation

Interactions

— CNS depressant effects of
dihydrocodeine enhanced by alcohol
and tranquillizers
— CNS depressant effects of
droperidol, haloperidol, trifluperidol,
MAO inhibitors and sedatives
enhanced by dihydrocodeine

Nursing points and note

— as for dextromethorphan

NORMETHADONE WITH HYDROXYEPHEDRINE

Action

— long-acting antitussive closely related
to methadone combined with the
sympathomimetic action of
hydroxyephedrine on the
tracheobronchial mucosa

Use

— relief of unproductive cough
— prevent coughing after surgery

Adult dose

1 tablet or 15–20 drops orally after food
mane and nocte

Paediatric dose

Not given to children under 3 years
3–13 years: ½ tablet or 10 drops orally
after food mane and nocte

Adverse effects

— euphoria, sedation, respiratory
depression

— bradycardia, hypotension,
bronchospasm, miosis
— nausea, vomiting, constipation,
hiccup
— addiction

Interactions

— adverse effects enhanced by alcohol,
sedatives, tranquillizers, narcotic
analgesics and MAO inhibitors

Nursing points

— administration and storage
precautions as for drugs of addiction
— drops may be taken on sugar or with
plenty of fluid
— warn patient against driving a vehicle
or operating machinery if drowsy
— must not be taken more than twice
within 24 hours unless otherwise
directed
— have naloxone or nalorphine available
to reverse respiratory depression

Note

— contra-indicated with or for 2 weeks
after MAO inhibitors

OXOLAMINE

Action

— peripherally acting antitussive agent

Use

— relieves cough associated with
inflammation and/or irritation of
respiratory tract

Adult dose

150 mg 4-hourly

Paediatric dose

Not given to infants under 3 months
3 months–2 years: 50 mg 4-hourly
3–9 years: 100 mg 4-hourly

Adverse effects

— slight, transient local anaesthetic action on oral mucosa

Interaction

— prolongs prothrombin time if used with anticoagulants

OTHER AGENTS USED TO SUPPRESS COUGH

See codeine phosphate

EXPECTORANTS, MUCOLYTICS, DECONGESTANTS

ACETYLCYSTEINE

Action

— mucolytic which disrupts sulphide bonds of mucoproteins thereby reducing the viscosity of the mucus

Use

— to liquefy and help remove thickened mucous secretions in bronchopulmonary disease
— mucoviscidosis (cystic fibrosis of the pancreas)
— paracetamol overdose (IV formulation) (see p. 299)

Adult dose

3–5 ml of a 20% solution by nebulization or intratracheal instillation 3–4 times daily, as a mucolytic

Paediatric dose

i) 2 ml per inhalation (not within 30 minutes of administration of antibiotics by inhalation); OR
ii) 2.5–5 ml of 20% solution well diluted with orange juice or cola soft drink 3–4 times daily for cystic fibrosis

Adverse effects

— nausea, stomatitis, rhinorrhoea
— bronchospasm

Nursing points

— warn patient of the unpleasant smell
— air from either a compressed air cylinder or compressor provides the pressure for nebulization
— oxygen may be used, but with caution if patient has carbon dioxide retention
— not used in heated nebulizer

— wash patient's face and mask to remove stickiness after nebulization
— watch asthmatic patient for signs of bronchospasm
— bronchospasm relieved quickly with sympathomimetic bronchodilator
— be ready to maintain airway with suction if cough inadequate
— after ¾ nebulized, the remainder may be diluted with an equal volume of sterile water or sterile isotonic saline
— the unused portion of the vial should be refrigerated and used within 96 hours to prevent bacterial overgrowth
— clean nebulizing equipment immediately after use to prevent fine orifices being blocked and metal parts corroding

Note

— nebulizers with certain metal or rubber components should not be used
— a parenteral preparation of acetylcysteine, Parvolex®, is available for treating paracetamol overdose (see p. 299)
— see note for mucolytics

BROMHEXINE

Action

— mucolytic which reduces the viscosity of mucus and promotes a flow of thin bronchial secretions

Use

— asthma, bronchitis and pulmonary emphysema

Dose

i) 8–16 mg t.d.s. as tablets; OR
ii) 4–8 mg t.d.s. as elixir

Adverse effects

— nausea, diarrhoea, indigestion, abdominal fullness

Nursing points

— warn patient to expect an initial increase in the flow of secretions

Note for mucolytics

— many proprietary cough preparations contain ammonium chloride, guaiphenesin, potassium iodide, or senega and ammonia, all of which have an expectorant action.
— nursing mothers should avoid taking cough preparations containing potassium iodide
— tinc. benz. co., when used in a steam inhalation, soothes mucous membranes and liquifies mucus

Note for decongestants

— decongestants are cough preparations which contain an antihistamine which decreases capillary permeability and a sympathomimetic agent which causes vasoconstriction, the combined action resulting in less congested mucous membranes

DRUGS USED IN THE TREATMENT OF BRONCHIAL ASTHMA

Several lines of treatment are often necessary, including sympathomimetic and/or xanthine derivative bronchodilators for bronchospasm, the reduction of the response to the antigen-antibody reaction with sodium cromoglycate or corticosteroids and the treatment of infection occurring either as a precipitation factor or complication

SYMPATHOMIMETIC BRONCHODILATORS

SALBUTAMOL

Action

— causes bronchodilatation by mainly stimulating β_2-adrenoceptors
— effective orally from 15 minutes to 4 hours
— effective by inhalation from 5 minutes to 4 hours
— effective within 2 minutes of IV injection (5–10 minutes IM or SC) and lasts 3 hours
— produces uterine relaxation (IV)

Use

— relief of reversible bronchospasm in asthma and chronic bronchitis
— prevention of premature labour

Adult dose

Oral

2–4 mg 3–4 times daily as tablets or syrup (prophylaxis)

Metered aerosol

— 1 or 2 inhalations (100–200 micrograms) from metered dose aerosol 4-hourly p.r.n.
— if 2 inhalations required, allow a 1-minute interval
— up to a maximum of 16 inhalations in 24 hours (8 treatments)

Rotahaler®

— 1 or 2 Rotacaps® (200–400 micrograms) inhaled 3–4 times daily
— if 2 inhalations required, allow a 5-minute interval
— up to a maximum of 12 inhalations in 24 hours
— breath-actuated device

Respirator solution 0.5%

i) 1 ml solution (5 mg) plus 1–10 ml diluent 4- to 6-hourly in nebulizer; OR

ii) 1 ml solution plus 100 ml isotonic saline continuously via nebulizer coupled to an intermittent positive pressure ventilator usually using oxygen-enriched air

Injection

i) 500 micrograms SC or IM 3- to 4-hourly; OR (rarely)
ii) 200–300 micrograms over 1 minute IV; OR (rarely)
iii) 5–20 micrograms/min IV infusion

Obstetrics

10–50 micrograms/min by IV infusion up to 48 hours using an infusion pump or burette then 4–8 mg orally q.i.d.

Paediatric dose

Oral

— 80–150 micrograms/kg/dose 6-hrly

Metered aerosol

— over 12 years 1 inhalation (100 micrograms) 6-hourly; OR 2 inhalations if required with a 1-minute interval between

Rotahaler®

— up to 12 years 1 Rotacap® 3–4 times daily up to a maximum of 6 in 24 hours

Respirator solution 0.5%

| under 8 years: | 0.25 ml 0.5% solution in 1.75 ml diluent 3–4 times daily in nebulizer |
| over 8 years: | 0.5 ml 0.5% solution in 1.5 ml diluent 3–4 times daily in nebulizer |

Adverse effects

— fine skeletal muscle tremor, especially in hands
— tachycardia, palpitations, peripheral vasodilatation, hypotension
— nausea, headache
— hypokalaemia

Interactions

— improves respiratory function markedly when used in conjunction with beclomethasone or theophylline
— bronchodilator action of sympathomimetic bronchodilators inhibited by beta-adrenoceptor blocking agents

Nursing points

General

— overdose avoided by instructing the patient thoroughly in the correct use of the metered aerosol and nebulizer and ensuring that the inhaler is not used if the patient is receiving salbutamol by other means
— warn patient that tremor and palpitation may be experienced when salbutamol given parenterally
— warn patient to seek medical advice if not obtaining adequate relief (where effect of each dose lasts for less than 3 hours)
— monitor vital signs noting that an elevation of heart rate may be a side effect and a reduced heart rate a sign of improvement
— symptoms of overdose eased by rest and reassurance
— patient may also be prescribed an inhaled corticosteroid, beclomethasone, in which case it is taken approximately 10 minutes after salbutamol

Metered aerosol

— manufacturer's instruction leaflet in inhaler packet
— demonstrate how the inhaler is loaded with the canister of salbutamol
— the mouthpiece cap is removed and the inhaler shaken
— after inserting a new canister, prime the apparatus by activating the aerosol 2 or 3 times into the air
— patient holds the inhaler vertically with the mouthpiece at the bottom and breathes out slowly and fully
— the mouthpiece is placed well into the mouth, the lips closed firmly

around it and the head titled back slightly

— patient inhales rapidly and deeply through the mouthpiece, at the same time administering a metered dose by pressing the canister downwards
— pressure is released on the canister and the inhaler removed, the breath being held as long as possible (10 secs)
— patient breathes out slowly through the mouth
— if 2 inhalations required, allow 1 minute before taking the second to allow better assessment of the first inhalation and deeper penetration of the second inhalation
— mouthpiece cap replaced
— an alternative method is to hold the inhaler 2 centimetres away and keeping the mouth open while administering the metered dose
— the inhaler may be cleaned by removing the drug canister, rinsing the actuator in warm water and drying thoroughly ensuring that the small hole in the actuator is clear
— patient can practise with placebo inhaler (contains air)
— advise the patient of the benefit of a small dose early in an attack before bronchospasm becomes too severe
— in an emergency, 6 puffs are taken immediately then 1 every 5 minutes while seeking medical attention
— warn patient that the pressurized container should be kept intact and away from heat
— canister is approximately $\frac{1}{4}$ full if floats at about 45° on surface of bowl of water (need to obtain new canister)
— extension tubes ('spacers') are designed for attachment to mouthpiece to increase lung deposition of inhaled drug if patient unable to master metered dose inhaler technique. Larger more bulky 750 ml pear-shaped spacer incorporates a one-way valve so patient can only inhale

Rotahaler

— breaks Rotacap in half and airflow

through the device during inspiration disperses the powder in the inspired air

— suitable for young children and others unable to co-ordinate actuation and inspiration of metered-dose inhaler, also in severe asthma where low inspiratory flow rate and patients sensitive to freon propellants
— remove Rotahaler from container and hold vertically by dark-blue mouthpiece with light-blue body uppermost
— turn the light-blue body as far as it will go in either direction
— push the Rotacap, clear end first, firmly into the square hole, forcing any previously used Rotacap shell into the Rotahaler
— holding the Rotahaler horizontally to prevent Rotacap contents from falling out, turn the light-blue body as far as it will go in the opposite direction to open the Rotacap
— patient breathes out slowly and fully
— keeping the Rotahaler level, the mouthpiece is gripped between the teeth, the lips closed firmly around it and the head tilted back slightly
— patient inhales rapidly and deeply through the mouthpiece
— remove Rotahaler, patient holds breath as long as possible, then breathes out slowly through the mouth
— after each use, pull the two halves of the Rotahaler apart and remove loose Rotacap shells
— reassemble and store in container
— Rotahaler may be cleaned once every 2 weeks by rinsing both halves in warm water and drying thoroughly (removing empty shell first)
— protect Rotahaler from heat and protect from dirt and damage by keeping in its container
— children should be supervised by a responsible adult

Nebulizer

— no substances other than the prescribed diluent to be added to the respirator solution
— respirator solution may be diluted in

isotonic saline or distilled water or propylene glycol spray diluent
— most nebulizers deliver 1 ml of solution over 3 minutes and 2 ml over 8–10 minutes
— small compressed air pump can be used at home to provide pressure for nebulization
— ensure adequate oxygenation to avoid hypoxia
— any solution remaining in nebulizer after therapy should be discarded
— solution remaining after the stock bottle has been opened for 3 months should be discarded

Obstetrics

— the contents of the ampoule (5 mg/5 ml) are diluted in 500 ml of isotonic saline or glucose 5%
— an infusion pump or burette is used to deliver 10–50 micrograms/min, being adjusted to avoid a maternal heart rate greater than 140 beats/min, or in some cases 120 beats/min to prevent the distress associated with palpitations
— infusion rate varied according to strength and frequency of contractions
— any prepared solution remaining after 24 hours is discarded

Note

— excessive inhalation of the aerosol should be avoided to prevent overdose of the active therapeutic agent and to reduce the risk of hazards from the propellant
— no more than 8 treatments (16 inhalations or puffs) should be taken in any 24-hour period without consulting a medical officer, except in an emergency when 6 puffs are taken immediately then 1 every 5 minutes while seeking medical assistance
— Rotacaps® are designed to be used with the Rotahaler® for patients unable to use the metered dose aerosol inhaler satisfactorily

FENOTEROL

Action and use

— as for oral and inhaled salbutamol (p. 71) but has a duration of 6 hours

Adult dose

Metered aerosol

— 1 or 2 inhalations (200–400 micrograms) from metered dose aerosol 3–4 times daily
— if 2 inhalations required, allow a 5-minute interval

Solution 0.1%

0.5–1 ml solution (0.5–1 mg) diluted to 2–3 ml with isotonic saline 3–4 times daily in nebulizer

Note

— see salbutamol (p. 71) for adverse effects, interactions and nursing points
— fenoterol and ipratropium inhalant solutions are compatible when prepared immediately prior to use

ORCIPRENALINE

— used similarly to salbutamol as a bronchodilator

Adult dose

1 or 2 inhalations (750–1500 micrograms) from metered dose aerosol 3–4 times daily effective immediately and lasts for 4–6 hours;

Paediatric dose

Metered aerosol

over 12 years: 1–2 doses 3–4 times daily

Nursing points

— see salbutamol (p. 71)

RIMITEROL

β_2-adrenoceptor stimulant causing bronchodilatation similar to salbutamol (p. 71) but of shorter duration

Dose

— 1 or 2 inhalations (250–500 micrograms) from metered dose aerosol
— if 2 inhalations required, allow a 1-minute interval
— sequence not repeated in less than 1 hour
— up to a maximum of 16 inhalations in 24 hours

Nursing points

— see salbutamol (p. 71)

Note

— discontinued in Australia

TERBUTALINE

— as for salbutamol (p. 71)

Adult dose

Oral

2.5–5 mg b.d. or t.d.s. as tablets or syrup

Inhalation (1% solution)

i) 0.25–0.5 ml (2.5–5 mg) made up to 3–5 ml with prescribed diluent and given 5- to 6-hourly via nebulizer (short term); OR
ii) 1 ml (10 mg) made up to 100 ml with prescribed diluent and given at a rate of 1–2 mg/hr (chronic administration)

Metered aerosol

— 1 or 2 inhalations (250–500 micrograms) 4-hourly p.r.n.
— if 2 inhalations required, allow a 2-minute interval
— up to a maximum of 8 inhalations in 24 hours

Injection

0.25 mg SC up to 4 times daily

Paediatric dose

Oral

75 microgram/kg/dose 2–3 times daily

Metered aerosol

over 14 years 1–2 doses q.i.d.

Injection

5 microgram/kg/dose SC up to 4 times daily

Note

— a Misthaler® attachment is available for patients with poor co-ordination of inspiration and canister actuation

EPHEDRINE

Action

— more prolonged but less potent than adrenaline
— acts directly by stimulating alpha- and beta-adrenoceptors
— acts indirectly to release noradrenaline from peripheral nerve endings
— CNS and respiratory centre stimulant

Use

— relief of bronchospasm in asthma
— nasal decongestant
— combat hypotension associated with spinal anaesthesia

Dose

i) 15–30 mg orally t.d.s.; OR
ii) 15–50 mg SC, IM or slowly IV

Adverse effects

— anxiety, nervousness, tremor, insomnia
— tachycardia, palpitations

Interactions

— reduces antihypertensive effects of bethanidine, bretylium, debrisoquine, guanethidine
— severe hypertensive reaction if used concomitantly with MAO inhibitors

Note

— ephedrine should not be given with or for 14 days following withdrawal of MAO inhibitors
— orally effective agent often combined with aminophylline or theophylline and barbiturates

ADRENALINE

— see sympathomimetic agents

ISOPRENALINE

— see sympathomimetic agents

ANTICHOLINERGIC BRONCHODILATOR

IPRATROPIUM

Action

— similar to atropine sulphate
— causes bronchodilatation by blocking vagal reflexes
— effective within 3–5 minutes, peak response at 1½–2 hours and duration of 4–6 hours

Use

— symptomatic relief of bronchospasm in chronic reversible airways obstruction especially chronic bronchitis

Adult dose

Metered aerosol:

i) 2 inhalations (40 micrograms) t.d.s. or q.i.d.; OR
ii) up to 4 inhalations (80 micrograms) as single dose for maximum benefit early in treatment then as for i) above

Inhalation: (0.025% solution)

1–2 ml (250–500 micrograms) made up to twice the original volume with isotonic saline and given 6-hourly via nebulizer
Inhalation may be repeated after 2 hours as required

Paediatric dose

Metered aerosol

under 6 years: 1 inhalation (20 micrograms) t.d.s.
6–12 years: 1–2 inhalations (20–40 micrograms) t.d.s. or q.i.d.

Inhalation (0.025% solution)

1 ml (250 micrograms) made up to 2 ml with isotonic saline and given 6-hourly via nebulizer
Inhalation may be repeated after 2 hours as required

Adverse effects

— dry mouth
— rarely, urinary retention, acute closed-angle glaucoma
— mild, reversible visual disturbances if accidentally enters eyes

Nursing points

— see salbutamol (p. 71) for nursing points on metered aerosol
— warn patient to seek medical advice if not obtaining adequate relief
— inhalation solution is hypotonic and so should be diluted with isotonic saline to at least twice the original volume before administration
— ipratropium and fenoterol inhalation solutions are compatible when prepared immediately prior to use
— any solution remaining in nebulizer after therapy should be discarded
— solution remaining after the stock bottle has been opened for 28 days should be discarded

Note

— may be used alone or in combination with other bronchodilator agents and corticosteroids

XANTHINE DERIVATIVE BRONCHODILATORS

AMINOPHYLLINE

Action

Inhibits the enzyme phosphodiesterase resulting in an increase in cyclic adenosine monophosphate (AMP) concentration which causes:
— smooth muscle relaxation especially bronchial muscle
— cardiac stimulation
— CNS and respiratory stimulation
— diuresis

Use

— bronchial asthma, prophylaxis and therapeutic
— bronchopneumonia, bronchitis
— cardiac, pulmonary or renal oedema
— paroxysmal dyspnoea (cardiac asthma)
— Cheyne-Stokes respiration
— biliary colic
— anaphylaxis

Adult dose

i) 250–500 mg by slow IV injection; OR
ii) 250–1000 mg diluted in 500 ml 5% glucose or 0.9% isotonic saline and given IV over 12–24 hours; OR
iii) 100–200 mg orally t.d.s. or q.i.d.; OR
iv) 100–400 mg rectally by suppository daily

Paediatric dose

i) 2.5 mg/kg slow IV injection or IV infusion followed by 3 mg/kg 6-hrly by slow IV injection or IV infusion to maximum 16 mg/kg/24 hours; OR
ii) 5 mg/kg/dose suppository up to maximum 20 mg/kg/24 hours

Adverse effects

— gastrointestinal disturbances and bleeding
— restlessness, insomnia, hyperventilation
— palpitation, tachycardia, dizziness

— hypotension after too rapid IV injection
— proctitis from suppositories
— convulsions (high dose)

Nursing points

— take oral preparations with or immediately following food to minimize gastric irritation
— suppositories inserted before evening meal if providing nocturnal protection
— watch closely for adverse effects in children especially when suppositories given because of unpredictable absorption
— warn patient about taking other xanthine derivatives concurrently
— monitor vital signs especially during IV administration
— record fluid intake and output

CHOLINE THEOPHYLLINATE

— as for aminophylline (p. 77)

Adult dose

100–200 mg q.i.d. during or after meals (tablets or syrup)

Paediatric dose

3–5 mg/kg/dose q.i.d. (tablet or syrup according to age)

CHOLINE THEOPHYLLINATE WITH GUAIPHENESIN

Dose

20 ml elixir q.i.d. p.c.

Note

— guaiphenesin stimulates expectoration

THEOPHYLLINE

Action

— as for aminophylline (p. 77)

Use

— relieves reversible bronchospasm associated with bronchial asthma, bronchitis, emphysema and related conditions
— neonatal apnoea

Adult dose (based on 13 mg/kg/24 hours)

i) 125–200 mg orally 6- to 8-hourly; OR
ii) ½–1 tablet 12-hourly SR 250 or SR 500; OR
iii) 150–450 mg 12-hourly (CR tablet)
iv) 200–400 mg 12-hourly (bead-filled capsule) either swallowed whole or contents sprinkled onto soft food, e.g., apple sauce, yoghurt or custard

Paediatric dose

Asthma

5 mg/kg orally 6-hourly; OR
8 mg/kg orally 12-hourly (SR)

Neonatal apnoea

6 mg/kg orally stat.; then
0–1 week: 2 mg/kg 12-hourly
1–2 weeks: 3 mg/kg 12-hourly
over 2 weeks: 4 mg/kg 12-hourly

Interactions

— theophylline blood levels increased by allopurinol (high doses) cimetidine, erythromycin, isoprenaline, oral contraceptives, propranolol, troleandomycin
— theophylline blood levels decreased by phenytoin, carbamazepine, rifampicin, isoniazid, sulphinpyrazone
— rate of theophylline elimination increased by cigarette smoking (> 10/day) and decreased by congestive cardiac failure, liver disease, obesity

Nursing points

— SR (sustained release) and (CRT) controlled release theophylline tablet may be broken along score line but are not to be crushed or chewed
— blood levels monitored by sampling blood immediately before morning dose (trough level) then 1–2 hours after dose (4–6 hours if sustained or controlled release) for peak level provided therapy established for 48 hours and no excess or missed doses. Xanthine-containing beverages, e.g., tea, coffee, cola, cocoa may interfere with the theophylline assay.

Note

— additional potassium iodide stimulates expectoration
— theophylline excreted in breast milk so dosage to mother minimized to avoid irritability and restlessness in infant
— dosage highly individualized, preferably on basis of blood level monitoring to achieve 10–20 mg/l
— should not be administered concurrently with other formulations of theophylline or its derivatives

CORTICOSTEROIDS

BECLOMETHASONE

Action

— high topical anti-inflammatory effect on the lungs but has low systemic activity
— effective in about 7–14 days

Use

— prophylaxis of symptoms of asthma

Adult dose

Metered aerosol:

— 2 inhalations (100 micrograms) t.d.s. or q.i.d.
— up to a maximum of 20 inhalations in 24 hours

Rotahaler®:

i) 1 or 2 Rotacaps® (100–200 micrograms) b.d.; OR
ii) 1 Rotacap® (100 micrograms) t.d.s. or q.i.d.

Paediatric dose

Metered aerosol:

— 1 or 2 inhalations (50–100 micrograms) 2–4 times daily depending on age and response
— up to a maximum of 10 inhalations in 24 hours

Rotahaler®:

— 1 Rotacap® (100 micrograms) 2–4 times daily according to response

Adverse effects

— hoarseness (occasionally)
— monilia infection of throat and mouth

Interactions

— improves respiratory function markedly when used in combination with a bronchodilator

Nursing points

— ensure patient is aware of the detailed instructions for loading the inhaler, administering the preparation and cleaning the inhaler (see manufacturer's instructions and nursing points on salbutamol p. 71)
— a plastic reed fitted into the Aldecin® inhaler gives the signal on inspiration to fire the actuator so improves synchronization of inhalation and actuation
— advise patient to clear as much mucus as possible before inhalation
— Rotacaps® used with Rotahaler®, a breath-actuated device
— it is essential that the patient understands that beclomethasone gives no relief in an acute distress situation as it is not a bronchodilator aerosol and should be used regularly
— patient may be prescribed a bronchodilator, in which case it is taken approximately 10 minutes before beclomethasone for maximum benefit
— advise patient to rinse mouth or drink liquids after inhaling beclomethasone to reduce the incidence of hoarseness and monilia infection
— warn patient that the pressurized container should be kept intact and away from heat
— advise patient to obtain 'Identicare' bracelet or pendant and enter relevant information

Note

— avoids the side effects associated with systemic corticosteroids
— also prepared as a nasal spray for prophylaxis and treatment of allergic rhinitis

ORAL CORTICOSTEROIDS

May be required if patient inadequately controlled on a bronchodilator and steroid aerosol.

PARENTERAL CORTICOSTEROIDS

High doses of IV steroids (hydrocortisone or methylprednisolone) may be required in status asthmaticus where the patient has been on long term inhaled or oral corticosteroid therapy.

ANTI-ALLERGY AGENT

SODIUM CROMOGLYCATE

Action

— rapidly absorbed powder which, when inhaled, stabilizes pulmonary mast cell membrane inhibiting the release of histamine and other allergic mediators

Use

— prophylactic treatment of bronchial asthma and rhinitis associated with allergy

Adult and paediatric dose

Asthma prophylaxis

i) 1 capsule (20 mg) by inhalation 4- to 6-hourly (Spinhaler® or Halermatic®); OR
ii) 1 ampoule (20 mg) inhaled via power-operated nebulizer 4- to 6-hourly
iii) 2 inhalations (2 mg) from metered dose aerosol q.i.d.

Allergic rhinitis prophylaxis

i) 1 capsule (10 mg) by nasal insufflator q.i.d. equally both nostrils; OR
ii) 2 drops of the nasal drop preparation into each nostril 6 times daily (if unable to use nasal insufflator); OR

iii) 2 squeezes of the nasal spray into each nostril 6 times daily

Adverse effects

— transient irritation of throat and trachea
— transient bronchospasm following inhalation

Nursing points

— ensure patient is aware of the detailed instructions for loading the inhaler, administering the preparation and cleaning the inhaler (see manufacturer's instructions)
— it is essential that the patient understands that sodium cromoglycate is not a bronchodilator and should be used regularly

— the capsule Spincap® is ineffective if swallowed and is administered by a specially designed inhaler, Spinhaler® or Halermatic®
— advise patient to clear as much mucus as possible before inhalation
— patient may require inhalation of a sympathomimetic agent e.g. salbutamol or isoprenaline 10 minutes before using the inhaler to prevent bronchospasm
— improvement will not be noted for 2 to 4 weeks after commencing therapy
— advise patient that drug therapy is best withdrawn over several days unless urgent need to stop abruptly
— sodium cromoglycate nebulizer solution can be mixed with salbutamol respirator solution removing the need for diluent for salbutamol so reducing nebulizing time

5 Drugs acting on the nervous system

GENERAL ANAESTHETIC AGENTS (INHALATION)*

HALOTHANE

Properties

— potent volatile liquid agent
— non-flammable and non-explosive

Action

— smooth, rapid induction of anaesthesia
— weak analgesic properties
— mild muscle relaxation properties
— suppresses secretions
— recovery usually rapid, with little nausea

Use

— maintain surgical anaesthesia usually with nitrous oxide and oxygen

Adverse effects

— bradycardia, hypotension, cardiac arrhythmias
— respiratory depression
— shivering during recovery (occasionally)
— malignant hyperpyrexia (rare)
— hepatitis, if multiple exposure

Interactions

— sensitizes myocardium to beta-adrenergic activity

Note

— malignant hyperpyrexia (hyperthermia) is usually an inherited condition in which there is a skeletal muscle hypermetabolic state leading to a high oxygen demand. The clinical syndrome which occurs during anaesthesia and is often fatal, includes muscle contracture, acidosis, hyperkalaemia, tachycardia, arrhythmias, tachypnoea, cyanosis, sweating, and unstable blood pressure. The body temperature rises at a rate of at least 2°/hour, but sometimes this is a late sign

ENFLURANE

Properties

— non-flammable potent volatile liquid agent

Actions

— as for halothane
— moderate muscle relaxation

Use

— as for halothane

Adverse effects

— hypotension
— convulsions
— respiratory depression
— nausea, vomiting, hiccup

Interactions

— sensitises myocardium to beta-adrenergic activity

---

* see summary at end of general anaesthetic section

ISOFLURANE

Properties

— non-flammable volatile liquid agent

Actions

— rapid induction and recovery
— produces unconsciousness
— analgesic properties
— excellent muscle relaxant properties
— peripheral vasodilatation
— stimulates secretions weakly
— profound respiratory depressant

Use

— induction and maintenance of surgical anaesthesia usually with nitrous oxide and oxygen

Adverse effects

— respiratory depression
— hypotension, cardiac arrhythmias
— shivering, nausea, vomiting, paralytic ileus during recovery (occasionally)
— malignant hyperthermia (in susceptible individuals)
— hepatotoxicity (rare)

Interactions

— potentiates muscle relaxant properties of all muscle relaxants especially non-depolarizing muscle relaxants

Note

— stored in amber glass bottle below 30°C and kept tightly closed

METHOXYFLURANE

Properties

— non-flammable volatile liquid agent

Actions

— slower induction and recovery than halothane
— good analgesic properties
— moderate muscle relaxation properties

Use

— maintenance of surgical anaesthesia usually with nitrous oxide and oxygen
— anaesthesia and intermittent analgesia in obstetrics (administered by specially designed inhaler)

Adverse effects

— mild hypotension, bradycardia
— impaired renal function
— drowsiness persists after consciousness returns

Interactions

— tetracycline increases risk of renal damage
— sensitizes myocardium to beta-adrenergic activity

Note

— damages PVC plastics
— soluble in rubber and soda lime

NITROUS OXIDE

Properties

— colourless gas
— although non-flammable, supports combustion

Action

— strong analgesic properties
— weak anaesthetic and muscle relaxant properties

Use

— used with other agents in induction and maintenance of surgical anaesthesia
— used with oxygen in dentistry
— used with oxygen in obstetrics by self-administration

Adverse effects

— hypoxia (unless adequate oxygen administered)
— bone marrow depression (prolonged administration)

Note

— supplied in blue metal gas cylinder

TRICHLOROETHYLENE

Properties

— clear pale liquid tinted blue for identification
— non-flammable and non explosive

Action

— potent analgesic
— poor muscle relaxant

Use

— short surgical procedures requiring light anaesthesia with good analgesia (often mixed with air, oxygen or nitrous oxide)
— dentistry
— self-administration in obstetrics from specially designed apparatus

Adverse effects

— increases rate, decreases depth of respiration
— bradycardia
— post-anaesthetic nausea, vomiting, headache, confusion
— prolonged contact may cause dermatitis, eczema, burns or conjunctivitis

Interactions

— sensitizes myocardium to beta-adrenergic activity

Note

— stored in light-tight container in a cool place
— liquid in anaesthetic apparatus should be changed every few days
— should not be used in a closed-circuit because it forms poisonous substances with soda lime

GENERAL ANAESTHETIC AGENTS (PARENTERAL)*

KETAMINE

Action

— short acting general anaesthetic agent
— induction of anaesthesia in 30 seconds (IV) and lasts 5–10 minutes
— induction of anaesthesia in 3–4 minutes (IM) and lasts 12–25 minutes
— marked analgesic properties

Use

— induction of anaesthesia
— diagnostic or short surgical operations
— treatment of severe burns
— avoided in children over 8 years because of incidence of hallucinations

Adverse effects

— emergence reactions (vivid dreams, hallucinations, irrational behaviour)
— temporary hypertension and tachycardia
— respiratory depression during induction requiring assisted ventilation
— post-anaesthetic nausea, vomiting, headache

Nursing points

— great care taken not to disturb patient during recovery to avoid vivid dreams and hallucinations

METHOHEXITONE

Action

— very short acting potent IV barbiturate
— anaesthesia induced in 30 seconds and recovery starts in about 0 minutes
— little muscle relaxant property

* see summary at end of general anaesthetic section

Use

— complete anaesthesia of short
  duration
— induction of anaesthesia
— dentistry

Adverse effects

— muscle twitching
— hiccup, coughing
— laryngospasm

MIDAZOLAM

Action

— short acting benzodiazepine with
  rapid onset
— induces sedation, hypnosis, amnesia,
  anaesthesia
— induces sedation in 15 minutes (IM)
  peak effect 30–60 minutes
— induces sedation in 30–90 seconds (IV)
— induces anaesthesia (IV). Induction
  time reduced with narcotic or
  sedative premedication
— approximately 2 hours required for
  full recovery

Use

— preoperative sedation, relief of
  anxiety and to impair memory of
  perioperative events (IM)
— conscious sedation prior to
  endoscopy, coronary angiography and
  cardiac catheterization (IV)
— induction of anaesthesia (IV)

Adverse effects

— respiratory depression, apnoea
— variation in heart rate, blood pressure
— hiccups (IV)
— amnesia
— nausea, vomiting
— tenderness, redness, induration,
  phlebitis at IV injection site

Interactions

— enhances central sedative of
  neuroleptics, tranquillizers, antidepressants, hypnotics, analgesics,
  anaesthetics

— mutual potentiation of alcohol and
  midazolam

Note

— patient to avoid alcohol for at least
  12 hours after administration as
  mutual potential can cause
  unpredictable reactions
— may be mixed in same syringe with
  morphine, pethidine, atropine or
  hyoscine
— compatible with 5% glucose, isotonic
  saline and lactated Ringer's solution

PROPOFOL

Action

— short acting IV agent
— recovery usually within 5–10 minutes
— no analgesic properties

Use

— induction and maintenance of
  anaesthesia in adults

Adverse effects

— respiratory depression, apnoea
— hypotension
— tremor, hypertonus, hiccup
— nausea, vomiting, headache,
  shivering during recovery
— thrombophlebitis at injection site

Note

— compatible with 5% glucose
— store below 25°C but do not freeze
— do not use if emulsion is separated or
  discoloured
— shake each ampoule before use
— discard remaining contents after use

THIOPENTONE

Action

— very short acting IV barbiturate
— poor analgesic and muscle relaxing
  properties

Use

— induction of anaesthesia
— anaesthesia of short duration
— control convulsions
— narco-analysis in psychiatry

Adverse effects

— laryngospasm or bronchospasm
  during induction
— hypotension
— respiratory depression
— post-anaesthetic drowsiness,
  confusion, amnesia
— thrombophlebitis at injection site
— tissue necrosis if extravasation at
  injection site
— gangrene of digits if inadvertent
  arterial injection

SUMMARY FOR GENERAL ANAESTHESIA

Requirements

— unconsciousness
— analgesia
— muscle relaxation

Premedication

— reduce anxiety, apprehension
— relieve pain
— assist induction of anaesthesia
— usually given ½–1 hour IM or SC
  beforehand or IV just prior to
  induction

Induction

— short acting barbiturate or
  benzodiazepine IV often with short
  acting muscle relaxant

Maintenance

— inhalation or parenteral agent
  together with supplementary
  analgesia and if necessary skeletal
  muscle relaxant

Recovery

— anticholinesterase to reverse the
  effects of non-depolarizing muscle
  relaxants

Note

— see narcotic analgesics,
  anticholinergic agents, sedatives,
  tranquillizers, muscle relaxants and
  anticholinesterases

LOCAL ANAESTHETIC AGENTS

Action

— blocks or diminishes nerve conduction reversibly by inhibiting depolarization and ion exchange
— does not produce loss of consciousness
— can cause analgesia, anaesthesia and paralysis
— addition of vasoconstrictor (usually adrenaline 1 in 50 000 to 1 in 400 000) decreases blood flow in the area and prolongs the anaesthesia by reducing absorption

Surface (topical) anaesthesia

— blocks sensory nerve endings in the skin, mucous membranes and the eye.

Agents

— amethocaine, benzocaine, butyl aminobenzoate, choline salicylate, cocaine, lignocaine, oxybuprocaine and prilocaine

Local (infiltration) anaesthesia

— solution injected into and around site

Agents

— etidocaine, lignocaine, mepivacaine, prilocaine and procaine

Regional nerve block anaesthesia

— sensory nerve pathways blocked by injecting into or around nerve trunks or ganglia supplying affected area (including epidural and caudal anaesthesia)

Agents

— bupivacaine, etidocaine, lignocaine, mepivacaine, prilocaine and procaine

Spinal anaesthetics

— regional anaesthesia blocking transmission in spinal nerves in contact with the anaesthetic agent
— injected intrathecally following lumbar puncture
— the somatic level of anaesthesia depends on the specific gravity of the anaesthetic solution and the position of the patient

Agents

— cinchocaine, etidocaine and prilocaine

Adverse effects of local anaesthetics

— CNS excitation (yawning, restlessness, nervousness, dizziness, blurred vision, tremors, convulsions) then
— CNS depression (drowsiness, respiratory depression, unconsciousness)
— peripheral vasodilatation, bradycardia, arrhythmias, hypotension, possible cardiac arrest
— pallor, sweating
— allergic reactions (rash, oedema, anaphylactoid-type symptoms)
— idiosyncrasy
— hypotension, headache (after spinal anaesthesia)
— cardiac arrhythmias

Interactions

— blood pressure unpredictable when local anaesthetic containing vasoconstrictor administered to patients receiving tricyclic antidepressants, MAO inhibitors or phenothiazines
— vasoconstrictor enhances hypertensive effects of oxytocic drugs
— adrenaline may enhance toxic effects of cardiac glycosides leading to arrhythmias

Nursing points

— monitor heart rate and blood pressure of patient for at least 4 hours following spinal anaesthesia
— nurse patient in recumbent position

— have equipment available for assisted ventilation, mucus extraction, also diazepam and/or thiopentone

Dangers of vasoconstrictors

— adrenaline must not be used when producing a nerve block in an appendage such as the digits, ears, nose or penis because these are supplied by end arteries and therefore subject to gangrene
— spinal cord may be damaged if spinal anaesthetic contains adrenaline

Note on local anaesthetics

— other topical agents with local anaesthetic actions are ethyl chloride and some chlorofluoromethanes, which evaporate rapidly causing sudden chilling of the skin

SKELETAL MUSCLE RELAXANTS

BACLOFEN

Action

— antispasticity agent which acts at spinal end of the upper motor neurone

Use

— suppresses skeletal muscle spasm in multiple sclerosis and spinal lesions

Dose

— 5–25 mg orally t.d.s. p.c.

Adverse effects

— nausea, vomiting, dyspepsia, diarrhoea
— muscle weakness, muscular incoordination
— drowsiness, dizziness, headache, hallucinations

Nursing points

— take with food to minimize nausea
— warn patient against driving a vehicle or operating machinery if drowsy

DANTROLENE

Action

— thought to interfere with release of calcium ions from skeletal muscle sarcoplasmic reticulum

Use

— relieves long-standing spasticity
— malignant hyperpyrexia

Dose

i) 25 mg orally daily increasing to 100 mg q.i.d. as required; or
ii) 1 mg/kg IV up to a total dose of 10 mg/kg (malignant hyperpyrexia) or until signs subside

Adverse effects

— drowsiness, dizziness, muscle
  weakness, fatigue
— diarrhoea
— hepatotoxicity
— photosensitivity

Nursing points

— warn patient against driving a vehicle
  or operating machinery if drowsy
— advise patient to avoid skin exposure
  to direct sunlight
— reconstitute vial for IV use with
  60 ml sterile water shaking solution
  until clear
— protect reconstituted solution from
  direct light and use within 6 hours

Interactions

— benzodiazepines increase muscle
  relaxing effects

METHOCARBAMOL

Action

— centrally acting muscle relaxant

Use

— relieve acute muscular spasm
— relieve spastic, hypertonic and
  hyperkinetic conditions

Dose

— 1.5 g orally q.i.d. then 1 g q.i.d.

Adverse reactions

— drowsiness, dizziness
— nausea
— allergic reaction

Nursing point

— warn patient against driving a
  vehicle or operating machinery if
  drowsy

ORPHENADRINE CITRATE

Use

— relieve pain due to spasm of
  voluntary muscle

Dose

i) 100 mg orally b.d. or t.d.s.; OR
ii) 30–60 mg IM or slow IV injection
   daily or b.d.

· Note

— brief dizziness may be experienced
  following IV injection
— see benzhexol
— combined with paracetamol for use
  in tension headache, occipital,
  headaches associated with skeletal
  muscle spasm, severe sprains,
  strains, whiplash injury, acute
  torticollis, prolapsed intervertebral
  disc

TUBOCURARINE

Action

— rapidly acting non-depolarizing
  skeletal muscle relaxant with a
  duration of 20–40 minutes
— competes with acetylcholine for
  receptor sites
— blocks impulses at neuromuscular
  junction by reducing response to
  acetylcholine
— effects reversed by
  anticholinesterases

Use

— adjuvant to anaesthesia in major
  surgical operations and orthopaedic
  manipulations
— to control muscle spasms of tetanus
— diagnosis of myasthenia gravis
  (rarely)

Adult dose

— 10–20 mg IV up to overall dose of
  40 mg

Paediatric dose

— 0.3–0.5 mg/kg IV

Note

— patients under 3 months of age have an increased sensitivity to non-depolarizing muscle relaxants
— see anticholinesterases

ALCURONIUM

— as for tubocurarine

Adult dose

5–15 mg IV

Paediatric dose

0.125–0.2 mg/kg IV

ATRACURIUM

— as for tubocurarine but approximately half the duration of action

Dose

0.3–0.6 mg/kg IV bolus initially, then 0.08–0.1 mg/kg IV (maintenance); OR 0.3–0.6 mg/kg/hour IV infusion

GALLAMINE

— as for tubocurarine

Adult dose

80–120 mg IV

Paediatric dose

1.5 mg/kg IV

PANCURONIUM

— as for tubocurarine

Adult dose

4–6 mg IV

Paediatric dose

0.08 mg/kg IV

VECURONIUM

— as for tubocurarine

Dose

0.1 mg/kg IV initially, then 0.02–0.06 mg/kg

SUXAMETHONIUM CHLORIDE

(known as succinylcholine in USA)

Action

— blocks neuromuscular transmission by producing a partial depolarization at the muscle end plate preventing response to acetylcholine
— effective within 30 seconds with a duration of 3–5 minutes
— effects reversed by endogenous plasma pseudocholinesterase (not anticholinesterase)

Use

— intubation
— endoscopy
— examination under anaesthesia
— orthopaedic manipulations including reduction of fractures
— cephalic version
— dental surgery
— electroconvulsive therapy

Adult dose

20–100 mg IV
(May be given by IV infusion for finer control of degree of relaxation.)

Paediatric dose

i) 1 mg/kg IV
ii) 2 mg/kg IM

Adverse effects

— transient painful muscle fasciculation (reduced by giving thiopentone beforehand)
— prolonged apnoea occurs in patients with atypical or low blood levels of pseudocholinesterase (rare)
— malignant hyperpyrexia (rare)

ANTICHOLINESTERASES

NEOSTIGMINE

Action

— inhibits enzyme hydrolysis of acetylcholine by cholinesterases allowing acetylcholine to accumulate prolonging and intensifying its actions

Use

— reverses effects of non-depolarizing skeletal muscle relaxants
— diagnosis and treatment of myasthenia gravis
— paralytic ileus
— post-operative urinary retention
— reduces intra-ocular pressure in glaucoma (eye drops)

Dose

Antidote to curariform drugs

i) adults: 1–5 mg IV preceded 10–15 minutes earlier by 0.4–1.25 mg atropine to prevent parasympathetic stimulation
ii) children: 0.025 mg/kg neostigmine with a suitable dose of atropine

Myasthenia gravis

i) 5–20 tablets (neostigmine bromide 15 mg) daily in several divided doses; or
ii) 1–2.5 mg SC, IM or IV (neostigmine methylsulphate) daily in several divided doses

Other indications

i) 15–30 mg orally; or
ii) 0.5–2.5 mg SC or IM as required

Adverse effects

— nausea, vomiting, diarrhoea, abdominal cramps
— increased bronchial secretion and salivation, miosis, sweating (usually counteracted by atropine)
— muscle cramps and fasciculation, weakness

Interactions

— muscarinic side effects blocked by atropine
— antagonizes the neuromuscular blockade of aminoglycosides but enhances decamethonium
— increases the intensity and duration of narcotic analgesia

Nursing points

— keep record of muscle strength variations in patients with myasthenia
— modify dosage regime as required e.g. oral neostigmine taken 30–40 minutes a.c. if patient has difficulty chewing and swallowing

AMBENONIUM

— as for neostigmine

Use

— myasthenia gravis

Dose

15–200 mg orally daily in divided doses as required

DISTIGMINE

Action

— as for neostigmine
— peak effect of IM dose in 9 hours with a duration of 24 hours

Use

— post-operative urinary retention (non-obstructive)
— neurogenic atony of urinary bladder with retention
— intestinal and urinary tract atony
— myasthenia gravis

Dose

Urinary retention:

i) 5 mg orally daily ½ hour before breakfast; OR
ii) 0.5 mg IM daily as required

Myasthenia gravis:

5–10 mg orally b.d. a.c.

Adverse effects

— salivation, sweating, lachrymation
— nausea, vomiting, abdominal pain

PYRIDOSTIGMINE

Action

— as for neostigmine but slower in onset and of longer duration

Use

— myasthenia gravis
— reverses effects of non-depolarizing skeletal muscle relaxants

Dose

Antidote to curariform drugs

— up to 5 mg mixed with 0.5 mg atropine given IV in 2 divided doses

Myasthenia gravis

i) 60–80 mg orally 2–4 times daily; OR
ii) 1–3 'Timespan' tablets 180 mg daily or b.d.; OR
iii) 2–5 mg SC or IM

Note

— may be given in combined therapy with neostigmine

EDROPHONIUM

Action

— as for neostigmine but rapid in onset and of short duration

Use

— diagnosis of myasthenia gravis

Dose

2–10 mg IV

Adverse effects

— as for neostigmine

Nursing points

— have atropine available

Note

— in patients with myasthenia gravis, there is immediate subjective improvement and muscle strength increases lasting only about 5 minutes after which clinical features return

NARCOTIC ANALGESICS

MORPHINE

Action

— depresses respiratory and cough centres
— stimulates vomiting centre and vagus nerve
— causes miosis
— increases smooth muscle tone in gastrointestinal tract, especially in sphincters
— reduces peristalsis and secretions
— may produce euphoria or dysphoria, drowsiness and raised intracranial pressure
— effective within 15–30 minutes (SC or IM) wth a duration of 4 hours
— effective within 1–2 minutes IV with peak effect in 3–6 minutes

Use

— relief of moderate and severe pain
— premedication with atropine or hyoscine
— supplementary analgesia during general anaesthesia
— reduces peristalsis
— relieve dyspnoea of acute pulmonary oedema
— relief of anxiety and apprehension

Adult dose

i) 8–20 mg SC or IM about 4-hourly; OR
ii) 15 mg by slow IV injection or infusion diluted to at least 5 ml with isotonic saline; OR
iii) dilute 45 mg in isotonic saline to make a solution of 45 ml, i.e. a concentration of 1 mg/ml, then using a syringe pump, deliver the solution IV at 0.5 mg/hr increasing to 4 mg/hr or more as required
iv) 15–30 mg orally 4- to 6-hourly (tablets or solution)

Paediatric dose

0.1–0.2 mg/kg up to a maximum dose of 15 mg, which should only be exceeded with caution

Adverse effects

— nausea, anorexia, constipation, confusion, sweating
— vomiting (occasionally), dry mouth
— difficulty with micturition
— antidiuretic effect
— renal or biliary colic
— drowsiness, euphoria or dysphoria, miosis
— bradycardia, postural hypotension
— allergic reactions
— raised intracranial pressure (occasionally)
— dependence
— respiratory and cough depression, circulatory failure and deepening coma (high doses)
— tolerance may develop

Interactions

— CNS depressant effects of morphine enhanced by alcohol, sedatives, hypnotics, tranquillizers, antidepressants and general anaesthetics
— enhances the CNS depressant effects of furazolidone
— analgesic effects enhanced by chlorpromazine or prochlorperazine
— doxapram antagonizes morphine-induced respiratory depression
— nalaxone antagonizes analgesic and respiratory depressant effects of morphine

Nursing points

— administration and storage precautions as for drugs of addiction
— analgesic more effective if given before onset of intense pain
— note effectiveness of morphine
— withhold drug and report to medical officer if respiratory rate showing marked decline and especially if 12/min or less
— even if initial doses cause vomiting, subsequent doses depress the vomiting centre
— plan to give analgesic 15–30 minutes before undertaking any procedure which will cause the patient pain or discomfort

— advise patient to deep breathe, cough and move frequently (if permitted)
— note urinary output, presence of bowel sounds and bowel pattern
— advise patient to walk with assistance after receiving the drug
— not normally mixed in the same syringe with other drugs but is compatible with chlorpromazine, metoclopramide, prochlorperazine or promethazine when mixed in the same syringe as long as the resultant solution is used within 15 minutes and there is no precipitation
— have naloxone available to reverse respiratory depression

Note

— doses as high as 600 mg have been required for pain control in terminal stages of cancer
— contra-indicated with MAO inhibitors or within 10 days of discontinuing treatment
— may be given with an anticholinergic for biliary or renal colic

MORPHINE WITH ASPIRIN

Dose

— 1–2 tablets dissolved in water 4- to 6-hourly

Note

— the combination dose is chosen to give analgesia for up to 6 hours for intractable pain

MORPHINE WITH TACRINE

Tacrine, an anticholinesterase and CNS stimulant is added to reduce respiratory depression, sedation and constipation

Dose

½–2 tablets 6-hourly

PAPAVERETUM

— as for morphine but fewer adverse effects (p. 93)
— preferred for renal and biliary colic

Adult dose

i) 10–20 mg orally; OR
ii) 20 mg SC, IM or slow IV injection
diluted to at least 5 ml isotonic saline

Paediatric dose

0.2–0.4 mg/kg/dose orally or IM

Note

— contains 50% morphine
— compatible with chlorpromazine,
prochlorperazine or promethazine
when mixed in the same syringe as
long as the resultant solution is
used within 15 minutes and there is
no precipitation

PAPAVERETUM WITH HYOSCINE

— premixed narcotic analgesic and
anticholinergic agent for
premedication

PETHIDINE (known as meperidine in
USA)

— as for morphine but of shorter
duration (p. 93)
— used in obstetrics

Adult dose

i) 50–100 mg orally 3- to 4-hourly; OR
ii) 25–100 mg SC or IM 3- to 4-hourly;
OR
iii) 25–50 mg by slow IV injection or
infusion diluted to at least 5 ml with
isotonic saline

Paediatric dose

— 1 mg/kg/dose orally or IM

Adverse effects

— as for morphine but less constipation
and urinary retention

Interactions

— as for morphine
— causes severe CNS depression and
hypotension when given with
phenothiazines

— delays absorption of paracetamol
— phenobarbitone in high doses
reduces analgesic effect and
increases CNS toxicity
— results in excitation, sweating,
rigidity, hypertension or hypotension
and coma when combined with
furazolidone (after 5 days of
furazolidone therapy)

Nursing point

— compatible with chlorpromazine,
metoclopramide prochlorperazine or
promethazine when mixed in the
same syringe as long as the
resultant solution is used within 15
minutes and there is no precipitation

BUPRENORPHINE

— as for morphine but longer acting
and also has weak narcotic
antagonist properties

Dose

0.3–0.6 mg IM or slow IV injection 6- to
8-hourly

Adverse efects

— as for morphine but less constipation

Note

— may cause withdrawal effects if used
in patients dependent on other
narcotic analgesics

CODEINE PHOSPHATE

Action and use

— as for morphine (p. 93) but much
less potent
— antitussive
— relief of diarrhoea
— relieves mild/moderate pain alone or
combined with aspirin or
paracetamol

Adult dose

i) 15–60 mg orally 4- to 6-hourly (pain relief or diarrhoea); OR
ii) 50–100 mg IM (pain relief); OR
iii) 2.5–5 ml linctus (5 mg/ml) 4-hourly, as antitussive

Paediatric dose

over 1 year: 3 mg/kg/day in 4–6 divided doses

Adverse effects

— constipation, nausea, vomiting
— dizziness, drowsiness

Nursing point

— if dose 20 mg or greater, warn about reduced alcohol tolerance and not driving or operating machinery if drowsy

Note

— no benefit gained by exceeding 60 mg/dose
— dependence rare
— contained in many OTC preparations

DEXTROPROPOXYPHENE

Action and use

— as for codeine but less potent
— relieves mild/moderate recurrent pain

Dose

100 mg orally 4-hourly as required

Adverse effects

— dizziness, drowsiness
— nausea, vomiting
— skin rash
— psychic dependence
— convulsions (high dose)

Interactions

— enhances effects of warfarin
— CNS depressant effects enhanced by concurrent use of other CNS depressants

Nursing points

— warn patient about reduced tolerance to alcohol
— warn patient against driving a vehicle or operating machinery if drowsy

Note

— combined with aspirin or paracetamol for synergistic effect

METHADONE

— as for morphine (p. 93) but causes less sedation
— used for pain control in terminal stages of cancer
— used as substitution therapy in the treatment of narcotic dependence

Dose

5–10 mg orally, SC or IM 6- to 8-hourly

Interactions

— as for morphine
— renal excretion rate of methadone increased by acidification of urine and decreased by alkalinization
— methadone withdrawal symptoms occur when rifampicin or phenytoin given concurrently

DEXTROMORAMIDE

— related to methadone
— used for severe pain
— effective within 20–30 minutes with a duration of about 2–3 hours

Dose

i) 5–20 mg orally a.c., SC or IM; OR
ii) 10 mg rectal suppository t.d.s. or q.i.d.

Adverse effects

— nausea, vomiting, sweating (occasionally)

DIAMORPHINE (HEROIN)

— as for morphine (p. 93) but more potent and of shorter duration
— used mainly for pain control in terminal stages of cancer

Dose

i) 5–10 mg SC or IM 3- to 4-hourly; OR
ii) 5 mg IV

FENTANYL

— potent analgesic related to pethidine but with morphine-like properties
— used to control pain during surgery

Dose

25–100 micrograms IM or IV

Note

— may be given with haloperidol, droperidol and/or phenoperidine and/or diazepam to produce neuroleptanalgesia, a state of calm mental detachment in which procedures can be effected with the cooperation of the patient

OXYCODONE

— as for morphine (p. 93) but less marked adverse effects
— effective within 20–25 minutes with a duration of 8–10 hours
— for pain relief following surgery and in the terminal stages of cancer

Dose

i) 5 mg orally 6-hourly; OR
ii) 10–20 mg IM 6- to 8-hourly; OR
iii) 1 rectal suppository (30 mg) 6- to 8-hourly

OXYCODONE WITH ASPIRIN AND PARACETAMOL

— effective within 5–15 minutes with a duration of 6 hours
— useful oral analgesic for a large range of moderately painful conditions

Dose

— 1 tablet 6-hourly (with milk or food)

PENTAZOCINE

— as for morphine (p. 93)
— effective within 5–30 minutes depending if oral, SC, IM or IV and has a duration of 3–4 hours
— used for premedication and relief of moderate to severe pain

Dose

i) 25–100 mg orally 3- to 4-hourly p.c.; OR
ii) 45–60 mg SC or IM 3- to 4-hourly; OR
iii) 30 mg IV 3- to 4-hourly

Interactions

— decreases absorption of tetracyclines and phenytoin
— precipitation if mixed with soluble barbiturates or diazepam in the same syringe
— smoking increases metabolism of pentazocine

Nursing points

— rotate injection site
— warn about reduced alcohol tolerance and not driving or operating machinery if drowsy
— duration of action of parenteral preparations may be only 2–3 hours

Note

— also has mild narcotic antagonist properties so may produce acute withdrawal in some patients

PHENOPERIDINE

— as for morphine (p. 93)
— used alone for analgesia or in combination with droperidol in neuroleptanalgesia (see note for fentanyl (p. 97))

Adult dose

1 mg IV bolus over 1 minute supplemented with 0.5 mg during surgery about every 30 minutes

Paediatric dose

10–20 micrograms/kg IV

Note

— higher doses may be given with assisted respiration as necessary
— nitrous oxide and oxygen may be given to produce light anaesthesia
— post-operative depression can occur following neuroleptanalgesia with phenoperidine mostly in patients with a history of severe depressive illness
— have nalorphine and atropine available

BROMPTON MIXTURE (BROMPTON COCKTAIL)

— relieves intractable pain
— contains morphine and cocaine plus chloroform water and ethanol (APF)

NARCOTIC ANTAGONISTS

Action

— reverse toxic effects of narcotic analgesics
— some reverse analgesic effects

Use

— treatment of overdose with narcotic analgesics
— asphyxia of newborn resulting from maternal narcotic analgesia
— diagnosis and treatment of narcotic dependence

Preparations and dose

NALOXONE
Adult dose

Narcotic overdose

0.4 mg IV, IM or SC repeated every 2–3 minutes as required

Narcotic-induced depression

0.1–0.2 mg IV repeated every 2–3 minutes until desired degree of reversal

Paediatric dose

Overdose or narcotic-induced depression

0.01 mg/kg IV, IM or SC (neonatal preparation)

NALORPHINE
Adult dose

Narcotic overdose

5–10 mg IV, IM or SC repeated every 10–15 minutes as required (maximum total dose 40 mg)

Obstetrics

10 mg IV 10 minutes prior to expected time of delivery

Paediatric dose

0.25–1 mg into umbilical vein, IM or SC (neonatal preparation)

Adverse effects of narcotic antagonists

— reversal of analgesia
— severe withdrawal syndrome in
  · narcotic addict or neonate, therefore given with caution
— respiratory depression, drowsiness when nalorphine given apart from narcotics
— nausea, vomiting if not affected by narcotics (naloxone)

Interactions

— analgesic and respiratory depressant effects of morphine antagonized

Nursing points

— cardio-pulmonary resuscitative measures may be required
— observe respiration and heart rate and blood pressure and for signs of reversal of analgesia such as nausea, vomiting, sweating, tachycardia and raised blood pressure

Note

— narcotic antagonists not effective against respiratory depression caused by non-opioid drugs
— repeat doses are required frequently because the duration of action of some narcotics outlasts that of the antagonist

NON-NARCOTIC ANALGESICS

ASPIRIN (Acetylsalicylic acid)

Action

— salicylate
— analgesic anti-inflammatory, antipyretic
— inhibits biosynthesis of prostaglandins, important mediators in the inflammatory process
— antipyretic action, possibly by increasing blood flow through skin and by causing sweating
— reduces platelet adhesiveness
— increases bleeding time
— uricosuric (in large doses and urine alkaline)

Use

— relief of mild to moderate non-visceral pain
— headache, migraine
— arthralgia, myalgia
— acute febrile illnesses (not for children under 12 years)
— dysmenorrhoea
— rheumatoid arthritis, osteoarthritis, spondylitis
— gout
— antiplatelet therapy

Adult dose

i) 0.3–1 g orally or rectal suppository 3- to 4-hourly as required up to 4 g/day (analgesic, antipyretic); or
ii) 4–8 g/day in 4–6 divided doses (arthritic conditions)
iii) 50–300 mg daily (antiplatelet therapy)

Paediatric dose

Note

— not recommended for infants under 12 months
— use with caution in children with influenza or chickenpox (varicella) See Reye's syndrome (p. 100)

Analgesic and antipyretic

Based on 60 mg/kg/day in 4–6 divided doses
  i) 1–2 years: 450 mg/day
 ii) 3–5 years: 600 mg/day
iii) over 6 years: 900 mg/day

Rheumatic fever

120 mg/kg/day in 4–6 divided doses, then 60 mg/kg/day after 3–4 days

Adverse effects

— early signs in children are ketosis, acidosis, hyperventilation
— nausea, vomiting, dyspepsia, gastric bleeding and ulceration
— tinnitus, dizziness, temporary and, rarely, permanent deafness
— sweating
— severe hypersensitivity reaction, especially asthmatics
— increased bleeding time
— iron deficiency anaemia (long term therapy)
— acid-base balance disturbances
— hypoprothrombinaemia (large doses)
— hepatotoxicity, nephropathy (long term large doses)

Interactions

— aspirin enhances the action of methotrexate, heparin, tricyclic antidepressants and sulphonylurea hypoglycaemic agents
— increases blood levels of valproic acid
— aspirin absorption increased by metoclopramide during migraine attack
— gastric ulcerogenic effects may be enhanced by taking aspirin, alcohol and/or corticosteroids concurrently
— high doses of aspirin enhance the action of oral anticoagulants and para-amino salicylic acid
— reduces the uricosuric effects of probenecid and sulphinpyrazone
— antagonizes the action of spironolactone
— reduces phenytoin blood levels but not therapeutic efffect

Nursing points

— ask patient if taking anticoagulants and if any history of aspirin allergy, peptic ulceration or bleeding
— taken with or immediately after food or with milk if on continuous therapy
— effervescent and soluble preparations are dissolved in ½–1 glass of water for more rapid absorption
— sustained release and enteric coated preparations are swallowed whole
— avoid aspirin within ½ hour of alcohol
— keep airtight

Note

— not recommended under 12 years
— soluble, effervescent, buffered and enteric coated salicylate preparations reduce gastric irritation
— enteric coated and sustained action preparations have delayed absorption useful for regular long term therapy
— contained in many OTC preparations
— analgesic nephropathy can occur after long term combined analgesic abuse
— a high fluid intake with high doses of aspirin for prolonged periods may protect the renal papilla
— blood donors should not take aspirin for the previous week
— blood should not be sampled for phenytoin assay when aspirin being taken because aspirin reduces phenytoin blood levels
— nursing mothers should avoid taking high doses of aspirin
— tinnitus (with normal hearing) is a reliable index of therapeutic plasma level but may not be detected in patients with hearing loss
— symptoms of salicylism, chronic salicylate intoxication, are dizziness, tinnitus, deafness, sweating, nausea, vomiting, headache, mental confusion
— Reye's syndrome, a rare but fatal disease, which includes fatty encephalopathy, fatty degeneration of the liver and severe metabolic disturbances, may be associated with the taking of aspirin by children under 12 years for viral illnesses such as influenza or varicella

PARACETAMOL (known as acetaminophen in USA)

Action and use

— as for aspirin (p. 99) but has less anti-inflammatory effects
— suitable alternative if aspirin allergy, dyspepsia or peptic ulceration

Adult dose

i) 0.5–1 g orally 3- to 4-hourly p.r.n. up to 4 g/day; OR
ii) 0.25–1 g rectal suppository 4- to 6-hourly p.r.n.

Paediatric dose

Based on 25 mg/kg/day
i) under 6 months: 20 mg q.i.d.
ii) 6–12 months: 50 mg q.i.d.
iii) 1–5 years: 100 mg q.i.d.
iv) 5–10 years: 200 mg q.i.d.
v) over 10 years: 200–500 mg q.i.d.
Children may take soluble tablets from 5 years, elixir or suspension from 6 months to 10 years and paediatric drops from under 6 months to 5 years

Adverse effects

— rarely, nausea, dyspepsia, allergic reaction
— hepatic necrosis (10 g or more)

Interactions

— absorption increased by metoclopramide
— absorption reduced by diamorphine, pethidine and propantheline

Nursing points

— effervescent and soluble preparations are dissolved in ½–1 glass of water for more rapid absorption

Note

— not recommended for infants under 1 month
— contained in many OTC preparations

— paracetamol overdose may be treated within 10 hours of ingestion, by IV acetylcysteine (Parvolex®) to protect against liver damage (p. 299)

DICLOFENAC

Action

— inhibits biosynthesis of prostaglandins
— analgesic, anti-inflammatory, antipyretic
— reduces platelet adhesiveness

Use

— rheumatoid arthritis, osteoarthritis

Dose

25–50 mg orally b.d. or t.d.s. a.c.

Adverse effects

— gastrointestinal disturbances
— headache, dizziness
— occasionally, rash, pruritus, peripheral oedema
— rarely, blood dyscrasias

Interaction

— increases blood lithium levels by reducing renal clearance

DIFLUNISAL

Action

— as for aspirin but longer acting
— uricosuric

Use

— acute pain of injury and post-surgical trauma
— rheumatoid arthritis, osteoarthritis (short term treatment)

Dose

i) 500 mg orally initially, then 250 mg b.d. (osteoarthritis); OR
ii) 250–500 mg b.d. as required (trauma)

Adverse effects

— gastrointestinal disturbances (usually mild)

Interactions

— absorption decreased by aluminium hydroxide
— enhances effect of the oral anticoagulant, nicoumalone
— increases indomethacin blood levels significantly

Note

— nursing mothers should not take diflunisal or should stop breast-feeding their infants

FLUFENAMIC ACID

Action and use

— as for mefenamic acid (see this section)

Dose

100–200 mg orally t.d.s. with meals

IBUPROFEN

Action

— inhibits prostaglandin synthesis
— analgesic, anti-inflammatory, antipyretic

Use

— rheumatoid arthritis
— osteoarthritis
— ankylosing spondylitis
— primary dysmenorrhoea

Dose

Arthritis

1200–2400 mg orally daily in 3–4 divided doses with food

Primary dysmenorrhoea

400–800 mg orally with food at the first sign of pain or menstrual bleeding, then 400 mg 4- to 6-hourly up to a maximum daily dose of 1600 mg

Adverse effects

— gastrointestinal disturbances
— tinnitus, dizziness, headache, visual disturbances
— fluid retention
— decreased appetite, rash

Interactions

— combining alcohol with ibuprofen will increase bleeding time

Nursing points

— take with food or milk if nausea troublesome
— note tablet size may be 200 mg or 400 mg

INDOMETHACIN

Action

— as for ibuprofen

Use

— rheumatoid arthritis
— osteoarthritis
— ankylosing spondylitis
— gout
— bursitis, tenosynovitis
— sprains and strains
— primary dysmenorrhoea
— medical closure of patent ductus arteriosus in neonatal infants

Adult dose

i) 25 mg orally 2–4 times daily with food increasing to 50 mg orally 2–4 times daily; OR
ii) 100 mg rectal suppository daily or b.d. if oral therapy not tolerated; OR
iii) in combination e.g. 25 mg orally 2–4 times daily and 100 mg rectal suppository nocte
iv) 25 mg orally t.d.s. with food at the first sign of pain or menstrual bleeding and continuing for as long

as the symptoms usually last (primary dysmenorrhoea)

Paediatric dose

Neonate: 0.2–0.3 mg/kg in 2–3 doses at intervals of 8–24 hours under close supervision in neonatal intensive-care unit

Adverse effects

— gastrointestinal disturbances including ulceration and/or bleeding, stomatitis
— headache, dizziness, lightheadedness, tinnitus, depression, drowsiness, confusion, insomnia, blurred vision
— oedema, weight gain, hypertension
— hypersensitivity reaction
— (suppository) irritation of rectal mucosa, tenesmus

Interactions

— absorption reduced by aluminium hydroxide
— increases lithium carbonate blood levels significantly
— increased indomethacin blood levels if patient already receiving probenecid
— combination of alcohol and indomethacin increases bleeding time significantly
— reduces anti-hypertensive action of beta-adrenoceptor drugs
— reduces response to frusemide
— reduces naturetic and anti-hypertensive action of frusemide and thiazide diuretics
— renal failure can result when diuretics given with indomethacin
— diflunisal increases indomethacin blood levels significantly

Nursing points

— taken with or after food or with milk to minimize gastric irritation
— advise patient to report to the medical officer any gastrointestinal disturbances, dizziness or persistent headache as this requires a dosage reduction

— warn patient against driving a vehicle or operating machinery if drowsy

Note

— not recommended during pregnancy or lactation

KETOPROFEN

Action and use

— as for ibuprofen (p. 102)

Dose

i) 50 mg orally 2–4 times daily with food; OR
ii) 100 mg rectal suppository nocte supplemented as required with 50 mg orally daily or b.d.

Adverse effects

— gastrointestinal disturbances including ulceration and/or bleeding, stomatitis
— headache, dizziness, tinnitus, depression, drowsiness
— palpitations, peripheral oedema, bruising
— hypersensitivity reactions

MEFENAMIC ACID

Action

— inhibits prostaglandin synthesis
— analgesic, anti-inflammatory, antipyretic

Use

— primary dysmenorrhea
— primary menorrhagia
— rheumatoid arthritis
— dental and soft tissue pain

Dose

500 mg orally t.d.s. with meals. For dysmenorrhoea, continue dose for at least 3 days after onset of menses. For menorrhagia, continue as advised by the medical officer

Adverse effects

— gastrointestinal disturbances including ulceration and/or bleeding
— headache, dizziness, drowsiness, insomnia, visual disturbances
— urticaria, rash
— blood dyscrasias especially haemolytic anaemia

Interaction

— enhances activity of oral anticoagulants

Nursing points

— taken with or after food or with milk to minimize gastric irritation
— drug discontinued promptly if diarrhoea or rash occurs

Note

— dose of oral anticoagulant adjusted by monitoring prothrombin activity

NAPROXEN

Action and use

— as for ibuprofen (p. 102)

Dose

i) 375–750 mg orally daily in 2 divided doses with food (up to 1250 mg daily for gynaecological conditions); OR
ii) 250 mg orally mane with food and 500 mg rectal suppository nocte
iii) 500 mg orally with food at the first sign of pain or menstrual bleeding, then 250 mg every 6–8 hours as required up to a maximum daily dose of 1250 mg (primary dysmenorrhoea)

Adverse effects

— gastrointestinal disturbances
— headache, dizziness
— decreases platelet aggregation and prolongs bleeding time

Interactions

— probenecid increases naproxen blood levels

— absorption reduced by antacids and increased by sodium bicarbonate
— enhances effect of oral anticoagulants, phenytoin, methotrexate, sulphonamides and sulphonylurea hypoglycaemic agents

Nursing points

— taken with food or milk to minimize gastric irritation
— advise patient to report gastrointestinal symptoms to the medical officer immediately

PIROXICAM

Action and use

— as for ibuprofen (see this section)

Dose

10–20 mg orally as single daily dose

Adverse effects and interactions

— as for indomethacin (see this section)

Note

— only once daily dose required because of long plasma half-life
— dose of oral anticoagulant adjusted by monitoring prothrombin activity

SODIUM AUROTHIOMALATE (GOLD SALT)

Action

— anti-inflammatory effect on collagen and synovial membranes

Use

— rheumatoid arthritis
— Still's disease
— chronic discoid lupus erythematosus

Adult dose

i) 1, 5, and 10 mg IM at weekly intervals to test tolerance then 50 mg/week to a total of 1 g; OR

ii) 50 mg/week IM for 20 weeks to a total of 1 g then following either i) or ii) 50 mg/month to a total of 3 g

Paediatric dose

10 mg/week IM increasing slowly to 25 mg/week to a total of 500 mg

Adverse effects

— rash, pruritus (early sign of intolerance)
— nephritis with proteinuria, haematuria
— stomatitis, glossitis, gingivitis
— keratitis, corneal ulceration
— bone marrow depression (rare but may be fatal)
— occasionally, anaphylactic shock, angioneurotic oedema

Interaction

— penicillamine increases incidence of rashes and bone marrow depression in patients who have previously received gold salts

Nursing points

— before injection given, inspect for rashes and test urine for protein
— advise patient to report sore throat, mouth or tongue bruising or unusual bleeding to the medical officer immediately
— if any of above adverse effects present, injection withheld
— ampoules of gold salts stored in cool place, protected from light and not used if darkened in colour

Note

— patient informed of possibility of toxic reactions and of the need to report promptly any symptoms suggesting toxicity, e.g., skin reactions, mouth ulcers, fever or any new or unusual symptom
— urinalysis and complete blood cell and platelet count before treatment started
— blood cell and platelet count every 2–4 weeks

— severe blood dyscrasias may occur with little warning
— erythrocyte sedimentation rate estimated every 2–4 weeks for first 8 months then every 1–2 months

AUROTHIOGLUCOSE (GOLD SALT)

Action, use, adverse effects, note

as for sodium aurothiomalate

Dose

10 mg IM weekly increasing gradually to 50 mg/week to a total of 1 g

Nursing points

— before injection given, inspect for rashes and test urine for protein and blood
— advise patient to report sore throat, mouth or tongue and any bruising or unusual bleeding to the medical officer immediately
— if any of above adverse effects present, injection withheld
— shake vial thoroughly in horizontal position before dose withdrawn
— syringe and needle must be dry
— heat vial to body temperature (by immersion in warm water) to facilitate drawing suspension into syringe
— give deeply IM preferably in buttock

AURANOFIN

Action, use

— as for sodium aurothiomalate

Dose

6 mg orally daily with food

Adverse effects

— diarrhoea
— anorexia, nausea, vomiting
— others as for injectable gold (see above) but less common

Nursing point

— tablets should be protected from sunlight

SODIUM SALICYLATE

Action, adverse effects and interactions

— as for aspirin (p. 99)

Use

— rheumatic fever
— rheumatoid arthritis

Dose

600–900 mg orally 4- to 6-hourly (enteric-coated tablets)

SULINDAC

Action

— inhibits biosynthesis of prostaglandins
— analgesic, anti-inflammatory, antipyretic

Use

— rheumatoid arthritis
— osteoarthritis
— ankylosing spondylitis
— acute gouty arthritis
— bursitis, tendonitis, tenosynovitis

Dose

100–200 mg orally b.d. with food or milk

Adverse effects

— as for indomethacin (p. 102)

OTHER DRUGS USED TO TREAT RHEUMATOID ARTHRITIS

See chloroquine, hydroxychloroquine (p. 226)

TOPICAL ANALGESICS

Applications to the skin in the form of liniments, ointments, lotions and creams are absorbed for the relief of pain. Care must be taken to apply the appropriate agent for intact or broken skin surfaces

IF SKIN INTACT

Action

— produces warmth, smarting and a local anaesthetic effect (counter-irritant effect) when applied to intact skin, which is comforting in painful conditions involving muscles, tendons and joints
— some are local coolants (counter irritants)

Use

— arthritic, rheumatic and neuritic pain
— bursitis, fibrositis, lumbago, sciatica
— sprains, muscular aches and pains

Ingredients

benzydamine, bufexamac, camphor, capsicum, clove oil, dichlorodifluoromethane, dichlorotetrafluoroethane, diethylamine salicylate, dimethisoquin, ethyl chloride, eucalyptus oil, indomethacin, isobornylacetate, menthol, methyl salicylate, phenylbutazone, thyme oil, trichloromonofluoromethane, triethanolamine, turpentine

Nursing points

— applied only to intact skin
— cream massaged into skin

IF SKIN NOT INTACT

Use

— rapid relief of surface pain in perineal suturing, haemorrhoids, pruritus vulvae, pruritus ani, wounds, burns, abrasions, insect bites, removal of adhesive tapes and dressings

Ingredients

benzocaine, lignocaine, menthol

Nursing points

— holding aerosol can upright 30 cm from affected area, spray in short bursts avoiding contact with eyes
— usually administered 2–3 times daily

DRUG TREATMENT OF CHRONIC GOUT INCLUDING URICOSURIC AGENTS

ALLOPURINOL

Action

— reduces uric acid formation by inhibiting xanthine oxidase

Use

— chronic gout
— hyperuricaemia resulting from leukemia, antineoplastic or thiazide diuretic therapy or radiotherapy

Dose

50–100 mg orally daily p.c. inceasing to 300 mg b.d. p.c.

Adverse effects

— rash
— nausea, diarrhoea, abdominal pain
— drowsiness

Interactions

— enhances effect of mercaptopurine and azathioprine
— enhances the response to oral anticoagulants
— increases theophylline blood levels

Nursing points

— taken with food or milk to minimize gastric irritation
— advise patient to report rash as this indicates the need to stop therapy
— fluid intake increased to maintain a urinary output of at least 2L/24 hrs and urine made alkaline to minimize stone formation
— warn patient against driving a vehicle or operating machinery if drowsy

Note

— colchicine or an anti-inflammatory agent may be given as well in the early stages of allopurinol therapy

PROBENECID

Action

— promotes uric acid excretion by inhibiting its renal tubular absorption (uricosuric)
— reduces renal tubular excretion of some anti-infective agents

Use

— chronic gout
— adjuvant to therapy with penicillins and most cephalosporins

Dose

i) 250 mg orally b.d. increasing after 1 week to 500 mg 2–4 times daily (gout); OR
ii) 500 mg orally q.i.d. (penicillin therapy); OR
iii) 1 g orally as single dose taken with the high single dose of amoxycillin

Adverse effects

— headache
— anorexia, nausea, vomiting
— urinary frequency
— hypersensitivity reaction
— exacerbation of gout

Interactions

— therapeutic effects reduced by salicylates
— increases blood levels of penicillins, some cephalosporins, indomethacin, para-aminosalicylic acid, methotrexate and rifampicin

Nursing points

— taken with food or milk to minimize gastric irritation
— risk of urinary lithiasis reduced by increasing fluid intake to maintain a urinary output of at least 2L/24 hrs and by alkalinizing the urine

SULPHINPYRAZONE

Action and use

— potent uricosuric agent for chronic gout

Dose

100 mg orally b.d. t.d.s. or q.i.d. then 200 mg t.d.s. reducing to 100 mg daily or b.d., each dose taken after a meal or with milk

Adverse effects

— gastric discomfort (uncommon)
— rarely rash, blood dyscrasias

Interactions

— therapeutic effects reduced by salicylates and oral diuretics
— enhances the effects of oral anticoagulants, insulin and oral hypoglycaemic agents
— decreases theophylline blood levels

Nursing points

— tablets swallowed whole to avoid bitter taste
— increased fluid intake and alkalinization of the urine reduces stone formation

Note

— concurrent treatment with phenylbutazone will minimize an exacerbation of acute gout in a dose of 200 mg orally b.d. or t.d.s. or 600 mg deeply IM daily for 3–4 days

DRUG TREATMENT OF ACUTE GOUT

COLCHICINE

Action

— inhibits leucocyte migration and phagocytosis in gouty joints so counteracts inflammatory response to urate crystals

Use

— acute and chronic gout

Dose

i) 1 mg orally initially, followed every 2 hours by 0.5 mg until relief obtained
ii) after acute episode and during first 3 weeks of allopurinol, 0.5 mg b.d. or t.d.s. p.c. or 0.5–2 mg nocte or alternate nights

Adverse effects

— nausea, vomiting, diarrhoea
— abdominal pain

Nursing points

— treatment continued during acute attack until relief, nausea, diarrhoea, or the total maximum dose of 10 mg has been taken

Note

— course should not be repeated within 3 days
— may be taken daily to prevent and treat attacks of Mediterranean fever

PHENYLBUTAZONE

Action

— analgesic, antipyretic, anti-inflammatory
— uricosuric

Use

— acute rheumatic diseases where less toxic drugs have failed

Dose

i) 400 mg orally initially with food, then 100 mg 4-hourly until pain subsides (acute gout); OR
ii) 100 mg orally 1–4 times daily with food; OR
iii) 1 rectal suppository (250 mg) 1–3 times daily; OR
iv) 600 mg slowly IM daily for 1 week, then 5 days/week
v) concurrently with sulphinpyrazone to minimize an exacerbation of acute gout in a dose of 200 mg orally b.d. or t.d.s. or 600 mg deeply IM daily for 3–4 days

Adverse effects

— transient gastrointestinal disturbance but if persists or increases, drug withdrawn
— gastrointestinal bleeding and/or ulceration, stomatitis
— sodium and fluid retention, rash
— rare but serious blood dyscrasias or skin disorders

Interactions

— enhances activity of oral anticoagulants, and oral hypoglycaemic agents
— reduces antihypertensive effect of bretylium, debrisoquine and guanethidine

Nursing points

— taken with food or milk to minimize gastric irritation
— enteric-coated tablets swallowed whole
— ensure slow and deep IM injection into gluteal muscle to avoid pain and subcutaneous tissue irritation
— rectal suppository nocte produces relief during the night and reduces morning stiffness
— advise patient to report epigastric discomfort, dark stools, swelling of the ankles or rash
— advise patient to report fever or persistent sore throat which are early signs of bone marrow depression
— may require salt-restricted diet

Note

— cinchocaine premixed with injectable preparation to reduce pain
— babies of nursing mothers should be monitored frequenty because of the serious nature of the adverse effects
— drug discontinued if no improvement within a week
— blood counts monitored closely during therapy

OTHER DRUGS USED TO TREAT GOUT

See indomethacin, naproxen and corticosteroids

SEDATIVES AND HYPNOTICS (BARBITURATES)

AMYLOBARBITONE

Action

— moderately long action (up to 8 hours)
— depresses CNS

Use

— sedative, hypnotic, premedication

Dose

i) 30–50 mg orally b.d. or t.d.s. (sedative); OR
ii) 100–200 mg orally nocte (hypnotic)

Adverse effect

— drowsiness, excitement, hangover
— allergic reaction
— dependence

Interactions

— CNS depressant effects of amylobarbitone significantly increased by other CNS depressants
— reduces effect of coumarin oral anticoagulants, phenothiazines, dexamethasone, prednisone, doxycycline, oral alprenolol

Nursing points

— warn patient against driving a vehicle or operating machinery if drowsy
— warn patient about the reduced tolerance to alcohol

AMYLOBARBITONE SODIUM

Action

— moderately long action (8–11 hours)

Use

— sedative, hypnotic, premedication and anticonvulsant

Dose

i) 30–50 mg orally b.d. or t.d.s. (sedative); OR
ii) 100–200 mg orally nocte (hypnotic); OR
iii) 200 mg orally (premedication); OR
iv) 0.3–1 g IV (convulsions)

Adverse effects and interactions

— as for amylobarbitone

BUTOBARBITONE

— intermediate-acting sedative and hypnotic (8 hours)

Dose

i) 100 mg orally daily or b.d. (sedative); OR
ii) 100–200 mg orally nocte (hypnotic)

Note

— see amylobarbitone

PENTOBARBITONE SODIUM

Action

— intermediate action (6–8 hours)

Use

— sedative, hypnotic, premedication
— amnesic in obstetrics

Dose

i) 50 mg orally daily or b.d. (sedative) OR
ii) 100–200 mg orally nocte (hypnotic); OR
iii) 100–200 mg orally (premedication); OR
iv) 200–300 mg orally once labour established (with hyoscine occasionally)

Note

— see amylobarbitone

PHENOBARBITONE

Action

— long acting barbiturate, onset within 1 hour, duration of action 6–10 hours
— depresses CNS
— anticonvulsant

Use

— anxiety states
— insomnia
— migraine
— anticonvulsant in grand mal epilepsy or psychomotor epilepsy often as combined therapy

Adult dose

i) 15 mg orally daily or b.d. (sedation) OR
ii) 30–60 mg orally nocte (hypnotic) OR
iii) 60–180 mg orally nocte (anticonvulsant)

Paediatric dose

1–2 mg/kg orally 8–12 hourly (sedation) (see p. 136 for doses in epilepsy, febrile convulsions prophylaxis)

Adverse effects

— respiratory depression, sedation
— irritability, hyperexcitability (children)
— confusion, restlessness, excitement (elderly)
— dependence, tolerance
— folate deficiency (prolonged therapy)
— rarely rash, blood dyscrasias
— high dose, ataxia, nystagmus, 'hangover'

Interactions

— CNS depressant effects of phenobarbitone increased by other CNS depressants
— phenobarbitone reduces the effect of dexamethasone, prednisone, tricyclic antidepressants, quinidine, coumarin oral anticoagulants, metronidazole, levodopa, oral griseofulvin, rifampicin, phenothiazines, doxycycline, frusemide, oral alprenolol, mianserin
— phenobarbitone reduces blood levels of calcium, folic acid and sodium valproate
— phenobarbitone reduces chloramphenicol blood levels significantly in children
— analgesic effect of pethidine reduced but CNS toxicity increased by phenobarbitone
— pyridoxine reduces phenobarbitone blood levels
— sodium valproate increases phenobarbitone blood levels
— phenobarbitone blood level increased by sulthiame

Nursing points

— wakefulness, excitement and delirium may occur in presence of pain
— bedsides may be required if patient shows confusion or excitement (children, elderly)
— warn patient against driving a vehicle or operating machinery if drowsy
— warn patient about reduced tolerance to alcohol
— warn patient about the need to continue therapy and warn against abrupt withdrawal of therapy
— advise patient to report fever or sore throat which are early signs of bone marrow depression

Note

— abrupt withdrawal of phenobarbitone may result in anxiety, insomnia, delirium, convulsions and status epilepticus (in epileptics)
— monitoring of blood levels often necessary to achieve correct dosage (blood sample taken midway between doses) therapeutic range 10–30 mg/L (45–130 micromol/L) toxicity > 35 mg/L (> 150 micromol/L)
— phenobarbitone poisoning treated by activated charcoal (p. 298)

QUINALBARBITONE SODIUM

— rapidly-acting barbiturate of short duration used as hypnotic, premedication and occasionally for sedation in obstetrics

Adult dose

i) 100–200 mg orally nocte (hypnotic);
OR
ii) 200–300 mg orally (premedication)

Paediatric dose

5 mg/kg (premedication)

Note

— see amylobarbitone

SEDATIVES AND HYPNOTICS (BENZODIAZEPINES)

NITRAZEPAM

Action and use

— actions similar to diazepam (see in section on anxiolytics)
— effective as an hypnotic within 30–60 minutes, with a duration of 6–8 hours
— used as hypnotic and anti-convulsant

Adult dose

2.5–10 mg orally nocte, occasionally 20 mg (hypnotic)

Paediatric dose

1.25–2.5 mg orally daily, increasing slowly to 5 mg 2–4 times daily (epilepsy)

Adverse effects

— drowsiness and light-headedness next day
— 'hangover' effect mainly in the elderly as a result of the accumulation of nitrazepam and its metabolites
— restlessness and confusion in the elderly

Interactions

— CNS depressant effects of nitrazepam increased by alcohol, barbiturates, tricyclic antidepressants, phenothiazines and morphine derivatives
— enhances effects of amitriptyline significantly
— antagonized by methylphenidate

Nursing points

— warn patient against driving a vehicle or operating machinery if drowsy
— warn patient about the reduced tolerance to alcohol
— advise patient that drug therapy is best withdrawn over several days or

weeks unless urgent need to stop abruptly

Note

— may lead to dependence

DIAZEPAM

Dose

5–40 mg orally daily

Note

— see anxiolytics (p. 116)
— 'hangover' effect mainly in the elderly as a result of the accumulation of diazepam and its metabolites

FLUNITRAZEPAM

Action and use

— related to nitrazepam, flurazepam and clonazepam
— used as hypnotic in severe cases of insomnia

Dose

0.5–4 mg orally nocte

Adverse effects, interactions, nursing points

— see nitrazepam

Note

— also has anxiolytic, muscle relaxant and anticonvulsant properties

FLURAZEPAM

Action and use

— has hypnotic properties similar to nitrazepam

Dose

15–30 mg orally nocte

Note

— see nitrazepam

TEMAZEPAM

Action and use

— short acting benzodiazepine with no long acting active metabolite and tends not to accumulate with long term therapy

Dose

10–30 mg orally nocte

Note

— see nitrazepam

SEDATIVES AND HYPNOTICS (OTHER)

CHLORAL HYDRATE

Action

— effective within 30 minutes with a duration of 5–8 hours

Use

— relatively safe for children and the elderly who tolerate barbiturates adversely

Adult dose

i) 250 mg orally t.d.s. p.c. (sedative); OR
ii) 0.5–1 g orally nocte (hypnotic)

Paediatric dose

i) 25 mg/kg/day orally in divided doses (sedative); OR
ii) 50 mg/kg orally (hypnotic)

Adverse effects

— gastric irritation
— rash
— rarely excitement, delirium, dependence

Interactions

— CNS depressant effects of chloral hydrate increased by other CNS depressants
— effects of oral anticoagulants increased

Nursing points

— note different elixir strengths 250 mg/5 ml of Dormel® and 500 mg/5 ml of Chloralix®
— minimize gastric irritation by taking mixture or capsules immediately after food or with a full glass of water, fruit juice or ginger ale; syrup or elixir requires half a glass of diluent
— see nitrazepam

CHLORMETHIAZOLE

— see page 118 in anxiolytic section

PARALDEHYDE

Action

— CNS depressant effects similar to those of alcohol, barbiturates and chloral hydrate
— effective within 15–30 minutes with a duration of 8 hours

Use

— sedative and hypnotic in acute agitation because of alcohol withdrawal
— control convulsions of tetanus, eclampsia and status epilepticus

Dose

i) 5–30 ml orally; OR
ii) 5–10 ml deep IM (rarely IV)

Adverse effects

— nausea, vomiting
— rash
— sterile abscess from IM injection
— phlebitis after IV injection

Nursing points

— solution *not* used if has brownish colour or smells of acetic acid
— gastric irritation reduced and taste and odour masked by diluting oral preparation in milk or fruit juice
— paraldehyde has a solvent action on most plastics so is drawn up into a glass syringe
— give only 5 ml deeply into any one IM site
— IM injection very painful
— rotate injection sites
— bedsides required
— patient's breath will have the unmistakable characteristic odour of the drug for several hours as it is partly eliminated by the lungs

Note

— the administration of partly decomposed paraldehyde will cause death by corrosive poisoning
— not given to patients receiving disulfiram

DOXYLAMINE

— see antihistamines

PROMETHAZINE

— see antihistamines

TRIMEPRAZINE (ALIMEMAZINE)

— see antihistamines

ANXIOLYTICS (Minor Tranquillizers)

DIAZEPAM

Action

— benzodiazepine derivative
— sedative allowing mental relaxation
— skeletal muscle relaxant
— anticonvulsant, when given IV

Use

— anxiety and tension states
— allay anxiety prior to surgery, cardioversion, endoscopy, orthopaedic and dental procedures
— relieve acute withdrawal symptoms of alcoholism
— status epilepticus
— tetanus
— premature labour
— drug-induced convulsions

Adult dose

i) 2–10 mg orally b.d. or t.d.s.; OR
ii) 2–10 mg IM or slowly IV (up to 20 mg IV for status epilepticus); OR
iii) 20 mg diluted in 500 ml isotonic saline or 5% glucose by IV infusion, rate adjusted as required

Paediatric dose

1–5 mg/day in divided doses, orally, IM or IV

Adverse effects

— drowsiness, fatigue, ataxia
— hypotension
— depression, confusion, dizziness, slurred speech, visual disturbances
— constipation, urinary retention/incontinence
— change in salivation and libido, rash
— rarely, blood dyscrasias, jaundice
— excitement, muscle spasticity, sleep disturbances
— risk of dependence

Interactions

— CNS depressant effects enhanced by alcohol and other CNS depressants

— enhances effects of phenytoin
— absorption rate of oral diazepam
  increased by metoclopramide
— diazepam blood level increased by
  cimetidine and isoniazid
— diazepam blood level reduced by
  aminophylline and rifampicin
— diazepam increases digoxin blood
  level
— enhances effects of amitriptyline
  significantly
— reduces effects of levodopa
— methylphenidate reduces effects of
  diazepam
— increases anticholinergic side-effects
  of tricyclic antidepressants mainly in
  elderly
— diazepam-induced drowsiness less in
  heavy smokers.

Nursing points

— injectable diazepam forms an
  incompatible precipitate when mixed
  with other drugs
— monitor vital signs when drug given
  IM or IV, noting hypotension,
  tachycardia, respiratory depression
  and muscle weakness
— note and report paradoxical reactions
  such as excitement, muscle
  spasticity and sleep disturbances
— warn patient against driving a vehicle
  or operating machinery if drowsy
— warn patient about reduced tolerance
  to alcohol
— warn patient against abrupt
  withdrawal of therapy as this may
  cause vomiting, muscle cramps and
  convulsions
— the medical officer may order the
  majority of the daily dose ($\frac{2}{3}$), at night
  and ($\frac{1}{3}$) in the morning to offset some
  of the side effects

Note

— 'hangover' effect mainly in the
  elderly as a result of the
  accumulation of diazepam and its
  metabolites
— not given to patients with narrow
  angle glaucoma or myasthenia gravis
— nursing mothers taking high or
  repeated doses of diazepam (more

than 10 mg/day) should discontinue
breast-feeding

ALPRAZOLAM

— as for diazepam

Dose

0.5–4 mg/day orally in 2–3 divided
doses a.c.

BROMAZEPAM

— as for diazepam

Dose

6–60 mg/day orally in 2–3 divided doses
a.c.

CHLORDIAZEPOXIDE

Action

— as for diazepam

Use

— anxiety and tension states
— premedication
— relieve acute withdrawal symptoms
  of alcoholism

Dose

5 mg orally b.d. to 25 mg q.i.d.

Adverse effects and interactions

— as for diazepam

Nursing points

— swallow capsules or tablets whole
— note and report excitement or acute
  rage
— warn patient against driving a vehicle
  or operating machinery if drowsy
— warn patient about reduced tolerance
  to alcohol
— warn patient against abrupt
  withdrawal of therapy as this may
  cause vomiting, muscle cramps and
  convulsions

CLOBAZAM

— as for diazepam

Dose

10–30 mg/day orally in 2 divided doses or single dose nocte

CLORAZEPATE

— as for diazepam

Dose

5–60 mg/day orally in 2–3 divided doses or single dose nocte

LORAZEPAM

Action

— sedation
— anticonvulsant

Use

— anxiety and tension states
— premedication

Dose

2–5 mg orally b.d.

Adverse effects

— nausea, vomiting, dry mouth
— drowsiness, dizziness, headache
— blurred vision

Interactions

— CNS depressant effects enhanced by alcohol and other CNS depressants
— enhances effects of amitriptyline significantly
— IV cimetidine increases lorazepam blood levels

Nursing points

— as for chlordiazepoxide

Note

— as for diazepam

OXAZEPAM

— as for diazepam, but has no active metabolite so is useful in elderly patients

Dose

7.5–30 mg 2–4 times daily

CHLORMETHIAZOLE

Action

— chemically related to vitamin B_1
— sedative, hypnotic
— anticonvulsant

Use

— sedation of elderly
— acute alcohol withdrawal symptoms
— status epilepticus
— pre-eclampsia, eclampsia
— IV sedation during regional anaesthesia

Dose

Geriatric sedation

i) 1 capsule (192 mg) b.d. or t.d.s. (sedation); or
ii) 2 capsules nocte repeated after 1 hour if required (hypnotic)

Alcohol withdrawal

2–4 capsules initially then 2 capsules at 1 hour intervals up to 8 capsules in 2 hours if required; followed by 2–3 capsules q.i.d. up to 10 days as required (maximum dose in 24 hours is 16 capsules)

Delerium tremens, status epilepticus, pre-eclampsia and eclampsia

i) 40–100 ml 0.8% prepared solution (320–800 mg) slowly IV over 3–5 minutes; or
ii) 0.8% prepared solution by IV infusion at 3–7.5 ml/min reducing to 0.5–1 ml/min to maintain shallow sleep and spontaneous breathing (maximum dose is 1000 ml over 12 hours)

Sedation during regional anaesthesia

0.8% prepared solution by IV infusion at 25 ml/min for 1–2 minutes to maintain shallow sleep (after premedication with atropine)

Adverse effects

— nausea, vomiting
— rhinitis with sneezing
— transient hypotension and tachycardia (if given rapidly IV)
— CNS depression (IV therapy)
— dependence

Interactions

— CNS depressant effects enhanced by alcohol and other CNS depressants

Nursing points

— nurse as for heavily sedated patient where appropriate
— monitor vital signs when drug given IV, noting the level of consciousness, tachycardia or hypotension
— IV drip flow can be interrupted periodically to check the level of consciousness and effect of treatment on symptoms
— no other infusion fluids or drugs to be added to IV solution
— change IV line with each new flask as drug is absorbed by and softens the general purpose PVC administration set
— a burette or infusion pump should be used to regulate the IV rate
— store IV solution stock in refrigerator but do not freeze
— have resuscitation equipment available when giving drug IV
— warn patient about reduced tolerance to alcohol

Note

— treatment should not exceed 10 days to reduce risk of dependence, except where used for sedation
— 5 ml of syrup is equivalent to 1 capsule
— 0.8% solution contains 8 mg/ml

BUSPIRONE

Action

— relieves anxiety without sedative or muscle relaxant effects

Use

— short term treatment of anxiety (up to 1 month)

Dose

5 mg orally t.d.s. initially, increasing gradually to 10–20 mg 2–3 times daily (not to exceed 60 mg/day)

Adverse effects

— dizziness, light-headedness, nervousness, insomnia, dream disturbances, drowsiness
— nausea
— headache, fatigue, chest pain

Interactions

— food increases bioavailability of unchanged drug
— causes elevated blood pressure in patients receiving MAO inhibitors

Nursing points

— patients advised that medical officer is to be informed about current or planned medications, pregnancy or if breast-feeding
— patient advised that if unplanned pregnancy during therapy, cease tablets and contact medical officer

NEUROLEPTICS (Major tranquillizers, antipsychotics)

HALOPERIDOL

Action

— butyrophenone derivative with some actions of the phenothiazines
— selective depressant action on CNS
— inhibits central action of dopamine and noradrenaline
— anti-emetic

Use

— antipsychotic
— premedication
— during alcohol withdrawal
— combined with anti-depressant therapy
— neuroleptanalgesia
— radiation sickness
— severely aggressive and hostile children
— Gilles de la Tourette syndrome

Adult dose

i) 1–15 mg orally daily as single dose or 2 divided doses; OR
ii) 1–20 mg IM or IV injection (up to 100 mg/day may be required)

Paediatric dose

1–3 mg orally daily, then 0.05 mg/kg/day maintenance (tablets or liquid)

Adverse effects

— extrapyramidal reactions
— anxiety, drowsiness, depression, hallucinations
— anorexia
— transient tachycardia and postural hypotension
— leucopenia

Interactions

— CNS depressant effects enhanced by alcohol and other CNS depressants
— increases adverse effect of tricyclic antidepressants
— increases blood level of lithium salts resulting in CNS lithium toxicity

Nursing points

— patient to be recumbent for at least an hour after injection to avoid postural hypotension
— advise patient about the need to continue therapy
— warn patient against driving a vehicle or operating machinery if drowsy
— warn patient about reduced tolerance to alcohol
— observe carefully so that distinction may be made between a return of psychotic behaviour and the onset of extrapyramidal reactions (p. 122)
— have noradrenaline and benztropine available

Note

— has been used with fluphenazine decanoate, *Modecate®* in Huntington's chorea
— may be combined with antidepressants where depression and psychosis co-exist
— see fentanyl (p. 96)

DROPERIDOL

— as for haloperidol

Adult dose

Psychiatry

10–25 mg IM 4- to 6-hourly as required then 10–25 mg orally daily as single dose or 2 divided doses

Neuroleptanalgesia

up to 15 mg IV in combination with a narcotic analgesic

Anaesthesia

i) 2.5–10 mg IM or IV 30–60 minutes before induction OR
ii) 0.25 mg/kg IV with a narcotic analgesic and/or general anaesthetic agent to provide a smooth induction

Paediatric dose

i) 0.1 mg/kg IV; OR
ii) 0.15 mg/kg IM 2 hours pre-
operatively

PIMOZIDE

— long acting diphenylbutylpiperidine
structurally similar to the
butyrophenones

Use

— acute and chronic psychoses, mainly
chronic schizophrenia

Dose

2–4 mg orally as single daily dose then
up to 12 mg daily as required, then
4–6 mg daily as maintenance

Adverse effects

— extrapyramidal reactions
— nervousness, irritability, insomnia
— drowsiness, weakness, dizziness

Nursing points

— advise patient about the need to
continue therapy
— warn patient against driving a vehicle
or operating machinery if drowsy
— warn patient about reduced tolerance
to alcohol
— observe carefully so that distinction
may be made between a return of
psychotic behaviour and the onset of
extrapyramidal reactions (p. 122)

Note

— may aggravate endogenous
depression, parkinsonism and
epilepsy

CHLORPROMAZINE

Action

— phenothiazine derivative
— depresses CNS
— alpha-adrenergic blocking agent
— weak anticholinergic activity

— dopamine inhibitor
— inhibits heat regulating centre
— anti-emetic
— serotonin antagonist
— weak antihistamine
— relaxes skeletal muscle

Use

— antipsychotic
— antineurotic
— nausea, vomiting associated with
disease, drugs and surgery
— premedication
— enhancement of analgesia
— anti-pruritic
— controlled hypotension and
hypothermia
— intractable hiccups
— antidote to lysergic acid and
mescaline
— adjuvant in ECT, treatment of tetanus
and acute intermittent porphyria

Dose

i) 25–100 mg orally t.d.s.; OR
ii) 25–50 mg deep IM 6- to 8-hourly; OR
iii) 100 mg rectal suppository 6- to 8-
hourly

Adverse effects

— drowsiness
— dry mouth, constipation
— blurred vision, nasal stuffiness
— agitation, excitement, photophobia
— postural hypotension, tachycardia
— hypothermia (hyperthermia, if
ambient temperature high)
— weight gain
— extrapyramidal reactions
— urticaria, dermatitis, photosensitivity
— jaundice
— blood dyscrasias (rare but fatal)
— menstrual irregularities
— gynaecomastia
— urinary retention, inhibition of
ejaculation
— hyperglycaemia ˙·

Interactions

— CNS depressant effects enhanced by
alcohol and other CNS depressants

— enhances CNS depressant effects of narcotic analgesics and most hypnotics and tranquillizers
— blood levels of phenothiazines increased by propranolol and may be increased by high doses of tricyclic antidepressants
— increases blood levels and adverse effects of tricyclic antidepressants
— reduces the effect of bretylium, debrisoquine, guanethidine and levodopa
— lithium reduces chlorpromazine blood levels
— barbiturates reduce blood levels of phenothiazines
— aluminium hydroxide and magnesium trisilicate reduce absorption of oral chlorpromazine
— affects stability of oral anticoagulant control

Nursing points

— tablets to be swallowed whole
— aluminium hydroxide or magnesium trisilicate given 1 hour before or 2 hours after chlorpromazine
— contact dermatitis may be avoided if injectable preparations handled using plastic or rubber gloves
— if drug to be prepared as admixture, consult pharmacist as chlorpromazine is incompatible with many drugs and solutions
— compatible with morphine, pethidine or papaveretum when mixed in the same syringe as long as the resultant solution is used within 15 minutes and there is no precipitation
— give IM injections slowly and deeply to avoid irritating subcutaneous tissues
— irritation may be reduced by dilution with isotonic saline or the addition of a local anaesthetic agent
— rotate injection sites
— patient to remain recumbent for at least an hour after injection to avoid postural hypotension
— advise patient to avoid postural hypotension by moving gradually to a sitting or standing position especially after sleep

— advise patient that postural hypotension is aggravated by prolonged standing, hot baths or showers, hot weather, physical exertion, large meals and alcohol
— warn about reduced alcohol tolerance
— warn patient against driving a vehicle or operating machinery if drowsy
— observe carefully so that distinction may be made between a return of psychotic behaviour and the onset of extrapyramidal reactions (see below)
— advise patient to report fever or sore throat which are early signs of bone marrow depression
— advise patient that constipation may necessitate increased fluid intake, added dietary roughage or a laxative
— advise patient to avoid skin exposure to direct sunlight
— advise patient to report sensitivity to cold
— advise patient about the need to continue therapy
— advise patient against abrupt withdrawal of therapy
— have on hand noradrenaline, metaraminol, benztropine and diphenhydramine
— protect drug from moisture and light

Note

— some psychotic patients may require up to 1 gm or more chlorpromazine daily
  extrapyramidal syndromes:
— parkinsonian: akinesia, rigidity, tremor at rest
— akathisia: motor restlessness
— acute dystonic reaction: facial grimacing, torticollis, oculogyric crisis
— tardive dyskinesia: exaggerated and persistent chewing movements, tongue protrusion

FLUPHENAZINE HYDROCHLORIDE

— as for chlorpromazine but of longer duration

Use

— antipsychotic
— senile confusion

Dose

i) 10 mg orally daily in 3–4 divided doses initially, to establish control; OR

ii) 1–2 mg orally daily increasing to 2.5–5 mg t.d.s. or q.i.d. then a maintenance single daily dose of 1–5 mg;

FLUPHENAZINE DECANOATE

— as for chlorpromazine but of much longer duration

Use

— schizophrenia mainly where non-compliance with oral therapy

Dose

12.5–25 mg IM at 3–4 weekly intervals, determined by response

Nursing point

— use dry syringe and 21 gauge needle

Note

— has been used with haloperidol for Huntington's chorea

PERICYAZINE

— as or chlorpromazine

Dose

10–75 mg orally daily in 2 unequal portions, the larger amount taken in the evening

PERPHENAZINE

— as for chlorpramazine, but slighty more stimulant effects

Dose

Hospitalized patient

8–16 mg orally 2–4 times daily

Outside hospital

4–8 mg orally t.d.s.

PERPHENAZINE WITH AMITRIPTYLINE

— phenothiazine tranquillizer combined with a tricyclic antidepressant for the management of anxiety associated with depression

Dose

1 tablet 3–4 times daily

PROMAZINE

— as for chlopromazine

Dose

i) 25–50 mg orally or IM 4- to 6-hourly (anti-emetic); OR

ii) 50–300 mg deep IM then 10–200 mg deep IM 4- to 6-hourly (psychosis); OR

by slow IV injection, in concentrations not exceeding 25 mg/ml

Note

— maximum daily dose may be as high as 1 g

THIOPROPAZATE

— as for chlorpromazine, but slightly more stimulant effects

Dose

5–10 mg orally t.d.s.

Note

— compression-coated tablet, therefore not divided

— also used in Huntington's Chorea

— may be used as alternative to haloperidol to minimize tardive dyskinesia

THIORIDAZINE

— as for chlorpromazine

Adult dose

10–200 mg orally t.d.s. (tablets, solution or suspension).

Paediatric dose

2 mg/kg/day orally

Note

— shake suspension vigorously for at least a minute for complete resuspension

TRIFLUOPERAZINE

—as for chlorpromazine, but has little effect on blood pressure

Use

— anxiety, tension, agitation
— antipsychotic
— behaviour disorders in mental deficiency states
— nausea, vomiting

Dose

Hospitalized patients

i) 2–5 mg orally b.d. initially, then increasing to 20–30 mg daily in divided doses over 2–3 weeks, later maintained on lower dose b.d.; OR
ii) 15 mg orally daily (spansule); OR
iii) 1–2 mg deeply IM 4- to 6-hourly

Outside hospital

i) 1–2 mg orally b.d.; OR
ii) 0.5–1 mg deeply IM 4- to 6-hourly for immediate control, then as in i)

TRIFLUOPERAZINE WITH TRANYLCYPROMINE

— phenothiazine tranquilliser combined with a MAO inhibitor antidepressant for the management of anxiety associated with depression
— see nursing points for phenelzine (p. 131)

Dose

1 tablet 1–3 times daily

THIOTHIXENE

Action

— thioxanthene derivative with properties similar to the phenothiazines

Use

— schizophrenia
— psychoneurosis
— other psychoses

Dose

3–60 mg orally daily
A dose of 30 mg or less is taken as single daily dose; over 30 mg is taken in 2–3 divided doses

Note

— a 10 mg 'rapid dispersal' tablet prevents drug hoarding

LITHIUM CARBONATE

Action

— lithium ions may compete with sodium ions thereby altering the electrophysiological characteristics of neurones
— antidepressant

Use

— prophylaxis and treatment of mania
— prophylaxis and control of manic episodes in manic-depressive psychosis
— depression

Dose

250–500 mg orally 1–4 times daily p.c.

Adverse effects

— (early) fine tremor, malaise, polydipsia, polyuria
— (serious) anorexia, nausea, vomiting, severe abdominal discomfort,

diarrhoea, drowsiness, ataxia, slurred speech, coarse tremor
— goitre (prolonged treatment)

Interactions

— toxic blood lithium levels can result when combined with indomethacin, thiazide diuretics, haloperidol, fluphenazine decanoate, thioridazine, spectinomycin and tetracycline
— therapeutic effects of lithium reduced by acetazolamide, aminophylline and sodium bicarbonate
— inadequate intake or excessive excretion of sodium increases blood lithium levels and vice versa
— reduces chlorpromazine blood levels significantly
— results in reversible polyuria, polydipsia and tremor when combined with phenytoin

Nursing points

— taken with food to minimize nausea
— ensure patient has normal diet with adequate salt intake and a fluid intake of up to 3 l/day
— warn patient against driving a vehicle or operating machinery if drowsy
— advise patient about the need to continue therapy usually for at least 6 months and to keep follow-up appointments
— warn patient never to compensate for an omitted dose by subsequently taking a double dose
— serious adverse effects requiring immediate cessation of therapy must be committed to memory by the patient, relatives and nurses
— the narrow margin between therapeutic and toxic blood levels determines the need for frequent estimations of blood lithium levels, thereby detecting toxicity early and checking compliance
— blood levels estimated twice a week initially, then weekly for a month, then monthly for a year
— blood samples taken 12 hours after administration of the last dose
— some medical officers advise the withholding of the drug for 24 hours

once a week
— have available acetazolamide, mannitol, aminophylline and sodium bicarbonate

Note

— therapeutic blood level ranges between 0.8–1.6 mmol/l above which toxic effects may be expected because of the narrow margin between the therapeutic and toxic lithium concentrations
— nursing mothers taking lithium carbonate should not breast-feed to avoid the infant becoming hypotonic, flaccid and difficult-to-feed
— tremor resulting from lithium therapy may be controlled by beta-adrenoceptor blocking drugs

LOXAPINE

Action

— tricyclic dibenzoxazepine distinct from any previous drug groups
— anticholinergic

Use

— antipsychotic

Dose

i) 10–25 mg orally b.d initially, then 20–100 mg daily in 2or 3 divided doses as maintenance; OR
ii) 25–50 mg IM 6- to 12-hourly for prompt control followed by oral administration

Adverse effects

— drowsiness
— extrapyramidal reactions
— rarely convulsions, hypotension, hypertension, respiratory depression

Interactions

— enhance CNS depressant effects of alcohol and sedatives
— enhances anticholinergic effects of anti-Parkinson drugs

Nursing points

— warn patient against driving a vehicle
   or operating machinery if drowsy
— warn patient about reduced tolerance
   to alcohol

TETRABENAZINE

Action

— depletes stores of dopamine,
   noradrenaline and serotonin in CNS

Use

— chorea
— tardive dyskinesia
— certain dystonic syndromes

Dose

25–100 mg b.d.

Adverse effects

— drowsiness
— extrapyramidal reactions
— hypotension, bradycardia
— anxiety, confusion
— (serious) depression, dysphagia with
   choking attacks (requires withdrawal
   of drug)

Interactions

— enhances effects of CNS
   depressants
— blocks central action of reserpine and
   levodopa if given with either of these
— causes restlessness disorientation
   and confusion if given with MAO
   inhibitors or immediately after their
   cessation

Nursing points

— warn patient against driving a vehicle
   or operating machinery if drowsy

TRICYCLIC ANTIDEPRESSANTS

AMITRIPTYLINE

Action

— prevents re-uptake of noradrenaline
   and serotonin
— marked anticholinergic and sedative
   effects

Use

— endogenous depression
— reactive and other types of
   depression occasionally
— nocturnal enuresis

Adult dose

i) 25–50 mg orally t.d.s.; OR
ii) 20–30 mg IM or IV q.i.d.; then
    10–25 mg orally 2–4 times daily as
    maintenance

Paediatric dose

Enuresis

4–10 years: 10–25 mg nocte
over 10 years: 50 mg nocte

Adverse effects

— tachycardia, palpitations, cardiac
   arrhythmias, postural hypotension,
   occasionally hypertension
— drowsiness, dizziness, tinnitus,
   fatigue, headache, insomnia,
   confusion, extrapyramidal reactions,
   numbness, tingling and paraesthesia
   of extremities
— dry mouth, blurred vision,
   constipation, urinary retention
— alopecia, sweating, inappropriate
   antidiuretic hormone secretion, rash
— either increase or decrease in
   weight, blood sugar, libido
— gynaecomastia, testicular swelling
— breast enlargement, galactorrhoea
— photosensitivity
— blood dyscrasias (rare)

Interactions

— the patient is warned to seek medical advice before taking any other preparations with tricyclic antidepressants as there is an extensive list of effects which may be encountered
— CNS depressant effects enhanced by alcohol and other CNS depressants
— amitriptyline blood levels increased by alcohol, aspirin, chloramphenicol, chlorpromazine, haloperidol
— enhances effects of noradrenaline, adrenaline and benzodiazepines
— enhances effects of anticholinergic drugs and increases atropine-like side-effects of amantadine, chlordiazepoxide, cyproheptadine, diazepam, diphenhydramine, meclozine, oxazepam and promethazine
— bethanecol minimizes anticholinergic side-effects
— phenothiazine blood levels increased by high doses of tricyclic antidepressants
— tricyclic antidepressant blood levels decreased by anticonvulsants
— amitriptyline increases CNS depressant effect but not anticonvulsant action of barbiturates
— amitriptyline blood levels reduced by phenobarb and oral contraceptives
— reduces hypotensive effect of clonidine, debrisoquine, guanethidine and methyldopa
— risk of serious cardiac arrhythmias caused by amitriptyline increased by derisoquine, guanethidine, levodopa and thyroid hormones
— results in hyperpyrexia, coma, convulsions and circulatory collapse when combined with furazolidone or MAO inhibitors and may be fatal

Nursing points

— advise patient about the need to continue therapy and to keep follow-up appointments
— response may take up to 4 weeks to develop adequately
— higher doses may be used in severely depressed hospitalized patients
— warn patient against driving a vehicle or operating machinery if drowsy
— entire daily dose may be given mane, nocte, or in divided doses depending on requirements
— advise patient to avoid postural hypotension by moving gradually to a sitting or standing position especially after sleep
— advise patient that postural hypotension is aggravated by prolonged standing, hot baths or showers, hot weather, physical exertion, large meals and alcohol ingestion
— warn patient to avoid alcohol and OTC drugs during and for 2 weeks following termination of therapy
— observe for a beneficial elevation in mood
— observe for mania, hallucinations, delusions and suicidal tendencies which will necessitate discontinuation of therapy
— advise patient to report fever or sore throat which are early signs of bone marrow depression
— advise patient that constipation may necessitate increased fluid intake added dietary roughage or a laxative
— advise patient to avoid skin exposure to direct sunlight
— advise patient against abrupt withdrawal of therapy
— have available diazepam, paraldehyde, neostigmine, propranolol and cardiac anti-arrhythmic agents

Note

— many OTC preparations contain alcohol or sympathomimetic amines which have their effects enhanced by tricyclic antidepressants
— treatment for nocturnal enuresis usually successful after 1 to 2 weeks and is continued until the child is dry for 3 months
— tricyclic antidepressant therapy should be discontinued for several days prior to elective surgery
— when substituting a tricyclic antidepressant for a MAO inhibitor, allow 14 days to elapse after discontinuing MAOI therapy

AMITRIPTYLINE WITH PERPHENAZINE

— tricyclic antidepressant combined
with a phenothiazine tranquillizer for
the management of anxiety
associated with depression

Dose

1 tablet 2–4 times daily

CLOMIPRAMINE

— as for amitriptyline

Dose

25–50 mg orally 1–3 times daily

DESIPRAMINE

— as for amitriptyline but has less
marked sedative effects
— principal active metabolite of
imipramine

Dose

25–50 mg orally 1–4 times daily

DOTHIEPIN

— as for amitriptyline

Dose

i) 25–50 mg orally t.d.s.; OR
ii) 25 mg orally t.d.s. plus 75 mg nocte

DOXEPIN

— as for amitriptyline

Dose

10–50 mg orally t.d.s.

IMIPRAMINE

— as for amitriptyline but has less
marked sedative effects

Adult dose

i)   25 mg orally t.d.s. increasing to
50 mg t.d.s. then 25 mg t.d.s. or
q.i.d.; OR
ii) 25 mg IM t.d.s. increasing to 50 mg
IM q.i.d.; OR
iii) 10 mg orally t.d.s. increasing to
20 mg t.d.s. then 10 mg t.d.s. or
q.i.d. (elderly)

Paediatric dose

Enuresis

4–10 years: 10–25 mg orally nocte
over 10 years: 50 mg orally nocte

NORTRIPTYLINE

— as for amitriptyline (p. 126)
— principal active metabolite of
amitriptyline

Dose

10–25 mg orally 3–4 times daily

PROTRIPTYLINE

— as for amitriptyline (p. 126)

Dose

5–15 mg orally t.d.s. or q.i.d.

Note

— **discontinued in Australia**
— if insomnia present, last dose taken
no later than mid-afternoon

TRIMIPRAMINE

— as for amitriptyline (p. 126)

Dose

25–100 mg orally midday and
50–200 mg 2 hours before bedtime

TETRACYCLIC ANTIDEPRESSANT

MIANSERIN

Action

— antihistamine, antiserotonin, sedative

Use

— endogenous and reactive depression
— involutional melancholia

Dose

30–40 mg orally daily initially, slowly
increasing to a maintenance dose of
30–90 mg daily. Up to 200 mg daily has
been used

Adverse effects

— lethargy, drowsiness
— dry mouth
— dizziness, weakness
— weight gain
— changes in blood sugar levels
— blood dyscrasias

Interactions

— CNS depressant effects enhanced by
  alcohol, sedatives and hypnotics
— mianserin blood levels decreased
  significantly by phenobarbitone,
  carbamazepine and phenytoin

Nursing points

— tablets swallowed whole between
  meals
— warn patient against driving a vehicle
  or operating machinery if drowsy
— warn patient about reduced tolerance
  to alcohol
— advise patient to report fever or sore
  throat which are early signs of bone
  marrow depression

Note

— MAO inhibitors stopped for 14 days before commencing mianserin
— thought to lower convulsive threshold in epileptics

MONOAMINE OXIDASE INHIBITOR ANTIDEPRESSANTS

PHENELZINE

Action

— may inhibit monoamine oxidase (MAO) resulting in an increase in endogenous adrenaline, noradrenaline, serotonin and dopamine

Use

— reactive and endogenous depression
— combined with a tranquillizer in the treatment of depression and anxiety

Dose

15 mg orally t.d.s. increasing to 30 mg t.d.s. as required then 15 mg daily or alternate days

Adverse effects

— drowsiness, dizziness, weakness, postural hypotension
— nausea, vomiting, dry mouth, constipation
— hypomania
— rare, but fatal, liver damage
— severe hypertensive crisis, possibly fatal, if given with some other drugs or certain foods

Interactions

— the patient is warned to seek medical advice before taking any other preparations with MAO inhibitors as there is an extensive list of effects which may be encountered when combined with alcohol, anticholinergics, antihypertensives, dextromethorphan, hypnotics, oral hypoglycaemics, insulin, levodopa, narcotic analgesics, some pressor agents, tricyclic antidepressants and tyramine-containing food
— the 'cheese reaction', a combination of tyramine-containing food and MAO inhibitors can result in severe

hypertension and subarachnoid haemorrhage even up to 2 weeks following discontinuation of MAO inhibitors

Nursing points

— advise patient about the need to continue therapy and to keep follow-up appointments
— response apparent in 2 to 6 weeks and persists for several weeks following termination of therapy
— advise patient to avoid postural hypotension by moving gradually to a sitting or standing position especially after sleep
— advise patient that postural hypotension is aggravated by prolonged standing, hot baths or showers, hot weather, physical exertion, large meals and alcohol ingestion
— warn patient to avoid alcohol and OTC 'cold cures' during and for 2 weeks following termination of therapy unless advised by the prescriber
— warn patient against driving a vehicle or operating machinery if drowsy
— observe for improvement in mental and physical state
— ensure patient aware of foods or drugs known to cause severe hypertensive crisis, 'cheese reaction' by enhancing pressor activity
— warn patient to avoid mature cheese, yeast or meat extracts, broad bean pods, large amounts of alcohol, aged meats, coffee substitutes, stock cubes, packet or canned soup, caviare, pickled herring, dehydrated food
— if narcotic analgesics required, a trial dose of $\frac{1}{10}$ to $\frac{1}{5}$ the usual dose is given, monitoring the vital signs closely for 2 to 3 hours
— advise patient to note and report headache or palpitations as these may indicate the onset of prolonged hypertension
— observe for hypoglycaemia in diabetics
— advise patient against abrupt withdrawal

— have available phentolamine and chlorpromazine

Note

— tricyclic antidepressants generally should not be given within 14 days of MAO inhibitors
— many OTC cold cures contain dextromethorphan, sympathomimetic agents or antihistamines
— MAO inhibitors discontinued 10 days prior to elective surgery

IPRONIAZID

— as for phenelzine

Dose

100–150 mg orally as single daily dose reducing to 25–50 mg daily

ISOCARBOXAZID

— as for phenelzine

Dose

10 mg orally t.d.s. or 30 mg orally as single daily dose reducing to 10 or 20 mg daily

TRANYLCYPROMINE

— as for phenelzine

Dose

10 mg orally b.d. or t.d.s. then 10 mg daily

TRANYLCYPROMINE WITH TRIFLUOPERAZINE

— an antidepressant combined with a phenothiazine tranquillizer for the management of depression complicated by anxiety
— see nursing points for phenelzine

Dose

1 tablet 1–3 times daily

ANTICONVULSANTS

PHENYTOIN ˙

Action

— abolishes or attenuates seizures without causing general depression of CNS
— antiarrhythmic

Use

— grand mal epilepsy
— psychomotor epilepsy
— status epilepticus
— cardiac arrhythmia (see p. 36)

Adult dose

i) 100 mg orally t.d.s. increasing to 200 mg t.d.s. then 150–200 mg b.d.; OR
ii) 12–15 mg/kg orally in 2 or 3 divided doses over about 6 hours (loading dose) then 100 mg t.d.s.; OR
iii) 4–7 mg/kg orally daily in 2 equally divided doses; OR
iv) 5–12 mg/kg slowly I (loading dose), then as in iii); OR
v) 150–250 mg slowly IV (status epilepticus) then 100–150 mg 30 minutes later as required; OR
vi) 250 mg slowly IV 6- to 12-hourly until oral dosage possible (neurosurgery prophylaxis)

Note

IV administration must not exceed 50 mg/min

Paediatric dose

Status epilepticus

5–10 mg/kg IV given over 15–30 minutes

Maintenance

3–8 mg/kg/day orally or IM

Adverse effects

— nausea, vomiting, constipation
— ataxia, slurred speech, blurred vision
— nystagmus, mental confusion, hallucinations
— headache, dizziness, tremor, insomnia
— tenderness and hyperplasia of gums (mainly children)
— rash
— bone marrow depression
— hirsutism

Interactions

— alcohol, phenobarbitone and phenylbutazone increase *or* decrease phenytoin blood levels
— phenytoin blood levels increased by dexamethasone, disulfiram, isoniazid, sulthiame, cimetidine, sulphamethizole
— phenytoin increases the effect of methotrexate, primidone, chloramphenicol
— phenytoin blood levels decreased by theophylline, pyridoxine
— aspirin, sodium valproate reduce phenytoin blood levels but not therapeutic effect
— phenytoin reduces blood levels of clonazepam, rifampicin, frusemide, quinidine, dexamethasone, digoxin, mexiletine, theophylline, pyridoxine, mianserin, sodium valproate, tetracyclines, oral contraceptives, calcium and folate
— food increases rate of absorption of phenytoin
— simethicone reduces absorption of phenytoin
— phenytoin reduces absorption of folic acid and frusemide

Nursing points

— taken with at least half a glass of water a.c. but if tendency to nausea, taken with food or p.c. (always taken in the same relation to food for consistent absorption)
— give IM injections deeply
— injectable solutions are strongly alkaline so avoid mixing with other drugs or IV solutions, or giving SC
— supplied as 'Ready-Mixed' solution for injection

— IV administration not to exceed 50 mg/min and patient requires constant heart rate, blood pressure and cardiac monitoring
— blood not sampled for phenytoin assay when aspirin also being taken
— simethicone taken 2 hours apart from phenytoin if possible
— children weighed regularly to detect weight loss, an early sign of phenytoin toxicity
— warn patient against driving a vehicle or operating machinery, particularly early in treatment
— advise patient that alcohol is restricted because of its unpredictable effects
— advise patient about the need to continue therapy and keep follow-up appointments
— advise patient to report fever or sore throat which are early signs of bone marrow depression
— advise patient to report any rash as this indicates the need to withdraw drug
— advise about careful teeth cleaning to reduce gingival hyperplasia
— advise patient that drug therapy is best withdrawn over several days or weeks unless urgent need to stop abruptly

Note

— sometimes combined with phenobarbitone and primidone
— changing to phenytoin from other anticonvulsants and vice versa is made gradually as sudden withdrawal may precipitate status epilepticus
— long term therapy requires adequate vitamin D and folic acid intake
— can be given IM during a crisis, but absorption slow and unpredictable
— breast-fed infants monitored carefully for methaemoglobinaemia
— IV paediatric dose may be calculated on basis of 250 mg/m^2
— therapeutic blood level range 10–20 micrograms/ml

CARBAMAZEPINE

Action

— anticonvulsant, some actions similar to phenytoin
— antineuralgic properties
— mild sedative, anticholinergic, muscle relaxant and antidiuretic properties

Use

— grand mal epilepsy
— psychomotor epilepsy
— trigeminal neuralgia
— phantom limb phenomena
— glossopharyngeal neuralgia
— tabes dorsalis

Adult dose

Epilepsy

100–200 mg orally daily or b.d. up to 400–600 mg b.d. with food or p.c.

Other

100–200 mg orally b.d. with food or p.c. increasing gradually for several days until pain controlled, usually 200–400 mg b.d., then reduced at least once every 3 months to a minimum effective level

Paediatric dose

1–5 years: 100–200 mg b.d.
5–10 years: 200 mg b.d. or t.d.s.
over 10 years: 200 mg t.d.s. or q.i.d.

Adverse effects

— drowsiness, dizziness, headache, ataxia
— diplopia, nystagmus
— gastrointestinal disturbances
— rash, necessitating discontinuation
— photosensitivity
— confusion, agitation (elderly)
— blood dyscrasias

Interactions

— effect of carbamazepine reduced by phenobarbitone

— reduces effect of warfarin, phenobarbitone, phenytoin and tetracyclines
— reduces blood levels of tetracyclines, theophylline, sodium valproate, phenytoin, mianserin,
— carbamazepine blood levels increased by erythromycin, propoxyphene, isoniazid
— effect of warfarin enhanced markedly when carbamazepine withdrawn

Nursing points

— elderly patients may become confused or agitated so will require bedsides
— advise patient against driving a vehicle or operating machinery if drowsy
— warn patient about reduced tolerance to alcohol
— advise patient about the need to continue therapy and keep follow-up appointments
— advise patient that drug therapy is best withdrawn over several days or weeks unless urgent need to stop abruptly

Note

— similar in chemical structure to phenothiazines and tricyclic compounds
— changing to carbamazepine from other anticonvulsants and vice versa is made gradually as sudden withdrawal may precipitate status epilepticus
— not given to patients during or within 14 days of stopping MAO inhibitor therapy
— full blood count weekly for first month, then monthly for first year
— examine periodically for eye changes
— therapeutic blood level range 4–12.5 micrograms/ml

CLONAZEPAM

Action

— benzodiazepine closely related to nitrazepam with anticonvulsant,

sedative and muscle relaxant properties

Use

— grand mal epilepsy
— petit mal epilepsy
— psychomotor epilepsy
— status epilepticus

Adult dose

1–2 mg orally q.i.d.

Status epilepticus

1 mg slow IV injection or infusion, repeated if required

Paediatric dose

up to 2 years: 0.125–0.25 mg q.i.d.
2–5 years: 0.5–1 mg t.d.s.
6–12 years: 1–2 mg t.d.s

Status epilepticus

0.5 mg slow IV injection or infusion, repeated if required

Adverse effects

— drowsiness, dizziness, fatigue, muscle weakness
— coordination disturbances, ataxia
— salivary or bronchial hypersecretion in infants and small children
— behavioural changes
— tolerance
— blood dyscrasias
— hypotension, tachycardia (if given rapidly IV)

Interactions

— CNS depressant effects of clonazepam enhanced by alcohol
— CNS depressant effects of drugs enhanced by clonazepam
— phenytoin causes reduced blood levels of clonazepam
— clonazepam added to combined sulthiame and phenytoin therapy results in increased blood phenytoin levels

— lowers carbamazepine blood levels
— primidone blood levels varied unpredictably by clonazepam

Nursing points

— distinguish between 0.5 mg and 2 mg tablets
— contents of ampoule to be mixed thoroughly with supplied diluent
— advise patient to avoid alcohol
— warn patient against driving a vehicle or operating machinery if drowsy
— supervision of infants and small children is required to ensure that airway remains clear of excess secretions
— advise patient that drug therapy is best withdrawn over several days or weeks unless urgent need to stop abruptly

ETHOSUXIMIDE

Action and use

— controls petit mal epilepsy possibly by depressing the motor cortex and elevating the convulsive threshold

Adult dose

250–750 mg orally b.d

Paediatric dose

commence with 125 mg b.d. increasing to 500 mg b.d. or t.d.s. until control obtained or unwanted effects appear

Adverse effects

— anorexia, nausea, vomiting, diarrhoea, epigastric pain
— drowsiness, dizziness, ataxia
— rash
— blood dyscrasias
— systemic lupus erythematosus

Nursing points

— warn patient against driving a vehicle or operating machinery if drowsy
— be aware of the possibility of increased frequency of grand mal

seizure when ethosuximide used alone in mixed types of epilepsy
— dose and medication changes made gradually
— advise patient that drug therapy is best withdrawn over several days or weeks unless urgent need to stop abruptly
— advise patient about the need to continue therapy and keep follow-up appointments

Note

— full blood count weekly for first month, then monthly for first year
— may be used in conjunction with other anticonvulsants where petit mal co-exists.

METHSUXIMIDE

— as for ethosuximide

Use

— petit mal epilepsy
— psychomotor epilepsy

Dose

300 mg as single daily oral dose increasing to 300 mg 2–4 times daily

Note

— drug withdrawn if any behaviour alteration especially aggressiveness or unusual depression

PHENOBARBITONE

Action

— long-acting barbiturate, onset within 1 hour, duration of action 6–10 hours
— depresses CNS
— anticonvulsant

Use

— long-acting sedative or hypnotic
— anticonvulsant in grand mal epilepsy or psychomotor epilepsy often as combined therapy

Adult dose

30–120 mg orally b.d. or t.d.s.

Paediatric dose

Status epilepticus

15 mg/kg IV or IM initially, then 5 mg/kg/24 hours in 2 divided doses 12 hours apart

Maintenance

1.5–2.5 mg/kg orally 12-hourly

Febrile convulsion prophylaxis

3–4 mg/kg orally nocte

Neonatal fitting

2 doses of 10 mg/kg IV 3–4 hours apart (loading dose), then 3–4 mg/kg/24 hours slowly IV or orally

Sedation

1– mg/kg orally or IM
8- to 12-hourly

Adverse effects

— respiratory depression, sedation
— irritability, hyperexcitability (children)
— confusion, restlessness, excitement (elderly)
— dependence
— folate deficiency (prolonged therapy)
— rarely rash, blood dyscrasias
— high dose, ataxia, nystagmus, 'hang-over'

Interactions

— CNS depressant effects of phenobarbitone increased by other CNS depressants
— phenobarbitone reduces the effect of dexamethasone, prednisone, tricyclic antidepressants, quinidine, coumarin oral anticoagulants, metronidazole, levodopa, oral griseofulvin, rifampicin, phenothiazines, doxycycline

frusemide, oral alprenolol, mianserin
— phenobarbitone reduces blood levels of calcium, folic acid and sodium valproate
— phenobarbitone reduces chloramphenicol blood levels significantly in children
— analgesic effect of pethidine reduced but CNS toxicity increased by phenobarbitone
— pyridoxine reduces phenobarbitone blood levels
— sodium valproate increases phenobarbitone blood levels
— phenobarbitone blood level increased by sulthiame

Nursing points

— wakefulness, excitement and delirium may occur in the presence of pain
— injection given deep IM
— bedsides may be required if patient shows confusion or excitement (children, elderly)
— warn patient against driving a vehicle or operating machinery if drowsy
— warn patient about reduced tolerance to alcohol
— warn patient about the need to continue therapy and warn against abrupt withdrawal of therapy
— advise patient to report fever or sore throat which are early signs of bone marrow depression

Note

— abrupt withdrawal of phenobarbitone may result in anxiety, insomnia, delirium, convulsions and status epilepticus (in epileptics)
— monitoring of blood levels often necessary to achieve correct dosage (blood sample taken midway between doses) therapeutic range 10–30 mg/L (45–130 micromol/L) toxicity >35 mg/L (>150 micromol/L)
— phenobarbitone poisoning treated by activated charcoal (p. 298)

METHYLPHENOBARBITONE

Action

— long-acting barbiturate with anticonvulsive properties similar to those of phenobarbitone which it may replace over a 10-day period

Use

— grand mal epilepsy
— petit mal epilepsy
— sedation

Dose

i) 400–600 mg orally daily (anticonvulsant); OR
ii) 30–100 mg t.d.s. or q.i.d. (sedative)

Adverse effects

— as for the phenobarbitone

Interactions

— CNS depressant effects increased by alcohol and CNS depressants
— dexamethasone and phenothiazine blood levels and coumarin anticoagulant activity reduced

Nursing points

— warn patient against driving a vehicle or operating machinery if drowsy
— advise patient that drug therapy is best withdrawn over several days or weeks unless urgent need to stop abruptly

PHENSUXIMIDE

— as for ethosuximide but less potent

Dose

0.5–1 g orally b.d. or t.d.s.

PRIMIDONE

— related to phenobarbitone, some being converted slowly to phenobarbitone in the body

Use

— grand mal epilepsy
— psychomotor epilepsy
— focal epileptic seizures

Adult dose

125 mg orally nocte increasing gradually to 125–750 mg b.d.

Paediatric dose

1–12 months: 62.5 mg b.d.
1–2 years: 125 mg b.d.
2–5 years: 125–250 mg b.d.
5–10 years 250 mg b.d.
over 10 years: 250 mg t.d.s

Adverse effects

— drowsiness, nausea, rash (initially)
— dizziness, ataxia, fatigue, visual disturbances
— megaloblastic anaemia (rare) .

Interactions

— blood calcium and folic acid levels reduced leading to calcium deficiency
— enhanced by phenytoin and sodium valproate
— primidone decreases sodium valproate blood levels and reduces effectiveness of oral contraceptives

Nursing points

— warn patient against driving a vehicle or operating machinery if drowsy
— advise patient about the need to continue therapy
— observe neonates for bleeding whose mothers have been on long term therapy
— advise patient that drug therapy is best withdrawn over several days or weeks unless urgent need to stop abruptly

Note

— may be taken alone or in combination with other anticonvulsants

— vitamin K_1 given prophylactically to pregnant patient during last month of pregnancy or at the time of delivery to both mother and neonate
— folic acid and/or vitamin B_{12} may be required during pregnancy

SODIUM VALPROATE

Action

— thought to raise brain levels of the inhibitory synaptic transmitter, gamma-amino-butyric acid (GABA).

Use

— petit mal epilepsy
— grand mal epilepsy
— adjuvant therapy in partial (focal) epilepsy

Adult dose

200 mg orally b.d. or t.d.s. with food or p.c. increasing to 500 mg b.d. or t.d.s. up to a maximum of 2500 mg/day

Paediatric dose

under 20 kg: 20 mg/kg/24hours
20 kg and over: 20–30 mg/kg/24 hours

Adverse effects

— anorexia, nausea, vomiting, diarrhoea
— increased appetite, weight gain
— drowsiness, fatigue
— rarely, bleeding and bruising
— rare but usually fatal hepatotoxicity, mainly in children

Interactions

— enhances effects of phenobarbitone, primidone and methylphenobarbitone
— sodium valproate blood levels increased by aspirin and reduced by carbamazepine, phenobarb, phenytoin and primidone

Nursing points

— tablets absorb moisture so are kept in protective foil until just before use
— store drug in dry place at less than 30°C away from direct sunlight
— take with or after food, but avoid taking with aerated water
— regular dosage at least 3 times a day avoids excessive fluctuations in blood and brain drug levels
— take with milk to avoid unpleasant taste
— may prolong bleeding time, especially in major surgery
— warn patient that effects of alcohol unpredictable
— advise patient that drug therapy is best withdrawn over several days or weeks unless urgent need to stop abruptly

Note

— liver function assessed before starting therapy then monitored monthly for 6 months, then less frequently
— platelet function monitored before major surgery
— spontaneous bruising or bleeding, or signs of liver dysfunction are indications for immediate cessation of sodium valproate
— changing to sodium valproate from other anticonvulsants and vice versa is made gradually as sudden withdrawal may precipitate status epilepticus

SULTHIAME

Action

— carbonic anhydrase inhibitor
— probably inhibits hepatic metabolism of some other anticonvulsants given concurrently

Use

— all forms of epilepsy except petit mal
— behavioural disorders associated with epilepsy
— usually taken in conjuction with other anticonvulsants
— hyperkinetic behaviour

Adult dose

100 mg orally b.d. or 50 mg orally t.d.s.,

initially, gradually increasing up to
200 mg t.d.s.

Paediatric dose

3–5 mg/kg orally daily in equal divided
doses increasing to 10–15 mg/kg daily
in equal divided doses

Adverse effects

— paraesthesia of face and extremities
  (usually disappears with continued
  treatment)
— anorexia, nausea
— ataxia
— headache, dizziness, loss of weight
— tachypnoea (children)
— psychic changes

Interactions

— increases blood level of
  phenobarbitone and phenytoin

Note

— phenobarbitone blood levels
  monitored if sulthiame added to
  stable regimen and phenobarbitone
  dose reduced if necessary

OTHER ANTICONVULSANT AGENTS

See clobazepam, diazepam, nitrazepam

ANTIPARKINSONIAN AGENTS

LEVODOPA

Action

— the immediate precursor of the
  synaptic neurotransmitter, dopamine;
  readily enters the CNS, undergoes
  transformation and so replaces the
  depleted brain dopamine in patients
  with parkinsonism

Use

— all types of parkinsonism except
  drug-induced parkinsonian symptoms
— controls akinesia and rigidity more
  effectively than tremor
— chronic manganese poisoning

Dose

0.1 g orally t.d.s. p.c. increasing to 2 g
t.d.s. p.c.

Adverse effects

— anorexia, nausea, vomiting
— postural hypotension, cardiac
  arrhythmias
— involuntary movements
— depression with suicidal tendencies

Interactions

— effects of levodopa enhanced by the
  peripheral dopa decarboxylase
  inhibitors, carbidopa and benserazide
— effects of levodopa enhanced by
  amantadine, anticholinergics,
  amphetamine
— large doses of tricyclic
  antidepressants added to established
  levodopa therapy increases risk of
  cardiac arrhythmias
— enhances hypotensive effects of
  bretylium, debrisoquine, guanethidine
— effects of levodopa reduced by
  phenothiazines, haloperidol,
  droperidol, reserpine, pyridoxine,
  tetrabenazine, diazepam, oxazepam,
  chlordiazepoxide, phenobarbitone
— combining levodopa with furazolidone
  or MAO inhibitors may cause

hypertensive crises even up to 14 days after stopping MAO inhibitors
— effects of sympathomimetic and antihypertensive agents enhanced by levodopa
— propranolol enhances action of levodopa on tremor and diminishes cardiac side-effects, also combination results in raised growth hormone blood levels
— food reduces and delays absorption of levodopa
— effects of levodopa reduced by avocado, beans, beef liver, dry skim milk, malted milk, oatmeal, pork, tuna, yams, yeast and wheat germ

Nursing points

— gastric irritation reduced by taking with or immediately after food
— advise patient about the need to continue treatment as it is long term replacement therapy, maximum improvement may take up to 6 months and is maintained only while therapy continues
— supine and standing blood pressure checked regularly for postural hypotension
— advise patient to avoid postural hypotension by moving gradually to a sitting or standing position especially after sleep
— advise patient to resume activities gradually to avoid injury
— observe depressed patient for suicidal tendencies
— advise patient to discuss taking any OTC preparations with the medical officer or pharmacist
— note instability in diabetics
— a reddish tinge in the urine is harmless
— the appearance of involuntary movements is a sign of levodopa toxicity

Note

— may be used in combination with anticholinergic agents
— combination with an inhibitor of dopa decarboxylase at peripheral sites e.g. benserazide or carbidopa enables the

dose of levodopa to be reduced and may diminish some adverse reactions
— ensure correct formulation selected
— levodopa therapy discontinued at least 8 hours prior to surgery
— levodopa should not be given to nursing mothers
— not given to patients during or within 14 days of stopping MAO inhibitor therapy
— fortified cereals have high pyridoxine content
— may activate a malignant melanoma, so not given if history of malignant melanoma or suspicious lesion
— monthly full blood count and monitoring of hepatic, renal and cardiovascular function during prolonged therapy
— sudden fluctuations of effectiveness of levodopa develop after about 2 years of therapy ('on-off' effect)

LEVODOPA WITH BENSERAZIDE

— see note above for levodopa

LEVODOPA-CARBIDOPA

— see note above for levodopa

AMANTADINE

Action

— thought to stimulate release of dopamine in the brain
— probably inhibits penetration of virus into host cell

Use

— parkinsonism, improves hypokinesia and rigidity but less effect on tremor
— drug-induced extrapyramidal reactions
— prophylaxis against influenza type A_2 (Asian)

Dose

Parkinsonism

100 mg orally mane p.c. for 1 week, then 100 mg orally mane and midday p.c.

Influenza

100 mg orally mane and midday p.c. and if necessary, increase mane dose to 200 mg

Adverse effects

— ankle oedema
— mottling of skin (livedo reticularis)
— postural hypotension
— nervous excitement
— dry mouth, blurred vision
— dizziness, difficulty in concentration
— allergic reaction, necessitating cessation of therapy
— rarely, psychosis, congestive cardiac failure, leucopenia

Interactions

— increases anticholinergic atropine-like unwanted effects of tricyclic antidepressants
— may enhance effects of benzhexol, benztropine and orphenadrine

Nursing points

— capsules taken at mealtimes with fluid
— advise patient to consult the medical officer immediately any rash appears or pregnancy occurs
— advise patient to avoid postural hypotension by moving gradually to a sitting or standing position especially after sleep
— advise patient that drug therapy is best withdrawn gradually to reduce risk of inducing parkinsonian crisis

Note

— amantadine should not be given to nursing mothers
— may take several weeks to achieve optimal effects

BENZHEXOL

Action

— anticholinergic agent similar to atropine but with less side effects

Use

— all types of parkinsonism including drug-induced extrapyramidal symptoms
— controls rigidity more effectively than tremor

Dose

1–5 mg t.d.s. a.c. or with food if causes nausea

Adverse effects

— dry mouth, blurred vision
— mild nausea
— nervousness
— rarely, anhydrosis, hyperthermia (hot weather)
— rarely, psychosis necessitating cessation of therapy
— other as for atropine sulphate

Interactions

— anticholinergic effects increased by tricyclic and MAO inhibitor antidepressants and some antihistamines

Nursing points

— thirst may be relieved by water, chewing gum or mints, or sucking hard sweets
— warn patient against driving a vehicle or operating machinery if drowsy
— avoid sudden cessation of the drug

Note

— used in conjunction with levodopa or amantadine
— intraocular pressure monitored regularly
— anticholinergic antiparkinson agents do not control tardive dyskinesia associated with *long term* phenothiazine or other antipsychotic therapy

BENZTROPINE

Action and use

— combination of active portions of atropine and diphenhydramine
— as for benzhexol but has more sedative effects, a longer action and cumulative effects

Dose

0.5–6 mg orally or IM as single dose nocte or in 3 divided doses

BIPERIDEN

— as for benzhexol
— nocturnal cramps

Dose

i) 1–4 mg orally t.d.s. or q.i.d. p.c. (parkinsonism)
ii) 1–2 mg orally nocte with food (nocturnal cramps)

ORPHENADRINE HYDROCHLORIDE

— as for benzhexol

Dose

50–100 mg t.d.s. p.c.

PROCYCLIDINE

— as or benzhexol

Dose

i) 2.5–10 mg t.d.s. p.c.; OR
ii) 5–10 mg IM or slowly IV

BROMOCRIPTINE

Action

— stimulates dopaminergic receptors
— inhibits release of prolactin

Use

— prevent or suppress lactation
— hyperprolactinaemia

— adjunctive therapy in acromegaly
— parkinsonism

Dose

Parkinsonism

1.25 mg orally daily or b.d. with food for 7 days, then increase gradually up to 10 mg t.d.s. or q.i.d. as required

Others

— see p. 175

Adverse effects

— nausea, vomiting, dizziness, headache
— postural hypotension, nasal congestion
— drowsiness, depression
— mania, ataxia
— rare, but fatal gastric haemorrhage (acromegaly)
— high doses (more than 15 mg/day) confusion, hallucinations, delirium psychosis
— pleural effusion (long term parkinsonism therapy)

Nursing points

— advise patient to take initial doses on retiring to reduce the incidence of hypotension and loss of consciousness
— gastric irritation reduced if taken with/or immediately after food
— warn patient that alcohol may cause nausea, abdominal pain and bloating during bromocriptine therapy
— dosage increases made gradually, usually over several days, to reduce incidence of adverse effects
— warn acromegalic patient to report any gastrointestinal side-effects immediately
— warn patient against driving a vehicle or operating machinery if drowsy
— supine and standing blood pressure checked regularly for postural hypotension
— advise patient to avoid postural

hypotension by moving gradually to a sitting or standing position especially after sleep

Note

— may be used alone or in combination therapy for parkinsonism
— see p. 175
— since bromocriptine prevents lactation it should not be given to women who elect to breast-feed

CENTRAL NERVOUS SYSTEM STIMULANTS

DOXAPRAM

Action

— respiratory stimulant causing an increase in tidal volume and respiratory rate
— slight vasoconstrictor properties
— effective for 5–10 minutes

Use

— respiratory depression following anaesthesia

Dose

— add the maximum total dose of 400 mg to 180 ml of isotonic saline or 5% or 10% glucose to make a concentration of 2 mg/ml
— a burette, infusion pump or micro-drip regulator is used to deliver the solution at 1–3 mg/min over about 2 hours

Note

— stock vial contains 400 mg/20 ml

Adverse effects

— sweating, flushing, pruritus
— restlessness, muscle twitching or rigidity
— nausea, vomiting, coughing
— laryngospasm, bronchospasm
— tachycardia, increase in blood pressure
— high doses, epileptiform convulsions

Interactions

— antagonizes morphine-induced respiratory depression
— forms a precipitate if mixed with alkaline solutions such as aminophylline, frusemide, potassium penicillin G, sodium bicarbonate, thiopentone

Note

— not used in conjunction with a mechanical ventilator
— arterial blood gases monitored $\frac{1}{2}$ hourly for oxygen and carbon dioxide levels
— have available diazepam, thiopentone and resuscitation equipment

METHYLPHENIDATE

Action

— sympathomimetic agent which stimulates CNS, elevating the mood and improving the powers of judgement and concentration

Use

— hyperkinetic syndrome in children over 5 years
— narcolepsy

Adult dose

i) 10–20 mg orally $\frac{1}{2}$ hour before breakfast and lunch; OR
ii) 10–20 mg SC, IM or slowly IV as required

Paediatric dose

0.25–1 mg/kg/24 hours

Adverse effects

— nervousness, insomnia
— dizziness, drowsiness
— dependence
— rarely, changes in pulse rate and blood pressure

Interactions

— enhances effects of phenytoin
— not to be given with vasopressor agents or tricyclic antidepressants
— not to be given with or within one week of MAO inhibitors

Nursing points

— avoid adding injectable solution to a syringe or IV infusion line containing a barbiturate or strongly alkaline solution, as a heavy precipitate forms
— check blood pressure before each IV injection
— packed with separate ampoules of solvent
— under control as for drugs of addiction

DEXAMPHETAMINE

Action

— sympathomimetic agent with alpha- and beta-adrenergic activity

Use

— control of hyperkinetic behaviour in brain-damaged children (produces a paradoxical sedative effect)
— narcolepsy

Adult dose

5–60 mg daily in divided doses $\frac{1}{2}$ hour a.c. (narcolepsy)

Paediatric dose (over 5 years)

2.5 mg orally daily mane initially, increasing according to response, up to 20 mg/day in 2 divided doses

Adverse effects

— restlessness, tremor, insomnia
— anorexia, dry mouth
— tolerance, dependence
— hypertension (high dose)

Interactions

— hypertensive crises when given in conjunction with or within 2 weeks of ceasing MAO inhibitors
— reduces hypotensive effects of bretylium, debrisoquine, guanethidine

Note

— under control as for drugs of addiction
— limited to above uses by law in many centres

APPETITE SUPPRESSANTS

Action

— anorectics are mainly sympathomimetic agents which suppress the sensation of hunger possibly by an effect on the hypothalamus

Use

— adjuvant in control of obesity

Preparations and dose

DIETHYLPROPION

i) 25 mg orally t.d.s. 1 hour a.c. and in mid-evening if required (Tenuate®); OR
ii) 75 mg swallowed whole mid-morning (Tenuate Dospan®)

FENFLURAMINE

i) 20 mg orally b.d. 1 hour a.c.; increasing gradually to 40 mg orally t.d.s. 1 hour a.c. (Ponderax®), OR
ii) 1 or 2 capsules before breakfast (Ponderax Pacaps®).

MAZINDOL

0.5–3 mg orally daily after breakfast

PHENTERMINE

15–40 mg orally daily before breakfast

Adverse effects of appetite suppressants

— dry mouth, constipation
— irritability, nervousness, insomnia
— tachycardia, hypertension
— palpitations
— tolerance

Interactions

— not to be taken in combination with MAO inhibitors
— antihypertensive effects of debrisoqine and guanethidine reversed

OTHER APPETITE SUPPRESSANTS

METHYLCELLULOSE

Action

— absorbs moisture and increases bulk in the gastrointestinal tract

Use

— obesity
— bowel dysfunction including chronic constipation, severe diarrhoea, colostomy and ileostomy control

Dose

Obesity

i) 5 tablets (0.5 g each) ½ hour a.c. or when hungry with 1 or 2 full glasses of water up to 24 tablets daily; OR
ii) 1 heaped teaspoon of granules ½ hour a.c. or when hungry with 1 or 2 full glasses of water

Bowel dysfunction

i) 1 level to heaped teaspoon of granules t.d.s. with 1 or 2 full glasses of water (chronic constipation); OR
ii) 1 heaped teaspoon of granules t.d.s with as little water as possible (severe diarrhoea); OR
iii) 1 level to heaped teaspoon of granules mane and nocte with as little water as possible (colostomy, ileostomy); OR
iv) 3 or 4 tablets t.d.s. p.c. with 1 or 2 full glasses of water reducing as required to 2–4 tablets 3–4 times/week (all types)

Note

— granules may be sprinkled on cereals
— may take up to 3 days for full effect

PROPYLHEXEDRINE

Action and use

— reduces appetite by depressing peristalsis, useful in all types of obesity

Dose

25–50 mg b.d. or t.d.s., last dose taken before 4 p.m.

Adverse effects

— moderate constipation, nausea
— malaise
— tachycardia
— mild CNS stimulation

PSYLLIUM

— see section on bulk laxatives (p. 21)

6 Drugs acting on the endocrine system

SYSTEMIC CORTICOSTEROIDS

HYDROCORTISONE (cortisol)

Action

— adrenal corticosteriod with glucocorticoid and mineralocorticoid properties
— increases gluconeogenesis
— decreases peripheral glucose utilization
— decreases anabolism causing muscle wasting
— depresses inflammatory and allergic response
— slows growth in children
— delays healing
— increases fat deposition in face, shoulders and abdomen
— sodium retention
— osteoporosis
— euphoria
— anti-vitamin D action
— increases urinary calcium excretion
— suppresses pituitary-adrenocortical system

Use

— replacement therapy in adrenocortical insufficiency
— suppress undesirable inflammatory or immune responses
— adjunctive therapy in severe shock

Dose

i) 100–500 mg IV injection or continuous infusion, repeated 3–4 times in 24 hours, depending on severity of the condition and the patient's response, OR
ii) 50–100 mg deeply IM 6-hourly

Adverse effects

— sodium and fluid retention, potassium and calcium depletion
— hypertension
— muscle wasting, weakness, osteoporosis
— gastrointestinal disturbances and bleeding
— increased appetite, delayed wound healing
— bruising, striae, hirsuitism, acne, flushing
— raised intracranial pressure, headache, depression, psychosis
— menstrual irregularities
— hyperglycaemia, glycosuria, activation of latent diabetes mellitus
— cataract, glaucoma
— development of latent infections including tuberculosis
— obesity, moon face, buffalo hump
— suppression of pituitary-adrenocortical systems
— growth retardation in children on prolonged therapy
— acute adrenal insufficiency may be precipitated by sudden withdrawal or reduction in dosage or an increase in corticosteroid requirements associated with stress caused by injury, surgery or infection

Interactions

— risk of hyperglycaemia caused by hydrocortisone increased by thiazide diuretics
— ascorbic acid protects against corticosteroid-induced osteoporosis and reduces impairment of polymorphonuclear neutrophils caused by corticosteriods
— rifampicin reduces activity of corticosteroids

Nursing points

— select correct corticosteroid preparation
— IV injection given slowly over 10 minutes
— IM preparation given deeply into buttock rather than the deltoid muscle to avoid subcutaneous atrophy
— reduce sodium intake
— check urine for glycosuria
— check weight frequently to detect fluid retention
— check blood pressure frequently for hypertension
— ensure all relevant medical and nursing personnel are aware that the patient is on corticosteroid therapy
— advise patient to take medication regularly and never to change the dose or stop the drug without medical instruction (this refers to oral medication)
— advise patient about the need to continue therapy and to keep follow-up appointments
— advise patient to report infection, inflammation, persistent backache, chest pain and changes in body shape
— advise patient to pay strict attention to personal hygiene
— patient advised to obtain 'Identicare' bracelet or pendant and enter relevant information
— relatives or other household member also to be aware of implications and precautions during corticosteroid therapy
— advise patient that long term drug therapy is withdrawn gradually over several days, weeks or months to allow return of adequate adrenocortical function, but it may be 1 or 2 years before normal function returns
— watch for corticosteroid withdrawal syndrome: fever, malaise myalgia, arthralgia

Note

— increased doses of corticosteroids are required in times of stress such as injury, surgery and infection

— potassium supplement may be necessary
— antacids between meals may help to prevent peptic ulcer

BECLOMETHASONE

— see respiratory system (p. 79)

BETAMETHASONE

— as for hydrocortisone

Dose

i) 0.5–4.5 mg orally daily with food to reduce gastric irritation; OR
ii) 6–12 mg IM then 6 mg/week
iii) 3–6 mg locally into bursae, joint capsules

CORTISONE ACETATE

Action

— as for hydrocortisone
— converted to hydrocortisone in the liver

Use

— replacement therapy in adrenocortical insufficiency (Addison's disease)
— replacement therapy in chronic adrenocortical insufficiency secondary to hypopituitarism

Adult dose

12.5–50 mg orally daily with food in 3 or 4 divided doses

Paediatric dose

i) 0.6 mg/kg/24 hours (20 mg/m^2/24 hours) orally with food in 3 divided doses (physiologic replacement therapy); OR
ii) 2.5–10 mg/kg/24 hours (75–300 mg/m^2/24 hours) orally with food in 3 or 4 divided doses pharmacologic dose); OR
iii) $\frac{1}{3}$–$\frac{1}{2}$ the quoted oral dose IM
iv) 0.5 mg/kg/24 hours (15 mg/m^2/24 hours) IM once daily (adrenogenital syndrome)

DEXAMETHASONE

— as for hydrocortisone
— lacks sodium and water-retaining
  properties
— reduces cerebral oedema
— neonatal respiratory distress
  syndrome (antenatal prophylaxis)

Adult dose

i) 0.5–10 mg orally daily with food in 3
   or 4 divided doses; OR
ii) 4–20 mg IM or IV repeated as
   required, then 2–4 mg 3- to 4-hourly
   up to a maximum of 80 mg/day, OR
iii) 0.4–4 mg for intrasynovial and soft-
   tissue injections, OR
iv) 2–6 mg/kg IV stat. repeated in 2–6
   hours either slowly IV or IV infusion
   until condition stabilizes and usually
   no longer than 48–72 hours (severe
   shock); OR
v) 5 mg IM 12-hourly for 4 doses 1–7
   days before estimated time of
   delivery (neonatal respiratory distress
   syndrome)

Paediatric dose

i) 1/30 dose quoted for cortisone
   acetate, OR
ii) 5–10 mg IV for cerebral oedema,
   which may be followed by 2–4 mg
   IV 6-hourly

FLUDROCORTISONE

— as for hydrocortisone but used in
  adrenocortical insufficiency, adrenal
  hyperplasia and post adrenalectomy

Dose

i) 0.05–0.2 mg orally daily with food
   (maintenance); OR
i) 1–2 mg orally daily with food (for
   adrenal supression in adrenal
   hyperplasia)

Note

— causes marked sodium retention and
  increases potassium excretion

METHYLPREDNISOLONE

— as for hydrocortisone

Dose

i) 30 mg/kg IV over 10 minutes (severe
   shock); OR
ii) 2–60 mg orally daily; OR
iii) 4–80 mg IM or intra-articular,
   depending on site

PREDNISOLONE

— as for hydrocortisone
— causes less sodium retention,
  oedema and electrolyte imbalance
— already in an active form

Adult dose

i) 5–80 mg orally daily, large doses
   being divided through the day while
   smaller doses are best given as a
   single daily dose in the morning so
   as to cause less pituitary suppression
ii) 10 mg by infiltration
iii) 2.5–20 mg by intra-articular injection
iv) contents of 1 disposable enema unit
   nocte as a retention enema for
   ulcerative colitis and Crohn's disease

Paediatric dose

1–3 mg/kg/day orally

PREDNISONE

— given orally as for prednisolone, but
  not to be given instead of
  prednisolone
— converted in the liver to its active
  metabolite, prednisolone
— less reliably absorbed than
  prednisolone

TRIAMCINOLONE

— as for hydrocortisone but has less
  sodium- and water-retaining
  properties so not used in adrenal
  deficiency states

Dose

i) 4–48 mg orally daily, large doses
   being divided through the day while

smaller doses are best given as a single dose in the morning so as to cause less pituitary suppression; OR

ii) 40–80 mg deeply IV into buttock (triamcinolone acetonide); OR

iii) 10–80 mg for intrasynovial and soft tissue injections (triamcinolone acetonide)

Adverse effects

— as for hydrocortisone but particularly anorexia, weight loss, flushing, depression, muscle wasting

Note

— not given IV because it is a suspension

INSULIN PREPARATIONS

Insulin preparations contain either bovine (from cattle pancreas), porcine (from pig pancreas) or human insulin.

Bovine insulin differs from human insulin in 3 amino acids while porcine insulin differs by only 1 amino acid. Insulin which has an amino acid sequence identical to that of human insulin is obtained by either enzymatically replacing alanine at the terminal position 30 in the B-chain of purified pork insulin with threonine (semi-synthetic), or by recombinant DNA techniques using E. coli bacteria (biosynthetic).

emp is the code used to designate human insulin produced by enzymatic modification of insulin obtained from the pig pancreas. Modification by the addition of zinc or protein (protamine) or both, delays absorption from SC or IM depot resulting in a slower action of prolonged duration. Premixed insulins contain a stable mixture of unmodified (neutral) and intermediate acting (isophane) insulins.

Insulins are classified by onset, peak and duration of action (in hours).

Action

— an endocrine hormone which causes a fall in blood sugar concentration and promotes the conversion of glucose to glycogen

Use

— insulin-dependent diabetes mellitus (IDDM; type I)

Adverse effects, nursing points, interactions

— see p. 153

CLASSIFICATION OF INSULIN

Insulin	Onset	Peak	Duration
Short acting			
Insulin injection (regular, soluble)	$\frac{1}{2}$–1	4	6–10
Neutral	$\frac{1}{2}$–1	4	6–10
Insulin zinc suspension (amorphous)	1–2	5–10	16
Intermediate acting			
Biphasic	$\frac{1}{2}$	4–12	24
Neutral and isophane (Premixed)	$\frac{1}{2}$	4–8	24
Insulin zinc suspension	2–3	7–15	24
Isophane	2–4	4–12	18–24
Long acting			
Insulin zinc suspension (crystalline)	4–6	10–30	24–36
Protamine zinc suspension	4–8	15–20	24–36

SHORT ACTING INSULIN PREPARATIONS

REGULAR INSULIN (soluble, unmodified)

Action

— onset 30–45 minutes
— maximum 4 hours
— duration 8 hours

Use

— diabetic ketoacidosis and coma
— insulin-dependent diabetic following surgery or with acute infection

Note

— a soluble acidic preparation
— may be mixed with isophane insulin (50% regular), or with an insulin zinc suspension (10% regular), the regular insulin being taken into the syringe first
— incompatible with protamine zinc insulin but may be given separately at the same time
— ineffective by mouth
— anticipate hypoglycaemia 4–5 hours after administration

NEUTRAL INSULIN

Action

— onset 30 minutes
— maximum 3–4 hours
— duration 6–7 hours

Use

— diabetic ketoacidosis and coma
— insulin-dependent diabetic following surgery or with acute infection

Note

— a soluble neutral preparation
— may be mixed with biphasic or isophane and occasionally with insuln zinc suspensions, neutral insulin being taken into syringe first (not mixed with protamine zinc insulin)

— anticipate hypoglycaemia 4–5 hours after administration

INSULIN ZINC SUSPENSION (amorphous)

Action

— onset $\frac{1}{2}$–1 hour
— maximum 3–6 hours
— duration 12–16 hours

Note

— a neutral depot preparation
— commercially mixed with insulin zinc suspension (crystalline, ultralente) to give an intermediate action
— may be mixed with other insulin zinc suspensions, neutral insulin or regular insulin, taking the neutral or regular insulin into the syringe first (see note, regular insulin and neutral insulin); injection is then given immediately
— anticipate hypoglycaemia late morning

INTERMEDIATE ACTING INSULIN PREPARATIONS

BIPHASIC INSULIN

Action

— onset 30 minutes
— maximum 4–12 hours
— duration 18–22 hours

Note

— a neutral depot preparation
— commercially prepared by combining short- and intermediate-acting insulins in a set ratio
— may be mixed only with neutral insulin
— anticipate hypoglycaemia in the afternoon

INSULIN ZINC SUSPENSION

Action

— onset 2 hours
— maximum 8–12 hours
— duration 24 hours

Note

— a neutral depot preparation
— commercially prepared by mixing 3 volumes of insulin zinc suspension (amorphous) with 7 volumes of insulin zinc suspension (crystalline)
— may be mixed with regular or neutral insulin, taking the soluble insulin into the syringe first (see note, regular insulin)
— anticipate hypoglycaemia late afternoon

ISOPHANE INSULIN

Action

— onset 2 hours
— maximum 8–12 hours
— duration 20–24 hours

Note

— a neutral depot preparation
— may be mixed with regular insulin or neutral insulin (see note, regular insulin)
— anticipate hypoglycaemia late afternoon or evening

NEUTRAL AND ISOPHANE INSULIN

Action

— onset 30 minutes
— maximum 4–8 hours
— duration 24 hours

Note

— a pre-mixed preparation of unmodified and intermediate acting insulin in a ratio of either 3:7 or 1:1, the combination having both a prompt and prolonged action
— anticipate hypoglycaemia in the afternoon

LONG ACTING INSULIN PREPARATIONS

INSULIN ZINC SUSPENSION
(crystalline)

Action

— onset 4 hours
— maximum 12–18 hours
— duration 36 hours

Note

— a neutral depot preparation
— may be mixed with regular or neutral insulin, taking the soluble insulin into the syringe first (see note, regular insulin)
— anticipate hypoglycaemia during the night or early morning

PROTAMINE ZINC INSULIN

Action

— see regular insulin
— onset 4–8 hours
— maximum 14–20 hours
— duration 24–36 hours

Note

— a neutral depot preparation
— a dose of regular insulin or neutral insulin is often given at the same time, but separately, to tide over the time required for the absorption of the protamine zinc insulin
— given separately to prevent unpredictable duration of action
— anticipate hypoglycaemia during the night or early morning

Adverse effects of insulin

— hypoglycaemia, early signs: tremor, sweating, hunger, palpitations, apprehension, dizziness, headache pallor, circumoral paraesthesia, tachycardia
— later signs: drowsiness, confusion, and if untreated, may lead to

convulsions and coma
— permanent brain damage may follow prolonged hypoglycaemia
— local allergic reaction at injection site
— general allergic reaction, urticaria, angioneurotic oedema or anaphylactic shock (may need to change from bovine to porcine insulin)
— lipodystrophy (lipoatrophy or hypertrophy) at injection site which disappears slowly if site changed
— insulin resistance (requiring a change to purified pork or human insulin)

Interactions

— alcohol and some beta-adrenoceptor blocking agents may increase the activity of insulin

Nursing points for insulin

Soluble insulin

— a clear solution, usually given SC but in emergencies such as diabetic ketoacidosis precoma and coma, may be given IV or IM
— used to stabilize diabetics
— cloudy solutions are discarded

Depot insulin

— appears white and cloudy
— contain zinc or protamine allowing slow absorption by slow release, in stablized insulin-sensitive diabetics
— given SC, *never* IM or IV or in emergency

Storage

— store stock on its side between 2 and 8°C, but do not freeze
— insulin in use can be stored at room temperature for 1 month before being discarded, provided the room temperature does not exceed 25°C
— mark date of opening vial on label
— avoid over-exposure to light
— discard any vial if the insulin has been frozen or exposed to high temperatures, if discoloured or if any

lumps or flakes present
— do not store Penfill® cartridges which are in use in the refrigerator

Preparation

— select correct preparation
— porcine insulin not given to Moslems
— not mixed with other drugs
— have insulin at room temperature
— check expiry date
— suspensions are rotated gently and inverted several times to ensure full dispersion and prevent frothing
— insulin of one brand should not be mixed with insulin of another brand
— the model and brand of syringe or needle are not changed without consulting the medical officer
— mixtures should be made in the syringe and injected immediately
— when mixing insulins, use the same procedure every time for accuracy and constant effect
— the shorter acting insulin is drawn up first to prevent its contamination in the vial by the long-acting insulin which contains zinc or protamine which binds soluble insulin so reducing the amount of soluble insulin available for immediate effect
— when mixing ensure that insulin is from the same species, i.e. bovine with bovine and porcine with porcine
— insulin available in 100 units/ml together with a standard insulin syringe marked in units for U100 insulin (dose ranges from 10–100 or more units depending on the severity of the diabetes)
— a 25 gauge 1.25 cm needle used for SC injections
— soluble insulin may be added to flasks of total parenteral nutrition solution to prevent or correct hyperglycaemia caused by the administration of large amounts of glucose

Administration

— given SC usually, intravascular injection being avoided by withdrawing syringe plunger before injecting
— given usually 30 minutes before breakfast, or if b.d., second injection given before evening meal
— injection sites include upper arms, thighs and abdomen, but as absorption rates vary so much it is advisable to rotate injection sites within the same anatomical site, preferably the abdomen
— injection sites rotated, taking 4–6 weeks before reinjection to prevent thickening and dimpling at site
— instructions enclosed with injection pen and cartridge vial must be followed carefully
— pumps provide a method of continuous SC insulin infusion (CSII)

General

— patient education on insulin self-medication begins several days prior to discharge
— advise patient about methods of sterilization, injection technique and site rotation
— allow patient to experience early mild hypoglycaemia so that it is recognized and treatment instituted, e.g. oral glucose carried at all times, jelly beans, Life-Savers or barley sugar
— anticipate the likely times for hypoglycaemia and work out a snack or meal pattern to overcome it
— a responsible household member or close workmate should be advised how to identify and deal with hypoglycaemia early
— teach patient how and when to test urine or blood
— hypoglycaemia likely if blood sugar concentration less than 3 mmol/l, convulsions if less than 2 mmol/l
— advise patient to obtain 'Identicare' bracelet or pendant and have relevant information entered
— advise patient that extra food is required before or during increased activity such as sport, etc.
— advise patient that if feeling ill, continue to take insulin, take food in liquid form as replacement and check

urine and/or blood for sugar and
ketones
— advise patient to consult medical
officer if unable to eat prescribed
diet or if urine or blood tests positive
for sugar and/or ketones
— have available 50% glucose and
glucagon

INSULIN ANTAGONIST

GLUCAGON

Action

— derived from alpha cells of islets of
Langerhans in beef or pork pancreas
— raises blood sugar concentration by
mobilizing hepatic glycogen
— causes relaxation of gastrointestinal
smooth muscle

Use

— treatment of insulin and
sulphonylurea-induced hypoglycaemia
when glucose unavailable or cannot
be given
— aid in radiological examination of
gastrointestinal tract

Dose

i) 0.5–1 unit SC; IM or IV
(hypoglycaemia) may be repeated
twice if required; OR
ii) 0.5–2 units SC or IM (termination of
therapeutic insulin coma); OR
iii) 0.2–2 units IV, IM (endoscopy and
radiography)

Adverse reactions

— nausea, vomiting

Interactions

— increases effect of oral
anticoagulants

Nursing points

— reconstitute with accompanying
diluent
— if patient does not awaken within 20
minutes seek medical assistance
— although an emergency drug, the
patient and family may be instructed
in its use

Note

— IV glucose must be given if patient fails to respond to glucagon
— may cause severe hypertension in phaeochromocytoma

SULPHONYLUREA HYPOGLYCAEMIC AGENTS

Action

— orally active agent which facilitates insulin release from the beta cells of the pancreas
— peak hypoglycaemic effect 2–6 hours, duration 10–24 hours

Use

— non-insulin-dependent diabetes mellitus (NIDDM; type II) unresponsive to diet alone and in whom insulin is unacceptable

Preparations and dose

CHLORPROPAMIDE

125–500 mg as a single daily dose with breakfast

GLIBENCLAMIDE

2.5–15 mg daily, up to 10 mg as a single daily dose with or immediately after breakfast, while amounts in excess of 10 mg are taken with the evening meal

GLICLAZIDE

40–160 mg daily or b.d. $\frac{1}{2}$–1 hour a.c.

GLIPIZIDE

2.5–5 mg daily $\frac{1}{2}$ hour before breakfast increasing gradually to 15 mg. Amounts in excess of 15 mg are taken before the evening meal up to a total daily dose of 30 mg. Maximum total daily dose is 40 mg

TOLAZAMIDE

125–250 mg daily as single dose with breakfast increased gradually as required to 1 g daily

TOLBUTAMIDE

0.5–1.5 g as a single daily dose with breakfast or in 2 divided doses

Adverse effects of sulphonylurea hypoglycaemics

— nausea, vomiting, epigastric pain
— weakness, paraesthesias, headache
— sensitivity reactions including fever,
  . rash and blood dyscrasias
— photosensitivity
— cholestatic jaundice (rare)
— prolonged hypoglycaemia (uncommon but serious)

Interactions

— hypoglycaemic action enhanced by alcohol, aspirin, sodium salicylate, clofibrate, fenfluramine, phenylbutazone, oxyphenbutazone, oral coumarin anticoagulants, beta-adrenoceptor blocking agents, MAO inhibitors, levodopa, chloramphenicol, sulphamethizole, sulphinpyrazone, sulphaphenazole, furazolidone
— hypoglycaemic effects reduced by adrenaline, corticosteroids and thiazide diuretics, $beta_2$-adrenoceptor agonists, oral contraceptives, barbiturates, rifampicin, alcohol
— combined with alcohol, may cause headache, dyspnoea, nausea, giddiness and flushing (disulfiram-like reaction) particularly with chlorpropamide

Nursing points

— advise patient of the need to adhere to the principles of management in diet, personal hygiene, avoidance of infection and to report to the medical officer if any signs of illness
— allow patient to experience early mild hypoglycaemia so that it is recognized and treated early with oral glucose
— warn patient about reduced tolerance to alcohol
— a responsible household member or close workmate should be advised how to identify and deal with hypoglycaemia early
— advise patient to obtain 'Identicare' bracelet or pendant and have relevant information entered

Note

— sulphonylureas are not oral insulins but are capable of increasing circulating insulin
— insulin may be required in times of stress such as injury, surgery and infection
— the warning symptoms of hypoglycaemia are often absent
— metformin 0.5–3 g daily may be combined with a sulphonylurea
— adverse effects more frequent with chlorpropamide

OTHER ORAL HYPOGLYCAEMIC AGENTS

METFORMIN

Action

— orally active biguanide derivative which probably increases the peripheral utilization of glucose
— hypoglycaemia effect lasts 4–5 hours

Use

— as for sulphonylurea agents but may be used as adjuvant therapy in obese poorly controlled insulin-dependent diabetics

Dose

0.5–1 g 2–3 times daily with or immediately after meals

Adverse effects

— minor transient anorexia, nausea, vomiting, diarrhoea
— occasionally metallic taste, urticaria
— serious and often fatal lactic acidosis, signs of which are nausea, vomiting, abdominal pain, diarrhoea, malaise, hyperventilation

Interactions

— lactic acidosis may occur when alcohol taken

Nursing points

— advise patient of the need to adhere to the principles of management in diet, personal hygiene, avoidance of infection and to report to the medical officer if any signs of illness
— warn patient about reduced tolerance to alcohol
— advise patient to obtain 'Identicare' bracelet or pendant and have relevant information entered

Note

— this preparation is not an oral insulin and only produces a reduction in blood sugar in the diabetic patient
— may be combined with a sulphonylurea agent
— insulin may be required if diabetes becomes unstable

THYROID HORMONES

THYROXINE

Action and use

— thyroid replacement in cretinism, juvenile hypothyroidism, Hashimoto's thyroiditis and myxoedema
— delayed response may take 14 days to become apparent

Adult dose

50–100 micrograms orally daily a.c. increased every 3–4 weeks by 50 micrograms until a maintenance dose of 200–300 micrograms reached

Paediatric dose

under 1 year: 25 micrograms orally daily increased every 3–4 days to a maximum of 200 micrograms depending on response
over 1 year: 50 micrograms orally daily increased every 3–4 days to a maximum of 300 micrograms depending on response

Adverse effects

— nervousness, tremor, sweating, flushing
— headache, insomnia
— tachycardia, palpitations, cardiac arrhythmias, angina pectoris
— excessive loss of weight

Interactions

— enhances effect of oral anticoagulants
— may upset stability of patient receiving antidiabetic drugs
— aspirin and phenytoin may enhance effect of thyroxine
— therapeutic and toxic effects of tricyclic antidepressants enhanced
— cholestyramine reduces absorption following oral administration

Nursing points

— usually given as a single daily dose before breakfast
— monitor heart rate, reporting if more than 100, any marked change in rate or rhythm
— note and report palpitations, dyspnoea or chest pain
— advise the patient that the replacement therapy is to continue for life and follow-up appointments need to be kept
— progress in children is monitored by serial height measurement

LIOTHYRONINE (triiodothyronine)

Action

— similar to thyroxine but much more potent and rapid in onset and is of briefer duration

Use

— hypometabolism and myxoedema if unresponsive to thyroxine
— myxoedema coma

Dose

i) 10–20 micrograms orally daily increased every 3–7 days by 10 micrograms to a daily dose of 80–100 micrograms usually in 2 or 3 divided doses; OR
ii) 10–20 micrograms by slow IV injection for myxoedema coma, repeated if necessary after 4 hours

Adverse effects

— palpitations, headache

Interactions

— activity of oral anticoagulants enhanced
— may be enhanced by phenytoin
— absorption reduced following oral administration if given with cholestyramine

Nursing points

— monitor heart rate, reporting tachycardia and palpitations
— advise the patient of the need to continue therapy and keep follow-up appointments
— if treating myxoedema coma, also require ECG monitoring, assisted ventilation and corticosteroids

ANTITHYROID DRUGS

CARBIMAZOLE

Actions and use

— depresses thyroid hormones synthesis in thyrotoxicosis

Adult dose

10–20 mg orally 8 hourly reducing to 5–20 mg daily

Paediatric dose

0.4 mg/kg/day orally in divided doses

Adverse effects

— rash, urticaria, fever, sore throat
— anorexia, malaise, joint pains
— agranulocytosis
— toxic neuropathy

Nursing points

— report immediately any rash, fever or sore throat, as these are early signs of agranulocytosis
— advise patient to keep appointments during initial therapy and report any rash, fever or sore throat immediately

Note

— therapy may be continued up to 2 years
— nursing mothers taking carbimazole should not breast-feed their infants

PROPYLTHIOURACIL

— as for carbimazole

Dose

200–600 mg orally daily in 3 divided doses preferably 8-hourly reducing to 50–200 mg daily in 3 divided doses

IODINE SOLUTION (Lugol's Solution)

Action

— essential trace element in diet
— causes short-term inhibition of thyroid hormone synthesis and release (high doses)
— reduces vascularity and friability of thyroid so lessens risk of haemorrhage during surgery

Use

— added to antithyroid treatment about 10–12 days before sub-total thyroidectomy for thyrotoxicosis
— thyrotoxic crisis (thyroid storm)

Dose

i) 0.1–0.3 ml orally t.d.s. with milk or water; OR
ii) 2–3 ml orally daily (thyrotoxic crisis)

Adverse effects

— pain and swelling of salivary glands, unpleasant taste
— conjunctivitis, rhinitis, gastritis
— headache
— rarely, drug fever, rash, thrombocytopenic purpura

Note

— patient rendered euthyroid with an antithyroid agent and iodine solution added to therapy prior to surgery

POTASSIUM PERCHLORATE

Action

— interferes with iodine binding in thyroid gland
— increases vascularity of thyroid gland

Use

— treatment of thyrotoxicosis

Dose

200 mg orally 3 or 4 times daily reducing to 100 mg 3 or 4 times daily

Adverse effects

— nausea, vomiting
— nephrotic syndrome
— aplastic anaemia
— pancytopenia

Note

— nausea, vomiting reduced by taking antacid simultaneously
— dose not to exceed 1 g/24 hours
— treatment may be needed for 12–18 months or longer

ANABOLIC STEROIDS

Action

— increases retention of nitrogen, calcium, sodium, potassium, chloride and phosphate leading to increased protein synthesis and skeletal weight
— increases water retention

Use

— diseases in which there is protein and bone wasting

Preparations and dose

ETHYLOESTRENOL

2 mg orally daily or b.d. (larger doses used in plasminogen activator deficiency)

METHENOLONE

i) 5–10 mg orally b.d.; OR
ii) 5 mg orally b.d. (underweight females); OR
iii) 100 mg deep IM every 2 weeks then every 3 or 4 weeks; OR
iv) 50 mg deep IM every 2 or 3 weeks (girls and young women)

NANDROLONE

i) 25–50 mg deep IM weekly or fortnightly (phenylpropionate); OR
ii) 25–50 mg deep IM every 3 weeks (decanoate)

OXANDROLONE

2.5 mg orally 2–4 times daily up to 20 mg daily may be required

OXYMETHOLONE

100–300 mg orally daily mainly for aplastic and primary refractory anaemias

Adverse effects of anabolic steroids

— as for androgens

Interactions

— enhances action of corticosteroids and may interfere with diabetic control
— enhances action of oral anticoagulants

Nursing points

— oral preparations taken immediately before or with meals to minimize nausea
— anabolic steroids are more effective when combined with a diet high in protein, kilojoules, vitamins and minerals
— check weight and urinary output frequently
— observe closely for hoarseness or voice deepening in females and note any menstrual irregularities
— note instability in diabetics
— note and report abnormal bleeding if also taking anticoagulants

ANDROGENS

Action

— controls development and maintenance of the male sex organs and the male secondary sex characteristics
— increases retention of nitrogen, calcium, sodium, potassium, chloride and phosphate leading to increase in skeletal weight, water retention, increased bone growth, increased erythropoiesis

Use

— replacement therapy in male for hypogonadism, eunichoidism and male climacteric
— gynaecomastia
— disseminated breast cancer in female

Preparations and dose

FLUOXYMESTERONE

2.5–30 mg orally as single daily dose or in 3 or 4 divided doses

Note

— also has anabolic properties

MESTEROLONE

25 mg orally t.d.s. reducing to 25 mg daily or b.d.

METHYLTESTOSTERONE

10–50 mg orally daily in divided doses p.c.

TESTOSTERONE ENANTHATE

50–250 mg deeply IM every 2–4 weeks

TESTOSTERONE ESTERS

i) 100 mg deep IM every 2–3 weeks;
   OR
ii) 250 mg deep IM every 4–6 weeks

TESTOSTERONE PROPIONATE

10–25 mg deep IM 2–4 times/week

TESTOSTERONE UNDECANOATE

120–160 mg orally daily for 2–3 weeks then 40–120 mg daily in 2 divided doses p.c.

Note

— used in treatment of thalassaemia

Adverse effects of androgens

— sodium and water retention, oedema, weight gain
— increased nitrogen retention
— increased bone growth and skeletal weight
— increased vascularity of skin
— hypercalcaemia
— cholestatic jaundice (methyltestosterone and anabolic steroids)
— closure of epiphyses if high doses given in early puberty
— suppression of ovarian activity and menstruation.
— virilism in female (high doses)
— suppression of spermatogenesis, degenerative changes in seminiferous tubules

Interactions

— enhance effects of oral anticoagulants
— effects reduced by barbiturates

Nursing points

— as for anabolic steroids
— oily IM formulations may be stored at room temperature

ANTIANDROGEN

CYPROTERONE

Action

— reduces stimulating effect of androgen-dependent structures and functions probably by competitive inhibition
— negative feedback effect on hypothalamic receptors resulting in reducing production of testicular androgens

Use

Women: signs of androgenization

— hirsutism
— androgenic alopecia
— acne and/or seborrhoea

Men

— reduction in drive in sexual deviations
— inoperable prostatic carcinoma (p. 269)

Children

— idiopathic precocious puberty

Dose

Women

100 mg orally at the same time each day with some liquid after a meal from 5th–14th day of the menstrual cycle;
PLUS
ethinyl oestradiol 50 micrograms orally daily from 5th–25th day of the cycle to ensure contraception and stabilize cycle

Men

25–100 mg orally 2–3 times daily

Children

dose determined by body surface area and severity of disorder based on 50–150 mg/m²/day

Adverse effects

— tiredness, inability to concentrate, headache, depression
— gastrointestinal disturbances
— increases body weight
— reduces libido
— mastodynia
— inhibits ovulation
— menstrual cycle irregularity
— impairs spermatogenesis
— gynaecomastia
— thrombotic phenomena
— reduces adrenal cortical function (children)

Note

— pregnancy must be excluded at commencement of treatment and ethinyl oestradiol taken as well to ensure contraception
— if unscheduled bleeding during the 3-week cycle in which the tablets are being taken, tablet taking should not be interrupted
— contraindicated during lactation
— one control spermatogram is made before start of treatment
— spermatogenesis may take 3–20 months to return to normal after discontinuing treatment
— sexual drive reduction can be somewhat reversed under the influence of alcohol

OESTROGENS

Action

— control development and maintenance of the female sex organs, the secondary sex characteristics, and the mammary glands
— influence sodium and water retention, metabolism of protein, fat, glucose, calcium and phosphorus
— influence hair growth and erythropoiesis

Use

— replacement therapy in female for primary amenorrhoea, delayed onset of puberty and menopausal syndrome
— palliative treatment of breast cancer in postmenopausal women and prostatic cancer
— functional uterine bleeding
— local application for senile vaginitis and vulvitis   .
— orally active oestrogen combined with an orally active progestogen for oral contraception

Preparations and dose

CONJUGATED OESTROGENS

i) 0.3–1.25 mg orally daily from 5th day of cycle for 3 weeks then repeated after a week (menopausal syndrome); OR
ii) 1.25–7.5 mg orally daily for 3 weeks supplemented during last 7 days by a progestogen (amenorrhoea); OR
iii) 1.25–2.5 mg orally t.d.s. (abnormal uterine bleeding); OR
iv) 25 mg IM or IV repeated as required after 6–12 hours, then as in ii) (functional uterine bleeding)
v) 2–4 g vaginal cream PV or topically daily (senile vaginitis, vulvitis)

ETHINYLOESTRADIOL

i) 0.01–0.05 mg orally t.d.s. for 2 weeks then 2 treatment-free weeks before recommencing (primary amenorrhoea); OR
ii) 0.01–0.05 mg orally t.d.s. throughout cycle supplemented during second fortnight by a progestogen (secondary amenorrhoea); OR
iii) 0.01–0.05 mg orally b.d. initially reducing to 0.01 mg daily or b.d. (menopausal syndrome)

FOSFESTROL (stilboestrol diphosphate)

— see antineoplastic drugs (p. 269)
— used for prostatic cancer

OESTRADIOL

20 or 100 mg as compressed pellet for subcutaneous implantation to give prolonged absorption

OESTRADIOL VALERATE

i) 1–2 mg orally daily for 21 days, then cease for 1 week before commencing another 21-day course
ii) 10–20 mg IM on designated days

OESTRIOL

i) 4 mg orally daily for first 5–7 days then 1–2 mg during next 1–3 weeks as required then taken continuously, but if intermittent treatment preferable, the patient has a tablet-free period of 5–7 days after each 3 weeks of treatment; OR
ii) 0.5 mg vaginal cream daily PV for 3 weeks then twice a week for 2–3 months (senile vaginitis, vulvitis, pruritus vulvae).
Discontinued for 4 weeks to assess necessity for further treatment; OR
iii) 0.5 mg vaginal cream daily PV for 2 weeks (pre vulvo-vaginal surgery)

PIPERAZINE OESTRONE SULPHATE

0.625–5 mg orally daily for 3 weeks then one week off therapy before recommencing

Adverse effects of oestrogens

— nausea, vomiting
— headache, dizziness, depression, migraine
— breast tenderness and enlargement
— spotting and breakthrough bleeding during or on withdrawal of therapy
— oedema, weight gain
— jaundice, urticaria, rash
— chloasma (skin pigmentation)
— hypercalcaemia
— premature closure of epiphyses (high doses in puberty)
— gynaecomastia

Interactions of oestrogens

— may enhance toxic effects of imipramine resulting in lethargy, hypotension, tremors and depersonalization
— may reduce effectiveness of anticoagulants

Nursing points on oestrogens

— advise patient to report promptly any breakthrough or withdrawal bleeding
— advise patient to report any weight gain or jaundice
— note and report increasing mental depression, visual disturbances or migraine
— advise patients not to smoke during oestrogen therapy
— see p. 194 for nursing points for vaginal preparations

Note

— there is evidence that the use of oestrogens as replacement therapy for more than one year may increase the risk of endometrial cancer
— low doses of estrogens may stimulate malignant neoplasms
— high doses can indirectly suppress neoplastic growth

PROGESTOGENS

Action

— converts endometrial proliferative phase to secretory phase in preparation for fertilized ovum
— suppresses uterine motility
— causes further breast development

Use

— alone or with oestrogen in menstrual disorders
— endometriosis
— breast and endometrial cancer
— oral contraception either alone or combined with an orally active oestrogen
— threatened abortion
— habitual abortion

Preparations and dose

ALLYLESTRENOL

i) 10–20 mg orally daily (threatened abortion; OR
ii) 10–20 mg orally daily 16th–26th day of cycle until conception established then 15 mg daily until past critical period (habitual abortion)
iii) 10–20 mg orally daily 16th–26th day of cycle until conception achieved then 10 mg daily for at least 16 weeks (failure of nidation)

DYDROGESTERONE

10–30 mg orally daily in 2 or 3 divided doses on designated days of the cycle.

Note

— does not inhibit ovulation

LEVONORGESTREL

i) 50–125 micrograms orally with ethinyloestradiol on designated days of the cycle; OR
ii) 30 micrograms orally on designated days of the cycle

Note

— inhibits ovulation
— has androgenic properties

PROGESTERONE

i) 5–25 mg deep IM on designated days; OR
ii) 250–500 mg deep IM on designated days (hydroxyprogesterone)

MEDROXYPROGESTERONE

i) 100 mg orally 2–4 times daily (malignancy); OR
ii) 2.5–20 mg orally daily on designated days of cycle (menstrual disorders); OR
iii) 600–1200 mg deep IM weekly reducing to 450–600 mg every 1–4 weeks (malignancy); OR
iv) 10 mg orally t.d.s. for 90 consecutive days beginning the first day of the menstrual cycle (endometriosis); OR
v) 50 mg IM weekly or 100 mg IM fortnightly for 6 months (endometriosis)

NORETHISTERONE ACETATE

i) 5–10 mg orally b.d.
ii) 10–20 mg orally t.d.s. (inoperable breast cancer)

Note

— powerful inhibitor of the pituitary

NORETHISTERONE

i) 10–20 mg orally daily on designated days of cycle, withdrawal bleeding usually occurs 1–3 days after discontinuation (amenorrhoea); OR
ii) 15 mg orally daily for 10 days (functional uterine bleeding); OR
iii) 10 mg orally daily initially, increasing to a daily maintenance dose of 20–30 mg for 9–12 months (endometriosis)

Note

— has weak oestrogenic and androgenic properties

Adverse effects of progestogens

— nausea, dyspepsia
— occasionally acne, oedema, weight gain, gynaecomastia, headache, depression
— virilization of foetus.

ORAL CONTRACEPTIVES

Oestrogens and progestogens may be in a fixed combination taken as one dose, with a sequentially increasing progestogen dose, or as a low-dose progestogen-only preparation, the 'mini-pill'.

Action

— oestrogens inhibit secretion of follicle stimulating hormone (FSH) preventing follicular development and release of luteinizing hormone (LH)
— progestogens, in combination, appear to inhibit pre-ovulatory rise of luteinizing hormone
— combination preparations decrease the likelihood of conception and implantation by causing changes in the cervical mucus and endometrium
— progestogen-only preparations alter the cervical mucus and endometrium without influencing ovulation

Adverse effects of oral contraceptives

— thrombo-embolic disorders
— hypertension
— leg cramps
— changes in carbohydrate and lipid metabolism
— nausea
— impaired liver function possibly with jaundice and increased risk of hepatic tumours
— mental depression, irritability, headache, migraine
— oedema, weight gain
— chloasma (skin pigmentation), acne
— spotting, breakthrough bleeding, amenorrhoea
— leucorrhoea, vaginal monilia
— breast engorgement often with suppressed lactation (except with 'mini-pill')
— loss of libido
— post-pill infertility

Interactions

— decreases effect of tricyclic antidepressants, hypoglycaemic agents, vitamins and anticoagulants
— increases theophylline blood levels
— rifampicin, barbiturates, carbamazepine and phenytoin may cause a possible failure of oral contraceptives and increase the incidence of breakthrough bleeding
— ampicillin, co-trimoxazole, tetracyclines may cause failure of oral contraceptives

Nursing points

— recommend a routine of taking the 'pill' at the same time each day so that it is taken regularly
— advise the patient to keep follow-up appointments so that the breasts may be examined and a Papanicolaou (cervical) smear taken
— teach the patient how to examine her own breasts immediately after each 'period'
— advise the patient to check her weight frequently
— advise the patient to report to the medical officer any mental depression, dizziness, blurred vision, leg or chest pain, respiratory distress or unexplained cough, also any vaginal irritation and itching or persistent vaginal bleeding
— advise the patient to contact her medical officer if she has missed taking a dose of the 'pill' or if, despite following the prescribed dose pattern, she has missed two consecutive 'periods'

Note

— heavy smokers run a higher risk of developing venous thrombosis than those who do not smoke
— oestrogens used in oral contraceptives are ethinyloestradiol and mestranol
— progestogens in the combined formulation are norethisterone, norethynodrel, lynoestrenol,

ethynodiol, levonorgestrel and norgestrel
— the progestogen-only preparations contain norethisterone or levonorgestrel

ANTERIOR PITUITARY HORMONES
(trophic hormones)

CORTICOTROPHIN (corticotropin, adrenocorticotrophin, ACTH)

Action

— naturally occurring anterior pituitary hormone which stimulates the adrenal cortex to secrete hydrocortisone, corticosterone and androgens

Use

— diagnostic test for adrenal cortical function
— as for corticosteroids, but not as replacement therapy

Dose

10–200 units IV, IM or SC on designated days

Adverse effects

— as for corticosteroids but causes hypertrophy and not atrophy of adrenal cortex

Nursing points

— dilutions and storage according to manufacturer's literature
— select correct preparation i.e. long-acting forms not for IV use
— stopped gradually to minimize symptoms of hypopituitarism
— see hydrocortisone

TETRACOSACTRIN

— synthetic polypeptide with properties and uses similar to corticotrophin

Dose

i) 0.25 mg as single dose deep IM or IV infusion (diagnosis); OR
ii) 1 mg daily or b.d. deep IM initially reducing to 0.5–1 mg every 2–3 days or 1 mg weekly (therapeutic)

Note

— tetracosactrin zinc phosphate complex is used therapeutically
— shake suspension of 'depot' complex until uniformly cloudy before use

HUMAN CHORIONIC GONADOTROPHIN (HCG)

Use

— improves function of corpus luteum in females
— hypogonadism, cryptorchidism in males

Dose

500–4000 units IM or SC 2–3 times weekly

Note

— preparation obtained from urine of pregnant women.

MENOTROPHIN

Use

— amenorrhoea, infertility in females
— increase spermatogenesis in males.

Dose

determined by medical officer and given IM
usually combined with human chorionic gonadotrophin

Note

— preparation contains follicle stimulating hormone and luteinizing hormone and is obtained from urine of menopausal women
— also prepared from human pituitary gland

SERUM GONADOTROPHIN (PMSG)

Use

— amenorrhoea in females
— infertility in males

Dose

— determined by medical officer and given IM
— usually combined with human chorionic gonadotrophin

Note

— preparation of the gonad-stimulating substance from the serum of pregnant mares

HUMAN GROWTH HORMONE (somatotrophin)

Action

— promotes skeletal, visceral and general body growth
— stimulates protein anabolism
— increases water excretion

Use

— pituitary dwarfism

Note

— choice of patient, dose and management is very specialized

THYROTROPHIN (TSH)

Action

— increases iodine uptake by thyroid
— increases formation and secretion of thyroid hormones

Use

— diagnosis of hypothyroidism
— evaluate thyroid medication
— increases uptake of radio-iodine by thyroid, so of use as adjunct in treatment of certain types of thyroid cancer

POSTERIOR PITUITARY HORMONES

OXYTOCIN

Action

— stimulates uterine contraction
— stimulates lactating breast to eject milk

Use

— induction and maintenance of labour
— control post-partum bleeding and uterine hypotonicity in third stage of labour
— promotes lactation by being effectively absorbed from nasal mucosa

Dose

Induction of labour

5 units diluted in 500 ml 5% glucose and given by IV infusion at 8–40 drops/min adjusted as required

Management of third stage of labour

5–10 units IM or 5 units slowly IV

Post-partum haemorrhage

5–10 units IV or IM

Lactation disorder

— one firm squeeze from upright nasal spray into one or both nostrils 3–5 minutes prior to infant feeding (1 squeeze delivers 2 units)

Adverse effects

— large doses may result in violent uterine contractions leading to uterine rupture and its attendant dangers
— severe hypertension and subarachnoid haemorrhage

Nursing points

— gently rotate IV container to distribute oxytocin evenly in admixture
— oxytocin may be infused via a Y-line infusion
— a burette or micro-drip regulator should be used to deliver the solution to prevent inadvertent overdose
— during infusion, monitor maternal heart rate, blood pressure, strength, duration and frequency of uterine contractions, also foetal heart rate and rhythm
— notify medical officer if contractions become prolonged and unduly strong and be ready to reduce rate or stop infusion
— store ampoules and nasal spray in refrigerator between 2° and 8°C
— protect from light

VASOPRESSIN (antidiuretic hormone, ADH)

Action

— direct antidiuretic action on distal renal tubule by increasing permeability to water reabsorption
— constricts peripheral vessels
— reduces hepatic blood flow and portal venous pressure
— causes contraction of smooth muscle of intestine, gall-bladder and urinary bladder

Use

— symptomatic control of diabetes insipidus
— prevention and control of abdominal distension
— dispelling gas shadows in abdominal X-rays
— occasionally, bleeding oesophageal varices

Dose

i) 0.25–0.5 ml (5–10 pressor units) IM or SC 3- to 4-hourly (aqueous preparation); OR
ii) 0.6–1 ml (3–5 pressor units) IM at 1–3 day intervals as required (tannate in oil preparation)

Adverse effects

— high doses may cause pallor, nausea, abdominal cramp
— water intoxication

Nursing points

— tannate in oil preparation *never* given IV
— ampoule of tannate in oil preparation should be shaken thoroughly and warmed to body temperature before administration
— monitor blood pressure, weight, urinary specific gravity and fluid intake and output
— note and report any chest pain as angina pectoris can result from constriction of coronary arteries
— store preparations in refrigerator between 2° and 8°C

ORNIPRESSIN

Action

— a powerful vasoconstrictor and haemostatic
— a synthetic derivative of vasopressin

Use

— used locally in surgery to produce a bloodless field

Dose

5 units in 20–60 ml isotonic saline depending on the concentration required for the particular type of surgery

Adverse effects

— generalized pallor
— slight rise in blood pressure
— may precipitate anginal symptoms in patients with ischaemic heart disease

DESMOPRESSIN

— as for vasopressin

Adult dose

i) 10–40 micrograms intranasally daily

or in 2 divided doses; OR
ii) 1–4 micrograms IM or IV daily or in 2 divided doses (cranial diabetes insipidus)

Paediatric dose

i) 2.5–20 micrograms intranasally daily or in 2 divided doses; OR
ii) 0.4 micrograms IM or IV daily or in 2 divided doses

Adverse effects

— occasionally, vomiting, headache water intoxication from overhydration

Interactions

— inhibited by glibenclamide

Nursing points

— one end of plastic rhinyle (catheter, supplied) is placed in mouth, the other end in the nostril, the dose delivered by blowing into the nasal cavity (blowing prevents inhaling)

Note

— a synthetic form of vasopressin also known as DDAVP
— used to evaluate renal concentrating capacity
— given to patients with haemophilia or von Willebrand's disease before surgery

LYPRESSIN

— as for vasopressin

Dose

1 firm squeeze from upright nasal spray into each nostril 3–6 times a day (1 squeeze delivers 5 units), repeated 3–7 times daily

Adverse effects

— occasionally, nasal congestion with ulceration of nasal mucosa

OTHER HORMONAL AGENTS

CLOMIPHENE

Action

— stimulates ovulation in some anovulatory women
— possibly acts by stimulating output of pituitary gonadotrophins
— has both oestrogenic and antioestrogenic properties

Use

— stimulate ovulation in infertile women

Dose

50 mg orally daily for 5 days starting on the fifth day of the menstrual cycle (anytime if amenorrhoea) then repeat after 30 days on 5 occasions

Adverse effects

— hot flushes, visual blurring
— reversible ovarian enlargement
— abdominal discomfort

Nursing points

— record weight
— keep basal temperature chart to determine day of ovulation

Note

— the dose may be increased to 100 mg if ovulation does not occur
— the risk of multiple pregnancy is increased when conception takes place during a cycle in which clomiphene has been given

DANAZOL

Action

— inhibits pituitary gonadotrophin
— some androgenic activity

Use

— proven endometriosis
— prophylaxis in hereditary angioedema

Dose

Endometriosis

200 mg orally 2–4 times daily for 3–6 months

Hereditary angioedema

200 mg orally 1–3 times daily

Adverse effects

— oedema, weight gain
— acne, hirsutism, rash, flushing
— oily skin and hair
— deepening of voice
— nausea
— vaginitis

PARATHYROID HORMONE

Action

— releases calcium from bone
— increases calcium absorption from gut
— decreases urinary calcium excretion
— blood calcium level rises in 4 hours

Use

— acute hypoparathyroidism with tetany

Dose

20–40 units 12-hourly usually IM, may be SC or IV

Adverse effects

— weakness, apathy, vomiting, diarrhoea

Interactions

— may enhance activity of oral anticoagulants

Nursing points

— promote non-stimulating environment to reduce frequency of tetanic spasms
— IV calcium gluconate may be given in

— emergency to cover the lag time of 4 hours
— since patients soon become refractory to parathyroid hormone, other treatment will be required e.g. vitamin D preparations

DIHYDROTACHYSTEROL

Action

— raises blood calcium level in the absence of parathyroid hormone and functioning renal tissue

Use

— hypocalcaemia and associated tetany resulting from hypoparathyroidism
— vitamin D-resistant rickets
— osteomalacia following gastrectomy, severe steatorrhoea or renal failure

Dose

i) 6–20 capsules or 3–10 ml of drops orally daily for several days, then 2–14 capsules or 1–7 ml of drops weekly; OR
ii) 2 capsules or 1 ml of drops following thyroid surgery until danger of tetany passed (1 capsule contains 0.125 mg, 1 ml contains 0.25 mg)

Adverse effects

— thirst, anorexia, nausea, vomiting, abdominal cramps, diarrhoea
— headache, tinnitus, dizziness
— polyuria, sweating
— ataxia, psychoses

Note

— may require daily oral calcium lactate or gluconate supplements

CALCITONIN (thyrocalcitonin)

Action

— lowers blood calcium level by decreasing rate of bone resorption and increasing urinary calcium excretion

Use

— Paget's disease (oesteitis deformans)
— hypercalcaemia
— severe juvenille osteoporosis

Dose

Paget's disease

i) 0.5–2 units/kg daily IM or SC initially (porcine calcitonin); OR
ii) 50 units 3 times/week to 100 units daily IM or SC initially (salcatonin); OR
iii) 0.5 mg IM or SC daily for 3 months then 0.5 mg 2–3 times/week as maintenance for 6 months or more

Hypercalcaemia

i) 4 units/kg IM or SC (porcine calcitonin); OR
ii) 50–100 units IV infusion (porcine calcitonin); OR
iii) 400 units IM or SC 6- to 8-hourly (salcatonin)
iv) 0.5 mg IM or SC daily for 3 months then 0.5 mg 2–3 times/week as maintenance for 6 months or more

Adverse effects

— nausea, vomiting

Nursing points

— reconstitute or dilute according to manufacturer's literature
— store salcatonin between 2° and 8°C

Note

— salcatonin is synthetic salmon calcitonin and is much more potent than porcine calcitonin
— treatment may be necessary for 3–6 months

BROMOCRIPTINE

Action

— stimulates dopaminergic receptors in the hypothalamus inhibiting release of prolactin
— suppresses elevated growth hormone levels in acromegaly

Use

— prevent or suppress lactation
— hyperprolactinaemia
— adjunctive therapy in acromegaly
— parkinsonism (see p. 142)

Dose

Lactation inhibition

2.5 mg orally b.d. with food for 14 days initial dose taken 4 hours after delivery if vital signs stable

Hyperprolactinaemia

1.25–2.5 mg orally b.d. or t.d.s. with food

Acromegaly

1.25 mg orally nocte initially then 2.5–7.5 mg t.d.s. or q.i.d. with food

Adverse effects

— nausea, vomiting, dizziness, headache
— postural hypotension, nasal congestion
— drowsiness, depression
— mania, ataxia
— rare, but fatal gastric haemorrhage (acromegaly)
— high doses (more than 15 mg/day) confusion, hallucinations, delirium, psychosis

Nursing points

— advise patient to take initial doses on retiring to reduce the incidence of hypotension and loss of consciousness
— gastric irritation reduced if taken with/or immediately after food.
— warn patient that alcohol may cause nausea, abdominal pain and bloating during bromocriptine therapy
— dosage increases made gradually, usually over 2–3 days to reduce incidence of adverse effects
— warn acromegalic patient to report any gastrointestinal side-effects immediately

— warn patient against driving a vehicle or operating machinery if drowsy
— supine and standing blood pressure checked regularly for postural hypotension
— advise patient to avoid postural hypotension by moving gradually to a sitting or standing position especially after sleep

Note

— female patients receiving bromocriptine for more than 6 months to have regular gynaecological assessment
— treatment for hyperprolactinaemia commonly restores fertility so need for contraception to be considered

GONADORELIN gonadotrophin releasing hormone)

Action

— hypothalamic releasing hormone which stimulates release of follicle stimulating hormone and luteinizing hormone from anterior pituitary lobe

Use

— diagnostic aid in assessing hypothalamic-pituitary-gonadal dysfunction

Dose

100 micrograms SC, IM or IV

Adverse effects

— nausea, abdominal pain
— menorrhagia

Note

— given with protirelin in assessment of pituitary function

PROTIRELIN (thyrotrophin releasing factor)

Action

— hypothalamic releasing hormone

which stimulates release of
thyrotrophin from anterior pituitary
lobe
— has prolactin-releasing activity

Use

— diagnostic aid in assessing
hypothalamic-pituitary-thyroid
dysfunction

Dose

i) 200 micrograms IV; OR
ii) 40 mg orally after fasting

Adverse effects

— following IV injection, nausea,
dizziness, flushing, strange taste,
desire to micturate

Note

— given with gonadorelin in
assessment of pituitary function

SOMATOSTATIN (growth hormone-release-inhibiting hormone)

Action

— hypothalamic release-inhibiting
hormone which inhibits release of
growth hormone from anterior
pituitary lobe
— inhibits secretion of gastrin, insulin
and glucagon

Use

— reduces growth hormone blood
levels in patients with acromegaly

Dose

100 micrograms by IV infusion

7 Drugs acting on the genitourinary system

THIAZIDE DIURETICS

CHLOROTHIAZIDE

Action

— chemically related to sulphonamides
— increases excretion of sodium and chloride ions and water principally in the distal tubule
— increases excretion of potassium ions and bicarbonate
— slight hypotensive effect
— reduces calcium excretion
— paradoxical antidiuretic effect in diabetes insipidus
— onset of action 2 hours, duration 6–12 hours

Use

— oedema
— hypertension
— pre-menstrual tension

Adult dose

Oedema

0.25–1 g orally mane daily or b.d. (mane and midday), later alternate days or on 3–5 days each week

Hypertension

0.5–1 g orally mane daily or b.d. (mane and midday)

Pre-menstrual tension

0.25–0.5 g orally daily or b.d. from the first morning of symptoms until onset of menses.

Paediatric dose

10–30 mg/kg/day orally in 2 doses (250–750 mg/m^2)

Adverse effects

— gastrointestinal disturbances
— dizziness, headache, paraesthesia, weakness, visual disturbances
— blood dyscrasias
— jaundice
— hypersensitivity
— postural hypotension
— hyperglycaemia, glycosuria
— hypokalaemia (drowsiness, weakness)
— hyponatraemia
— photosensitivity
— hyperuricaemia
— electrolyte imbalance (see nursing points)

Interactions

— the risk of hyperglycaemia caused by corticosteroids and diazoxide is increased by chlorothiazide
— toxicity of cardiac glycosides increased by chlorothiazide-induced hypokalaemia
— increases blood lithium levels
— propranolol has an additive effect on thiazide-induced increase in blood urate and triglyceride levels
— postural hypotension enhanced when thiazides taken in conjunction with alcohol, barbiturates, narcotics, other CNS depressants or antihypertensive agents.
— indomethacin reduces effects of chlorothiazide

Nursing points

— taken with or following meals to minimize nausea
— taken early in the day to avoid nocturia
— if b.d., second dose taken around midday
— advise patient of the expected diuresis
— monitor fluid intake and output and patient's weight
— note increase or reduction in oedema
— supine and standing blood pressure checked regularly for postural hypotension
— see clonidine (p. 40) for ways of avoiding postural hypotension
— observe for features of electrolyte imbalance which include anorexia nausea, vomiting, dry mouth, thirst, excessive diuresis, oliguria, weakness, lethargy, hypotension, tachycardia
— observe for features of hypokalaemia (drowsiness, muscle weakness and cramps, paraesthesia) in patients on digitalis therapy as this may cause digitalis toxicity
— encourage high-potassium foods if prolonged high dose therapy, e.g. apricots, avocados, bananas, cantaloupe, dates, grapefruit, oranges, prunes, raisins, strawberries, watermelon, also orange, grapefruit, prune and pineapple juice
— note instability in diabetics

Note

— may need potassium supplement during prolonged therapy
— used alone or in conjunction with the antihypertensives methyldopa or timolol
— nursing mothers taking thiazides should not breast feed their infants

BENDROFLUAZIDE

— as for chlorothiazide but effective for 18 hours

Dose

Oedema

5–10 mg orally mane daily or alternate days then 5–10 mg mane 3 times/week

Hypertension

2.5–10 mg orally mane daily then 2.5–5 mg mane daily

CHLORTHALIDONE

— as for chlorothiazide but effective for 48–72 hours

Adult dose

Oedema

50–200 mg orally mane daily then 50 mg mane daily or 100 mg mane 3 times/week

Hypertension

25 mg orally mane daily

Paediatric dose

2 mg/kg orally mane 3 times/week

Note

— combined with atenolol for antihypertensive effect (see p. 54)

CLOPAMIDE

— as for chlorothiazide but effective for 24 hours

Dose

Oedema

40–80 mg orally mane daily then 10–20 mg daily or 20 mg alternate days

Hypertension

20–40 mg orally mane daily then 5–20 mg daily

Note

— combined with pindolol for antihypertensive effect (see p. 55)

CLOREXOLONE

— as for chlorothiazide but effective for 24–48 hours

Dose

Oedema

i) 25–100 mg orally mane daily or alternate days; OR
ii) 10 mg orally mane daily or 25 mg 3 times/week (premenstrual syndrome)

Hypertension

i) 10 mg orally mane daily or b.d.; OR
ii) 25 mg orally mane daily

Diabetes insipidus

10–20 mg orally mane daily

CYCLOPENTHIAZIDE

— as for chlorothiazide (p. 177)

Dose

i) 0.5–1 mg orally mane daily reducing to 0.25–0.5 mg daily or 0.5 mg on alternate days (oedema); OR
ii) 0.25–0.5 mg orally mane daily (hypertension)

HYDROCHLOROTHIAZIDE

— as for chlorothiazide (p. 177) but effective in smaller doses

Dose

Oedema

50–100 mg mane daily or b.d. May also be given on alternate days or 3–5 times/week

Hypertension

25–50 mg daily or b.d.

HYDROCHLOROTHIAZIDE WITH AMILORIDE

The potassium-conserving agent amiloride enhances the natriuretic and diuretic effect of hydrochlorothiazide but prevents excessive potassium loss thereby eliminating the need for a potassium supplement

Dose

1 tablet mane daily gradually increasing to·2 tablets b.d. if required

Note

Hyperkalaemia can occur (blood level over 5.5 mmol/1) so watch for fatigue, muscular weakness, flaccid paralysis of extremities, paraesthesia, bradycardia, shock or ECG changes

HYDROCHLOROTHIAZIDE WITH TRIAMTERENE

— as for hydrochlorothiazide with amiloride

Dose

Oedema

1–2 tablets b.d. p.c. reducing to 1 tablet mane daily or alternate days

Hypertension

1–2 tablets b.d. p.c. then adjusted as required

MEFRUSIDE

— as for chlorothiazide (p. 177) with some structural similarity to frusemide

Dose

25–100 mg mane daily then 25–50 mg on alternate days

METHYCLOTHIAZIDE

— as for chlorothiazide (p. 177) but effective for 24 hours

Dose

Oedema

2.5–10 mg mane daily then 2.5–5 mg mane daily

Hypertension

2.5–5 mg mane daily

METOLAZONE

— as for chlorothiazide (p. 177) but effective for 24 hours and excretes less potassium

Dose

Oedema

5–20 mg orally mane daily then at intervals of 2–3 days as maintenance

Hypertension

2.5–5 mg orally mane daily for 3–4 weeks then reduced or given on alternate days as maintenance

QUINETHAZONE

— as for chlorothiazide (p. 177) but effective for 24 hours

Dose

50–100 mg orally daily or b.d.

INDAPAMIDE

— as for chlorothiazide (p. 177) but effective for 36 hours

Dose

2.5mg orally mane daily

HIGH-CEILING (LOOP) DIURETICS

FRUSEMIDE (known as furosemide in USA)

Action

— potent diuretic which inhibits sodium, potassium and chloride reabsorption in the proximal and distal renal convoluted tubules, but mainly in the ascending loop of Henle
— oral dose effective within 1 hour and lasts for 4 hours
— IM dose effective within 10–15 minutes (IV, 5 minutes) IM and IV doses having a duration of 2 hours

Use

— cardiac, hepatic, renal, cerebral and pulmonary oedema
— acute and chronic renal failure
— nephrotic syndrome
— mild, moderate hypertension

Adult dose

i) 20–80 mg orally daily, b.d. or alternate days; OR
ii) 20–40 mg IM or slow IV injection or infusion repeated as required.
iii) 500 mg daily (chronic renal failure)

Paediatric dose

i) 1–5 mg/kg/day (20–100 mg/m^2/day) as single daily morning oral dose up to a maximum of 40 mg; OR
ii) 0.5–1 mg/kg/dose IM or IV

Adverse effects

— anorexia, thirst, drowsiness, dizziness
— fatigue, leg muscle cramps
— hyponatraemia, hypovolaemia
— hypokalaemia, hyperuricaemia
— hyperglycaemia
— rash, blood dyscrasias
— anaphylaxis after parenteral administration
— tinnitus and deafness in presence of renal insufficiency

Interactions

— effects of antihypertensive agents enhanced
— risk of toxicity of cardiac glycosides increased by frusemide-induced hypokalaemia
— ototoxicity of aminoglycosides increased when given with frusemide in presence of renal failure (conflicting reports on effect on gentamicin blood level, therefore not given in combination)
— blood levels of cephaloridine and beta-adrenoceptor blocking agents increased
— phenobarbitone, phenytoin and indomethacin reduce effects of frusemide
— increases risk of salicylate toxicity if high dose salicylate therapy
— may result in excessive potassium loss when given with corticosteroids

Nursing points

— not mixed with other drugs for injection or infusion
— add only to isotonic saline or compound sodium lactate for infusion
— maximum injection and infusion rate 4 mg/min to avoid hearing impairment
— monitor vital signs if given parenterally
— have available adrenaline, noradrenaline, isoprenaline and IV corticosteroids
— watch for dehydration especially in hot weather
— taken early in the day to avoid nocturia
— if b.d., second dose taken around midday
— advise patient of the expected diuresis
— monitor fluid intake and output and patient's weight
— note increases or reduction in oedema
— observe for features of electrolyte imbalance which include anorexia, nausea, vomiting, dry mouth, thirst, excessive diuresis, oliguria, lethargy, hypotension, tachycardia
— observe for features of hypokalaemia (drowsiness, muscle weakness and cramps, paraesthesia) in patients on digitalis therapy as this may cause digitalis toxicity
— encourage high-potassium foods if prolonged high dose therapy, e.g. apricots, avocados, bananas, cantaloupe, dates, grapefruit, oranges, prunes, raisins, strawberries, watermelon, also orange, grapefruit, prune and pineapple juice
— note instability in diabetics

Note

— in renal failure, large doses given in form of Lasix High Dose® and Urex Forte®

BUMETANIDE

— as for frusemide

Dose

i) 1 mg orally mane daily; OR
ii) 1 mg orally mane and midday daily; OR
iii) 1 mg IM or IV

Adverse effects

— fluid and electrolyte imbalance
— dizziness
— nausea, vomiting, abdominal discomfort
— rash, blood dyscrasias
— muscle cramps (severe with high dose)
— gynaecomastia

Interactions

— increases blood levels and toxicity of lithium

Note

— may require up to 20 mg/day

ETHACRYNIC ACID

— as for frusemide (p. 180) and chlorothiazide (p. 177)

Dose

50–150 mg orally daily or alternate days after breakfast up to a maximum of 400 mg/day

Note

— drug ceased immediately if profuse watery diarrhoea

ALDOSTERONE INHIBITOR DIURETIC

SPIRONOLACTONE
Action

— competitive inhibitor of aldosterone in distal renal tubule
— increases sodium and water excretion but decreases potassium excretion
— takes 3 days for maximum response and effect lasts 3 days after discontinuation

Use

— oedema and ascites associated with congestive cardiac failure, hepatic cirrhosis, nephrotic syndrome and hyperaldosteronism
— hypertension associated with hyperaldosteronism
— diagnosis and treatment of hyperaldosteronism
— adjunctive therapy in myasthenia gravis and malignant hypertension

Adult dose

25–100 mg orally 2–4 times daily with or immediately after food

Paediatric dose

1.5–3 mg/kg/day in divided doses mainly in patients with hepatic insufficiency

Adverse effects (high doses)

— mental confusion, drowsiness, headache
— rash
— abdominal pain
— hyponatraemia (tachycardia, hypotension, oliguria)
— hyperkalaemia (confusion, weakness, paraesthesia)
— hirsuitism, menstrual disturbances, deepening of voice
— gynaecomastia, impotence

Interactions

— inhibits gastric ulcer healing properties of carbenoxolone
— sodium excretion effect inhibited by aspirin
— reduces effect of warfarin
— increases blood digoxin levels
— hyperkalaemia may occur if spironolactone given with potassium supplements

Nursing points

— taken with food or immediately after to increase absorption
— advise patient that diuresis occurs 2–3 days after drug commenced and will continue 2–3 days after drug stopped
— monitor fluid intake, output and weight
— note increase or decrease in oedema
— check blood pressure at outset then regularly during therapy
— advise patient to avoid high potassium foods (see chlorothiazide (p. 177)) once hypokalaemia corrected
— observe for features of hyponatraemia and hyperkalaemia

OSMOTIC DIURETIC

MANNITOL

Action

— raises osmotic pressure of glomerular filtrate producing an osmotic diuresis by inhibiting tubular reabsorption of solutes and water
— excreted rapidly by kidneys
— increases plasma osmolality

Use

— promote renal function after severe injury or surgery
— reduce intracranial and intraocular pressure
— salicylate, barbiturate and bromide overdose
— measure glomerular filtration rate

Adult dose

50–200 g/day IV infusion

Paediatric dose

IV infusion over 30 minutes
under 2 years: 0.5–1 g/kg
over 2 years: 0.25–0.5 g/kg

Adverse effects

— fluid and electrolyte imbalance
— marked diuresis, urinary retention
— hypotension, hypertension
— tachycardia
— nausea, vomiting, thirst
— headache, dizziness, blurred vision
— rash

Nursing points

— crystals which may have formed in the 20% supersaturated solution may be redissolved by warming the bottle to about 50°C in a water bath then allowing to cool to body temperature before administration
— infusion rate regulated to maintain a urine output of 30–50 ml/hr or as directed

— monitor vital signs during infusion noting changes in heart and respiratory rate and blood pressure
— monitor fluid intake and output carefully noting signs of circulatory overload or excessive diuresis

POTASSIUM-SPARING DIURETICS

AMILORIDE

Action

— increases excretion of sodium, chloride and water in the distal renal tubule but conserves potassium
— effective in about 2 hours with a duration of 24 hours

Use

— mainly in conjunction with thiazides or other more potent diuretics to conserve potassium
— oedema

Dose

5–10 mg orally mane daily or b.d.

Adverse effects

— fluid and electrolyte imbalance
— thirst, dizziness, muscle cramp
— nausea, vomiting, diarrhoea or constipation
— postural hypotension
— hyponatraemia, hyperkalaemia
— rash
— hyponatraemia and hypokalaemia if used with other oral diuretics

Interactions

— hyperkalaemia may occur if amiloride given with potassium supplement

Nursing points

— taken with or immediately after food to minimize nausea
— taken early in day to avoid nocturia
— advise patient of expected diuresis
— monitor fluid intake, output and patient's weight
— advise patient to avoid high potassium foods (see chlorothiazide p. 177) once hypokalaemia corrected
— observe for features of hyponatraemia and hyperkalaemia

Note

— not given with other potassium-sparing diuretics

AMILORIDE WITH HYDROCHLOROTHIAZIDE

— see hydrochlorothiazide with amiloride (p. 179)

TRIAMTERENE

— as for amiloride

Dose

100 mg orally daily, b.d. or alternate days

Note

— may stain urine blue

TRIAMTERENE WITH HYDROCHLOROTHIAZIDE

— see hydrochlorothiazide with triamterene (p. 179)

URINARY ALKALINIZING AGENTS

Action and use

— enhances the action of clindamycin, erythromycin, gentamicin, lincomycin, streptomycin and the sulphonamides
— discourages growth of some micro-organisms e.g. *E. coli*
— increases excretion of some drugs e.g. salicylates, barbiturates
— reduces crystalluria by increasing the solubility of sulphonamides and uric acid in urine
— relieves dysuria in cystitis

Preparations and dose

SODIUM ACID CITRATE
Adult dose

40 ml orally q.i.d.

Paediatric dose

2–6 years: 5 ml orally 4–5 times daily
6–12 years: 10–15 ml orally 3–4 times daily

SODIUM BICARBONATE
Dose

1 capsule (840 mg) daily increasing as required

Note

— used in chronic renal failure as a bicarbonate source
— enhances the excretion of methotrexate

SODIUM CITROTARTRATE
Adult dose

4–8 g (1–2 teaspoonsful) in half a glass of cold water t.d.s. or q.i.d.

Paediatric dose

2–4 g ($\frac{1}{2}$–1 teaspoonful) in half a glass of cold water t.d.s.

Interactions of alkalinizing agents

— sodium citrate, sodium citrotartrate
and sodium bicarbonate reduce
doxycycline blood levels, reduce
activity of hexamine by making urine
alkaline and enhance the effects of
dexamphetamine, fenfluramine,
quinidine and pseudoephedrine
— sodium bicarbonate reduces
absorption of oral iron and
tetracycline and increases blood
levels of mexiletine, methadone and
diethylcarbamazine

PARASYMPATHOMIMETICS

BETHANECOL

Action

— a parasympathomimetic agent which
produces the effects of stimulation
of the parasympathetic nervous
system, but is not inactivated by
acetylcholinesterase
— produces rapid but transitory increase
in tone and motility of the urinary
bladder, stomach and intestine
— oral dose effective within 30–60
minutes and persists for about an
hour
— SC dose effective within 5–15
minutes and persists for about 2
hours

Use

— post-operative and post-partum
urinary retention (non-obstructive)
— neurogenic atony of urinary bladder
with retention
— post-operative abdominal distention
— reduce anticholinergic side effects of
tricyclic antidepressants

Dose

i) 5–30 mg orally 3 or 4 times daily
a.c.; OR
ii) 2.5–5 mg SC repeated at 15- to 30-
minute intervals to a maximum of 4
doses until satisfactory response

Adverse effects

— salivation, sweating, flushing
— nausea, abdominal discomfort
— high dose, colicky abdominal pain,
hypotension

Nursing points

— taken on an empty stomach to
prevent nausea and vomiting
— aspirate before giving SC injection to
ensure not in blood vessel to avoid
severe cholinergic (parasympathetic)
stimulation

— a small test dose may be given to check response
— monitor heart rate and blood pressure if high dose or SC dose
— monitor fluid intake and output
— have atropine available

ANTISPASMODIC AGENT

FLAVOXATE

Action

— smooth muscle relaxant

Use

— dysuria, frequency, urgency, nocturia, incontinence
— cystitis, prostatitis, urethritis

Dose

100–200 mg orally t.d.s.

Adverse effects

— nausea, vomiting, dry mouth
— drowsiness, vertigo, confusion, visual disturbances
— increased intraocular pressure
— anaphylactic shock, blood dyscrasias (rare)

Nursing points

— no other drugs 1 hour before or after flavoxate to avoid interference with their absorption
— warn patient against driving a vehicle or operating machinery if drowsy

ION-EXCHANGE RESINS

SODIUM POLYSTYRENE SULPHONATE

Action

— cation exchange resin
— removes potassium ions from body by exchanging sodium ions for potassium ions in the large intestine

Use

— hyperkalaemia mainly associated with acute renal failure

Dose

i) 15 g orally as a suspension in 100 ml water 3 or 4 times daily; OR
ii) 30 g mixed with 10% glucose and/or water up to 200 ml as retention enema daily or b.d.

Adverse effects

— gastrointestinal disturbances
— faecal impaction

Nursing points

— not given in fruit juices which have a high potassium content
— observe for features of electrolyte imbalance which include anorexia, nausea, vomiting, dry mouth, thirst, excessive diuresis, oliguria, weakness, lethargy, hypotension, tachycardia
— a mild laxative would relieve constipation and avoid faecal impaction

Note

— small amounts of magnesium and calcium ions can be lost during therapy along with potassium ions
— treatment stopped when potassium blood level falls to 5 mmol/l

SODIUM CELLULOSE PHOSPHATE

Action

— binds dietary calcium ions within intestines reducing amount of calcium available for absorption so decreasing urinary calcium excretion

Use

— calciuria associated with recurrent calcium-containing renal calculi

Dose

5 g t.d.s. in half a glass of cold water or sprinkled onto food

Adverse effects

— diarrhoea
— hyperoxaluria

Interactions

— take 2 hours apart from dietary mineral supplements so mineral absorption not reduced

Nursing points

— as daily sodium intake is increased, monitor for hypertension, weight gain and clinical features of cardiac disease

Note

— used in conjunction with restricted calcium diet (not more than 400–600 mg calcium per day)
— avoid vitamin C supplements during treatment to prevent hyperoxalaemia
— magnesium gluconate supplement is recommended during prolonged therapy

PHOSPHATE BINDING AGENT

ALUMINIUM HYDROXIDE

Action and use

— reduces blood phosphate levels in patients with renal failure by binding dietary phosphate in the bowel and preventing its absorption

Adult dose

600–1200 mg orally q.i.d. (tablets)

Paediatric dose

i) 300–1200 mg orally 2 to 4 times daily; OR
ii) 5–20 ml (320 mg/5 ml) in water orally 3 to 4 times daily (gel); OR
iii) 300–1200 mg 2–4 times daily (tablets)

Adverse effects

— constipation

Interactions

— reduces absorption of tetracyclines, chlorpromazine, digoxin, chlordiazepoxide, ethambutol, salicylic acid, indomethacin, propranolol, cimetidine, ranitidine and oral iron compounds

Nursing point

— if constipation occurs, discontinue medication and consult medical officer

URINARY TRACT ANALGESIC

PHENAZOPYRIDINE

Action

— exerts topical analgesic effect on urinary tract mucosa

Use

— symptomatic relief of pain, burning, frequency or urgency arising from irritation of urinary tract mucosa

Dose

200 mg orally t.d.s. p.c.

Adverse effects

— gastrointestinal disturbances (occasionally)

Nursing points

— inform patient that the urine will acquire a harmless reddish-orange discolouration
— stains to clothing removed while fresh

URINARY ANTISEPTICS

HEXAMINE MANDELATE

Action and use

— yields formaldehyde which is bactericidal
— acidifies urine which is bacteriostatic
— used as urinary antiseptic in long term treatment of chronic or recurrent urinary tract infections

Dose

1 g orally q.i.d.

Adverse effects

— occasionally, nausea, dyspepsia, rash

Interactions

— effects reduced when combined with alkalinizing agents and sulphonamides
— ascorbic acid or ammonium chloride increase acidification of urine

Note

— only active if urinary pH less than 6, therefore check pH frequently
— not given with sulphonamides to avoid crystalluria

HEXAMINE HIPPURATE

— as for hexamine mandelate

Dose

1 g orally b.d.

AMMONIUM CHLORIDE

Action

— absorbed from gastrointestinal tract and converted to urea in the liver with the release of hydrogen and chloride ions which cause a mild metabolic acidosis resulting in a reduced urinary pH and a transient diuresis

— aids excretion of basic drugs
— effective for only a few days

Use

— urinary tract infections when low urinary pH required
— correct hypochloraemic alkalosis
— promote excretion of basic drugs

Dose

500 mg orally b.d. or t.d.s. p.c.

Adverse effects

— high doses, nausea, vomiting, thirst, headache, hyperventilation, drowsiness, acidosis, hypokalaemia

Interactions

— reduces blood levels of mexiletine, methadone and diethylcarbamazine

Nursing points

— check urinary pH and specific gravity frequently
— note dyspnoea, increase in respiratory rate

Note

— bacterial growth in urine usually inhibited when pH falls below 5.5

TOPICAL URINARY ANTISEPTIC

SODIUM OXYCHLOROSENE

Action

— a topical chlorine-releasing germicidal compound useful for local infections
— dissolves necrotic tissue

Use

— urinary bladder instillation for interstitial cystitis

Administration

— 1 treatment every 5–7 days
— each treatment consists of 2–3 instillations at intervals of several minutes
— bladder filled to maximum tolerated capacity and retained for a maximum of 3 minutes

Adverse effects

— instillation of 0.2% solution into the bladder frequently causes severe discomfort, bladder irritation and soreness of pubic region for 12–48 hours
— post-irrigation chills, fever, macroscopic haematuria
— intolerance to therapy

Nursing points

— reconstitute 2 g of powder with 2 litres of sterile cool or lukewarm water or isotonic saline (0.1% solution) or with 1 litre (0.2% solution)
— mix contents thoroughly for 2 minutes, allow to stand 2–3 minutes, then mix for further 2–3 minutes
— not mixed with other solutions
— 0.1% solution used initially to avoid severe discomfort, 0.2% solution used subsequently
— solution retained in bladder for a maximum of 3 minutes, as longer contact with bladder wall inactivates the solution
— compound more effective when pH 6–7

URINARY TRACT INFECTIONS

See specific anti-infective agents amoxycillin, cephalexin, gentamicin, nalidixic acid, nitrofurantoin, norfloxacin, trimethoprim with or without sulphamethoxazole

CHELATING AGENT

See penicillamine

DRUGS ACTING ON THE UTERUS

ERGOMETRINE MALEATE

Action

— causes firm prolonged uterine contraction
— effective within 2–3 minutes IM (6–15 minutes orally) and lasts for 2–3 hours

Use

— prevent or reduce post partum and postabortal haemorrhage as a result of uterine atony

Dose

i) 0.2–0.4 mg IM after infant born; OR
ii) 0.2 mg IV in emergency; OR
iii) 0.2–0.4 mg orally 6- to 12-hourly for about 48 hours after delivery

Adverse effects

— nausea, vomiting
— increased blood pressure (rare)

Nursing points

— IM ergometrine immediately infant born will cause uterine contraction, separation of placenta and prevent blood loss
— monitor pulse, blood pressure and uterine state frequently post partum for about 2 hours
— ergometrine 0.25 mg is given in some centres IV after infant born but not if mother is pre-eclamptic or has a cardiac condition

Note

— not to be confused with ergotamine

ERGOMETRINE MALEATE WITH OXYTOCIN

Action

— combines rapid oxytocic properties of oxytocin and the more sustained oxytocic action of ergometrine

Use

— management of third stage of labour
— prevention and treatment of post-partum haemorrhage

Dose

1 ml IM at birth of anterior shoulder

Note

— ergometrine maleate 0.5 mg with 5 units of oxytocin in each ml

OXYTOCIN

— see posterior pituitary hormones (p. 171)

RITODRINE

Action

— selective β_2 adrenoceptor stimulant
— uterine muscle relaxant

Use

— inhibition of premature labour
— inhibition of uterine contractions for the relief of acute foetal distress resulting from either extreme uterine contraction or compression of the umbilical cord

Dose

— dilution according to manufacturer's literature
— IV infusion rate as ordered by medical officer
— a burette or microdrip regulator should be in the infusion line for close control
— oral administration of 10–20 mg 4- to 6-hourly may be commenced 30 minutes before ceasing IV infusion

Adverse effects

— maternal sinus tachycardia, palpitation, hypotension, nausea, vomiting, hand tremors
— foetal tachycardia

Nursing points

— monitor maternal heart rate, blood pressure and uterine contraction frequency, duration and intensity frequently, reporting heart rate over 135 beats/min
— monitor foetal heart rate frequently
— to prevent hypotension due to aortocaval compression, the patient should lie on her left side during ritodrine infusion

Note

— continued for 12–48 hours after contractions cease

SALBUTAMOL

— see bronchodilators, sympathomimetic (p. 71)

DINOPROST TROMETAMOL
(PROSTAGLANDIN F_2 alpha)

Action

— causes uterine contraction (oxytocic action)

Use

— therapeutic termination of pregnancy during the first or second trimester
— missed abortion
— hydatidiform mole
— foetal death *in utero*

Dose

the medical officer injects the suitably diluted product into the uterus, transabdominally, or occasionally via the extra-amniotic route through the cervix, after establishing the foetal size using ultrasound equipment

Adverse effects

— nausea, vomiting, diarrhoea
— transient flushing, shivering, headache and dizziness
— rarely, convulsions, bronchospasm

Nursing points

— note and report the onset of uterine contractions
— an IV infusion of oxytocin is commenced once uterine contractions are evident
— stored in a refrigerator at less than 8°C, but not frozen

Note

— laminaria, a type of seaweed is introduced into the vagina the evening prior to induction to 'ripen the cervix'

DINOPROSTONE (PROSTAGLANDIN E_2)

— as for dinoprost trometamol

MAGNESIUM SULPHATE
Action

— when given IV, depresses CNS and abolishes uterine contractions

Use

— prevention of premature labour

Dose

4–6 g diluted in at least 250 ml of 5% glucose and given by IV infusion over 15–20 minutes, then 1–3 g/hr

Adverse effects

— thirst, flushing, hypotension, cardiac arrhythmias
— drowsiness, loss of tendon reflexes, weakness, respiratory depression
— coma, cardiac arrest

Note

— hypermagnesaemia may be corrected by 10–20 ml of 10% calcium gluconate IV

VAGINAL ANTI-INFECTIVE AGENTS

Introduced into the vagina to treat infections caused by bacteria, fungi and protozoa.

Agents

amphotericin, bacitracin, clotrimazole, dequalinium, diiodohydroxyquinoline, econazole, hydrargaphen, isoconazole, miconazole, neomycin, nystatin, oxyquinoline, povidine-iodine, sulphabenzamide, sulphacetamide, sulphathiazole

VAGINAL HORMONAL AGENTS

Introduced into the vagina to treat senile vaginitis, vulvitis and kraurosis vulvae.

Agents

dienoestrol, conjugated oestrogens, oestrone

Nursing points for vaginal preparations

— the medication may be in the form of ovules, vaginal tablets, foaming vaginal tablets, pessaries, foaming pessaries, cream pessaries and cream, all of which need applicators except ovules
— applicator only used during pregnancy on advice of medical officer
— draw patients attention to the instruction leaflet accompanying the preparation
— show the patient how to load the applicator and to insert it into the vagina in an upward and backward direction
— most preparations can be introduced deep into the vagina in the dorsal or in a squatting position
— creams and foaming preparations are best introduced in the dorsal position, the patient remaining recumbent for 10 minutes
— advise the patient on hygiene and storage of applicator after use
— advise the patient to continue treatment through menstruation unless otherwise instructed by the medical officer
— pessary preparations to be stored below 15°C

Note

— acetic acid and/or lactic acid are used in some formulations to restore vaginal acidity

8 Anti-infective agents

HAZARDS OF THERAPY

— development of resistant strains of microorganisms
— severe gastrointestinal irritation
— superinfection
— allergy and hypersensitivity reaction

THE NURSE'S ROLE

Reduce the chance of resistant strains of micro-organisms developing

— maintain activity of drug by correct storage conditions and correct reconstitution procedures according to the manufacturer's literature or check with pharmacist
— ensure adequate dose given
— ensure administration at regular intervals to maintain adequate blood drug concentration
— maintain asepsis where required during patient care
— ensure that drugs are handled carefully to avoid spillage and spraying into the air
— ensure course completed, usually 7–10 days
— discourage self-medication of anti-infective agents

Adverse reactions

— note and report gastrointestinal disturbances, especially diarrhoea
— note and report signs of superinfection, such as stomatitis, 'black tongue' and diarrhoea
— if patient receiving anti-infective therapy is breast-feeding, check if alternative feeding method necessary to prevent adverse effects in the infant

Superinfection (suprainfection)

— overgrowth by non-susceptible microorganisms, e.g. *Candida albicans* during antibiotic therapy
— more common with the use of broad spectrum antibiotics which eliminate more of the natural microbial flora
— diarrhoea can be a symptom of superinfection in the bowel

Allergy and hypersensitivity

— note if history of allergy, cross-allergy and hypersensitivity; then after adminisration of drugs, especially penicillins, cephalosporins and streptomycin, absderve closely for bronchospasm, urticarial rash, cardiovascular collapse or angioneurotic oedema

Intravenous administration of anti-infective agents

— reconstitute dry powders with Water for Injection
— the recommended method of administration is by slow infusion which is prepared by diluting the reconstituted drug in 50–100 ml of compatible infusion fluid and infusing over 30 minutes via a burette
— where a slow bolus injection is necessary, the drug is reconstituted with or diluted to 10–20 ml in Water for Injection and injected over 1–3 minutes into the side arm (injection port) of a flowing administration set
— consult manufacturer's literature for detailed information

PENICILLINS

Action

— selectively suppress the formation of
  a rigid bacterial cell wall
— high internal osmotic pressure results
  in cell rupture and lysis
— bactericidal

Preparations and dose

BENZYLPENICILLIN (pencillin G,
crystalline penicillin)

300–900 mg 6-hourly IM, IV injection or
infusion

Note

— active against most Gram-positive,
  some Gram-negative bacteria and
  some spirochaetes
— not acid stable
— not penicillinase resistant
— much higher doses can be given for
  serious infections
— 1 megaunit (1 Mu) is equivalent to
  600 mg (mega means million)
— gives high blood levels quickly

PROCAINE PENICILLIN

i) 1–1.5 g IM daily; OR
ii) 4.8 g as single IM dose (gonorrhoea)

Note

— must NOT be given IV
— slowly absorbed and maintains
  antibacterial blood levels for up to
  24 hours but level reached lower
  than for benzyl penicillin
— may be given with probenecid 1 g to
  increase and prolong penicillin blood
  level

BENZATHINE PENICILLIN

Syphilis

i) 1.8 g as single deep IM injection; OR
ii) 1.8 g deeply IM weekly for 3 weeks

Prophylaxis

i) 0.9 g deeply IM once each month; OR
ii) 0.45 g deeply IM evey 2 weeks

Note

— used for syphilis, the dose depending
  on the stage
— used for prophylaxis in rheumatic
  fever, rheumatic heart disease and
  acute glomerulonephritis
— swirl container to resuspend
  contents (do not shake vigorously)

BENZATHINE PENICILLIN WITH PROCAINE PENICILLIN AND POTASSIUM PENICILLIN

Adult dose

i) 2.4 mega units deeply IM (1.2 into
   each buttock) twice weekly for 5
   injections (syphilis); OR
ii) 1.2 mega units deeply IM for 2 or 3
    injections at 48 hour intervals

Paediatric dose

1.2 mega units deeply IM repeated after
24 hours

Note

— after a single IM injection,
  therapeutic blood levels persist up to
  10 days
— suspension prepared with 2 ml
  diluent supplied
— also used for prophylaxis in
  rheumatic fever, rheumatic heart
  disease and acute glomerulonephritis

PHENOXYMETHYLPENICILLIN
(penicillin V)

i) 250–500 mg orally 4- to 6-hourly 1
   hour a.c.; OR
ii) 250 mg orally b.d. 1 hour a.c.
    (prophylaxis)

Note

— also used for prophylaxis in
  rheumatic fever, rheumatic heart

disease and acute glomerulonephritis
— not penicillinase resistant
— acid stable

PHENETHICILLIN

i) 250–500 mg orally 6-hourly 1 hour
a.c.; OR
ii) 2 g orally ½–1 hour before procedure,
then 500 mg orally 6-hourly for 8
doses (prophylaxis)

Note

— acid stable

CLOXACILLIN

i) 250–500 mg orally 6-hourly 1 hour
a.c.; OR
ii) 500 mg 4- to 6-hourly IM, IV injection
or infusion (dilutions according to
manufacturer's literature)

Note

— may also be given by intrathecal,
intrapleural or intra-articular injection
— acid stable and penicillinase resistant

FLUCLOXACILLIN

i) 250 mg orally 6-hourly 1 hour a.c.; OR
ii) 250 mg IM 6-hourly; OR
iii) 250 mg–1.0 g 6-hourly IM, IV
injection or infusion (dilutions
according to manufacturer's literature)

Note

— may also be given by intrapleural or
intra-articular injection
— acid stable and penicillinase resistant

MEZLOCILLIN

i) 2 g made up to 20 ml and injected
slowly IV over 3–5 minutes 8-hourly;
OR
ii) 5 g made up to 50 ml and infused IV
over 30 minutes 8-hourly

Note

— not penicillinase resistant
— the prepared solution may show a
harmless yellowish tinge

AMPICILLIN

i) 250–500 mg orally 6-hourly 1 hour
a.c.; OR
ii) 250–500 mg IM 4- to 6-hourly; OR
iii) 250–500 mg 4-hourly IV injection or
infusion
iv) 3.5 g as single oral dose (gonorrhoea)

Note

— may also be given by intrathecal, intraperitoneal, intrapleural or intra-articular injection
— dilutions according to manufacturer's literature
— broad spectrum, acid stable penicillin
— not penicillinase resistant
— may be given with probenecid 1 g to increase and prolong penicillin blood level
— may cause failure of oral contraceptives

AMOXYCILLIN

i) 250–500 mg orally 6- to 8-hourly; OR
ii) 3 g as single oral dose (gonorrhoea); OR
iii) 250–500 mg IM 6- to 8-hourly, OR
iv) 1 g 6- to 8-hourly IV injection or infusion (dilutions according to manufacturer's literature)

Note

— select correct syrup concentration
— doses over 500 mg not given as single IM injection
— a transient pink colouration or slight opalescence may appear during reconstitution
— add the 3 g dispersible tablet to 40–50 ml of water, swirl until dispersed and take immediately
— broad spectrum, acid stable penicillin
— not penicillinase resistant
— may be given with probenecid 1 g to increase and prolong penicillin blood level

AMOXYCILLIN WITH CLAVULANIC ACID

250–500 mg orally t.d.s. p.c. (dose calculated on amoxycillin content)

Note

— each tablet contains 250 mg of amoxycillin and 125 mg clavulanic acid or 500 mg of amoxycillin and 125 mg of clavulanic acid

— clavulanic acid is a potent inhibitor of penicillinase (β-lactamase), so enhances the activity of penicillins and cephalosporins against many resistant strains

PIPERACILLIN

i) 2–3 g IM or slowly IV 6- to 12-hourly; OR
ii) 3–4 g by IV infusion 4-, 6- or 8-hourly; OR
iii) 2 g as single IM dose (gonorrhoea)

Note

— not more than 2 g given into single IM injection site
— IM injection given deeply into buttocks
— pain of IM injection may be reduced by adding lignocaine (without adrenaline) when reconstituting drug (see manufacturer's literature)
— may be used as combined therapy with an aminoglycoside or cephalosporin in certain life-threatening infections but NOT mixed in the same solution
— broad spectrum antibiotic
— not penicillinase resistant except against gonococci

TICARCILLIN

i) 1–3 g IM or slowly IV 6-hourly; OR
ii) 150–300 mg/kg/24 hours by continuous IV infusion or in divided doses by intermittent injection or infusion at 3-, 4- or 6-hourly intervals

Note

— broad spectrum penicillin
— not penicillinase resistant
— see note under piperacillin

AZLOCILLIN

i) based on 225 mg/kg/24 hours under 40 kg and 80–200 mg/kg/24 hours over 40 kg in 2 or 3 divided doses IV; OR
ii) 3 g IV after each haemodialysis, then 12-hourly

Interactions

— incompatible in the same solution with cephalosporins, prednisolone, tetracyclines, aminoglycosides, suxamethonium, procaine

Note

— reconstituted with water for injection 10 ml per gram
— use freshly prepared solutions but can be stored for at least 6 hours at not more than 25°C

Adverse effects of penicillins

— glossitis, stomatitis
— allergic reactions, rash, fever, serum sickness
— may impair blood coagulation
— anaphylactic shock (rare)
— convulsions (very high dose)
— after oral administration, transient diarrhoea, occasional nausea and pruritus ani

Interactions

— penicillins affect stability of anticoagulant control
— probenecid increases and prolongs penicillin blood levels
— effect of penicillins is reduced by the bacteriostatic agents chloramphenicol, erythromycin and the tetracyclines
— oral neomycin reduces phenoxymethyl penicillin blood levels
— incidence of skin rash with ampicillin or amoxycillin increased when combined with allopurinol
— ampicillin may cause failure of oral contraceptives

Nursing points for penicillins

— a careful routine history is taken to exclude previous penicillin reactions to avoid anaphylaxis
— the medical officer and all relevant staff must be informed of the penicillin allergy and the history and patient labelled suitably

— advise the patient to obtain an 'Identicare' bracelet or pendant and enter the relevant information concerning the allergy
— advise the patient to inform any other medical or nursing personnel of the allergy
— advise the patient to ask if penicillin is being administered
— oral preparations are taken 1 hour before or 2 hours after meals to avoid delayed absorption by food and to reduce destruction by gastric acid (except amoxycillin)
— avoid taking oral preparations with acidic fruit juices or liquids as these may accelerate drug decomposition
— penicillin should be handled carefully by staff to prevent self-sensitization
— reconstitute drugs according to manufacturer's literature
— when only part of a vial contents required, add stated amount of diluent to give a specific final concentration
— needle blockage is less likely if a small bore syringe and 20 gauge needle are used
— when giving IM avoid intravascular injection by withdrawing syringe plunger
— reconstituted penicillin stored at 2–8°C (not frozen) and used within 7 days, but if stored at about 20°C used within 24 hours
— have available adrenaline, aminophylline, antihistamines, hydrocortisone and resuscitation equipment

CARBAPENEM

IMIPENEM

Action

— inhibits bacterial wall synthesis
— bactericidal against most aerobic and anaerobic Gram-negative and Gram-positive microorganisms
— administered in combination with cilastatin, the specific inhibitor of the renal enzyme that metabolizes the active drug

Dose

i) 250–500 mg 6- to 8-hourly IV; OR
ii) 1 g 6- to 8-hourly IV (severe infection)

Adverse effects

— nausea, vomiting
— diarrhoea (may begin several weeks after cessation of therapy)
— rash, urticaria, pruritus
— hypotension, dizziness, convulsions, somnolence
— phlebitis, thrombophlebitis
— pseudomembranous colitis (rare but often fatal)

Nursing points

— a careful routine history is taken to exclude allergy to penicillin, cephalosporin and aztreonam to avoid cross reaction
— medical officer and all relevant staff must be informed of the allergy and the history and the patient labelled suitably
— advise the patient to obtain an 'Identicare' bracelet or pendant and enter the relevant information about the allergy
— advise the patient to inform any other medical or nursing personnel of the allergy
— advise the patient to ask if cephalosporin, penicillin, aztreonam or imipenem is being administered
— no other drugs are mixed in the same syringe or IV infusion container

— reconstitute the powder with water for injection and dilute in 100 ml of compatible infusion fluid, mixing solution well until clear and infuse over 30 minutes via a burette (a 1 g dose is infused over 60 minutes)
— colour of solution will vary from colourless to yellow but does not affect potency of the product
— if patient develops, nausea, slow rate of IV infusion
— reconstituted drug can be maintained at room temperature for 4 hours and 24 hours under refrigeration at 4°C
— have available adrenaline, aminophylline, antihistamines, hydrocortisone and resuscitation equipment

Note

— dose refers to imipenem content

MONOBACTAM

AZTREONAM

Action

— synthetic monocyclic beta-lactam
— inhibits bacterial cell wall synthesis
— bactericidal against the majority of aerobic Gram-negative bacteria
— resists the action of beta-lactamase (penicillinase, cephalosporinase)

Dose

i) 2 g 6- to 8-hourly, slow IV injection or infusion (dilutions according to manufacturer's literature; OR
ii) 1 g as single deep IM dose (gonorrhoea, acute cystitis)

Adverse effects

— nausea, vomiting, diarrhoea, abdominal cramps, mouth ulcers, altered taste
— rash
— hypotension, dizziness, vertigo, confusion, headache, malaise
— weakness, muscle aches
— diaphoresis, fever
— candidiasis
— breast tenderness, vaginitis
— halitosis
— sneezing, nasal congestion
— phlebitis, discomfort at IV injection site

Nursing points

— a careful routine history is taken to exclude any form of allergy, particularly to drugs, to avoid anaphylaxis
— medical officer and all relevant staff must be informed of the allergy and the history and patient labelled suitably
— advise the patient to obtain an 'Identicare' bracelet or pendant and enter the relevant information about the allergy
— advise the patient to inform any other medical or nursing personnel of the allergy
— advise the patient to ask if penicillin, cephalosporin, imipenem or aztreonam is being administered
— no other drugs are mixed in the same syringe or IV infusion container
— reconstitute the powder with water or isotonic saline and shake contents immediately and vigorously
— colour of solution may vary from colourless to pale yellow with a slight pink tint on standing
— discard any unused solution
— solutions prepared for IV use should be used immediately
— solutions prepared for IM use must be used within 48 hours and stored below 25°C
— have available adrenaline, aminophylline, antihistamines, hydrocortisone and resuscitation equipment

CEPHALOSPORINS

Action

— selectively interfere with bacterial cell wall synthesis, as does penicillin
— bactericidal
— resists the action of penicillinase (β-lactamase)

Preparations and dose
CEFACLOR

250 mg orally 8-hourly

CEFOPERAZONE

50–100 mg/kg/24 hours IM or IV in 2 divided doses, or if severe infection, 200 mg/kg/24 hours in 2, 3 or 4 divided doses

CEFOTAXIME

i)   100–150 mg/kg/24 hours IM or IV in 3 or 4 divided doses, or if severe infection, 6 divided doses; OR
ii) 1 g as single IM dose or 0.5 g as single IM dose plus probenecid, 1 g orally, taken 1 hour earlier (gonorrhoea); OR
iii) 1 g IM ½–1 hour before surgery, repeated on completion of surgery then 8-hourly for 24 hours, or for Caesarian section, 1 g IV after cord clamped, then at 6 and 12 hours (prevention of post-operative infection)

Note

— dilutions according to manufacturer's literature
— 0.5% or 1% lignocaine without adrenaline may be added to reduce pain at IM site
— not more than 1 g given into single IM injection site
— 1 g of drug reconstituted with 4 ml Water for Injection is stable up to 24 hours under refrigeration

CEFOXITIN

i)   50–100 mg/kg/24 hours IM or IV in 3 or 4 divided doses, or if severe infection, 150 mg/kg/24 hours in 4 divided doses; OR
ii) 2 g as single IM dose plus probenecid, 1 g orally, taken stat or 1 hour earlier (gonorrhoea); OR
iii) 2 g IM 1 hour before surgery or IV just before, then 2 g IM or IV at 6 and 12 hours after first dose, or for Caesarian section, 2 g after cord clamped, then 2 g IM or IV at 4 and 8 hours after first dose (prevention of post-operative infection)

Note

— dilutions according to manufacturer's literature
— 0.5% or 1% lignocaine without adrenaline may be added to reduce pain at IM site
— reconstituted drug is stable for 24 hours below 25°C and 1 week under refrigeration

CEFTAZIDIME
Adult dose

0.5–2 g IM, IV bolus or infusion 8- to 12-hourly

Paediatric dose (over 1 year)

30–100 mg/kg/24 hours IM or IV in 2 or 3 divided doses

Note

— dilution according to manufacturer's literature
— vials as supplied are under reduced pressure and as the product dissolves, carbon dioxide is released, causing effervescence and a positive pressure develops
— 0.5% lignocaine without adrenaline may be added to reduce pain at the IM site, but stable for only half the time compared with addition of Water for Injection

— reconstituted drug is stable for 12 hours below 25°C and 1 week under refrigeration (2–8°C)
— colour of solution may vary from pale yellow to amber

CEFTRIAXONE

Adult dose

i) 1–2 g IM or IV daily or in equally divided doses 12-hourly: OR
ii) 250 mg as single IM dose (gonorrhoea): OR
iii) 1 g IM or IV ½–2 hours before surgery (prevention of post-operative infection)

Paediatric dose

50 mg/kg/24 hours IM or IV in a single daily dose or in equally divided doses 12-hourly (not to exceed 2 g/day)

Note

— dilution according to manufacturer's literature
— 1% lignocaine without adrenaline may be added to reduce pain at IM site
— reconstituted drug is stable for 6 hours at below 25°C and 24 hours under refrigeration (2–8°C)
— colour of solution may be yellowish and have a slight opalescence

CEPHALEXIN

Adult dose

250–500 mg orally 6-hourly without regard to meals

Paediatric dose

25–50 mg/kg/24 hours in 4 divided doses

CEPHALOTHIN

Adult dose

0.5–1 g IM, IV bolus or infusion 4- to 6-hourly, or if severe infection, up to 2 g 4-hourly

Paediatric dose

40–80 mg/kg/24 hours IM or IV in 4 divided doses

Note

— daily dose of 4–12 g may be given continuously IV but for prolonged infusions replace at least every 24 hours
— may be added to peritoneal dialysis fluid (6 mg/100 ml)
— IM injection very painful
— dilutions according to manufacturer's instructions
— reconstituted drug is stable for 48 hours under refrigeration and 6 hours at room temperature
— precipitate in solutions can be redissolved by warming to room temperature with constant agitation

CEPHAMANDOLE

i) 0.5–1 g IM or IV 4- to 8-hourly, or if severe infection, 2 g 4-hourly; OR
ii) 1–2 g IM 1 hour before surgery or IV ½ hour before, then 1–2 g IM or IV 6-hourly for 24 hours (prevention of post-operative infection)

Note

— daily dose of 3–12 g may be given continuously IV
— dilutions according to manufacturer's literature
— 0.5% lignocaine without adrenaline may be added to reduce pain at IM site

CEPHAZOLIN

Adult dose

750 mg–3 g daily IM, IV injection or infusion in 2, 3 or 4 divided doses, or as continuous IV infusion

Paediatric dose

25–50 mg/kg/24 hours IM or IV in 3 or 4 divided doses

Note

— dilutions according to manufacturer's literature

LATAMOXEF

100–150 mg/kg/24 hours IM or IV in 3 divided doses, or if severe infection, 200 mg/kg/24 hours in 4 divided doses

Note

— dilutions according to manufacturer's literature
— reconstituted drug is stable for 24 hours at 25°C and 96 hours under refrigeration
— note and report any bleeding immediately as clotting mechanism can be disturbed
— bleeding time monitored in patient who has received more than 4 g/day for longer than 3 days
— vitamin K_1 10 mg given weekly as prophylaxis
— warn patient against taking alcohol or alcohol-containing preparations during/or for 48 hours after ceasing latamoxef to prevent a disulfiram-alcohol-like reaction of nausea, vomiting and hypotension

Adverse effects of cephalosporins

— allergic reactions, rash, urticaria, fever, serum sickness
— blood dyscrasias
— bleeding (latamoxef)
— disulfiram-alcohol-like reaction (latamoxef)
— dizziness, headache, drowsiness (cefaclor)
— diarrhoea which may begin several weeks after therapy (ceftazidime, cefotriaxone)
— rare but often fatal pseudomembranous colitis (ceftazidime, cefotriaxone)
— superinfection
— anaphylactic shock (rare)
— IM injections painful
— thrombophlebitis (if high doses IV)
— after oral administration, transient diarrhoea, nausea, vomiting and dyspepsia

Interactions

— cephalosporins affect stability of oral anticoagulant control
— probenecid increases and prolongs blood levels of most cephalosporins
— increased risk of renal damage if used in conjunction with other potentially nephrotoxic agents such as the aminoglycosides
— disulfiram-alcohol-like reaction with latamoxef

Nursing points

— a careful routine history is taken to exclude allergy to cephalosporins, imipenem or penicillin to avoid anaphylaxis
— cephalosporins are sometimes used in patients hypersensitive to penicillin, but about 3–8% of patients with penicillin hypersensitivity will have cross reactions with cephalosporins and imipenem
— the medical officer and all relevant staff must be informed of the allergy and the history and patient labelled suitably
— advise the patient to obtain an 'Identicare' bracelet or pendant and enter the relevant information about the allergy
— advise the patient to inform any other medical or nursing personnel of the allergy
— advise the patient to ask if imipenem, aztreonam, cephalosporin or penicillin is being administered
— food or gastric acid has no effect on the amount of oral preparation absorbed
— no other drugs are mixed in the same syringe or IV infusion container as a precipitate will form
— if cephalosporins are being administered by a Y-line infusion method, the primary or main container is stopped to avoid incompatibility
— when giving IM, avoid intravascular injection by withdrawing syringe plunger
— urine from a patient on cephalosporins may give a false positive reaction for glycosuria with

Clinitest® tablets (not Clinistix® or Tes-Tape®)
— have available adrenaline, aminophylline, antihistamines, hydrocortisone and resuscitation equipment

AMINOGLYCOSIDES

Action

— interferes with bacterial protein synthesis
— bactericidal
inhibits wide range Gram-negative organisms and some Gram-positive

Preparations and dose

AMIKACIN

i) 5 mg/kg IM or IV infusion 8-hourly; OR
ii) 7.5 mg/kg IM or IV infusion 12-hourly IV infusion prepared by adding 500 mg to at least 200 ml isotonic saline or 5% glucose and give separately over ½–1 hour

Note

— toxic blood level, trough >5, peak >20 micrograms/ml

FRAMYCETIN

i) 500 mg sterile powder dissolved in 0.5–1 ml of Water for Injection and given by subconjunctival injection daily for 3 days (infections of cornea, anterior chamber): OR
ii) 200–500 mg sterile powder dissolved in 50 ml isotonic saline and retained in urinary bladder for 3–4 hours, repeated 3 times in 24 hours for up to 10 days

GENTAMICIN

Adult dose

i) 1 mg/kg IM 8-hourly (based on 60 mg if under 60 kg or 80 mg if over 60 kg); OR
ii) 1 mg/kg IV 8-hourly (as for IM dose) diluted in 100–200 ml isotonic saline or 5% glucose and infused separately over 1–2 hours; OR
iii) 1 mg IT daily combined with IM therapy; OR
iv) 10–20 mg undiluted or mixed with equal volume isotonic saline injected into conjunctival sac

v) acrylic beads containing gentamicin threaded onto surgical wire and implanted to treat bone infections

Paediatric dose

i) 3–7.5 mg/kg/day IM or IV in 2 or 3 divided doses
ii) 1 mg IT daily combined with i)

Note

— toxic blood level, trough >2, peak >8 micrograms/ml

KANAMYCIN

i) 0.5 g IM 12-hourly or 0.25 g IM 6-hourly; OR
ii) up to 15 mg/kg/24 hours IV infusion diluted in 200 or 400 ml of isotonic saline or 5% glucose to 2.5 mg/ml and run at a rate of 60–80 drops/min
iii) 2 g as single IM dose (gonorrhoea); OR
iv) 250–500 mg orally 6-hourly (bacterial enteric infection); OR
v) 1 g orally hourly for 4 hours, then 1 g 6-hourly for 36–72 hours (pre-operative bowel steriliztion)

Note

— not more than 1 g given into single IM injection site
— may also be given by intraperitoneal catheter and nebulization

NEOMYCIN

1 g orally hourly for 4 hours then 4-hourly for 4 doses (pre-operative bowel sterilization)

Note

— may also be used in patients with neutropenia, or to suppress ammonia-forming bacteria in gut, so reducing blood ammonia levels in hepatic coma
— 100 ml of solution instilled in bladder for 20–30 minutes b.d. via indwelling catheter after bladder surgery

NETILMICIN

4–6 mg/kg/24 hours in 2 divided doses, or if severe infection, 7.5 mg/kg/24 hours in 3 divided doses deeply IM or IV bolus or diluted in 50–200 ml isotonic saline or glucose 5% and infused over $\frac{1}{2}$–2 hours

Note

— therapeutic blood level range 3–5 microgram/ml

STREPTOMYCIN

i) 0.5 g IM 12-hourly; OR
ii) 50–100 mg IT daily (tuberculous meningitis combined with i)

Note

— contact dermatitis may occur in persons handling streptomycin
— patients over 40 years old should not exceed 750 mg daily and those over 60 years old should not exceed 500 mg, because of the greater risk of vestibular disturbance

TOBRAMYCIN

i) 1–1.5 mg/kg IM 8-hourly; OR
ii) 1–1.5 mg/kg IV 8-hourly diluted in 50–100 ml isotonic saline or 5% glucose and infused separately over 20–60 minutes

Note

— toxic blood level, trough >2, peak >8 micrograms/ml

Adverse effects of aminoglycosides

— ototoxicity, auditory and vestibular
— nephrotoxicity
— hypersensitivity, rashes, fever
— superinfection
— blood dyscrasias (rare)

Interactions

— ototoxicity of aminoglycosides increased when given with bumetanide, ethacrynic acid or frusemide in presence of renal failure

— cross allergenicity with other
aminoglycosides
— streptomycin enhances effects of
pancuronium

Nursing points

— note and report headache, dizziness,
nausea, vomiting, ataxia, nystagmus
— note and report oliguria
— encourage fluid intake
— urine kept alkaline if treating urinary
tract infection
— no other drugs mixed in the same
syringe or IV infusion container
— dilute and give by IV infusion
according to manufacturer's
literature, not given by IV injection
— IM injection given deeply into
buttocks

TETRACYCLINES

Action

— interferes with bacterial protein
synthesis
— bacteriostatic
— broad spectrum antibiotic
— concentrates in developing teeth and
bone

Preparations and dose

TETRACYCLINE

250–500 mg orally 6-hourly 1 hour a.c.
or 2 hours p.c.

TETRACYCLINE WITH NYSTATIN

i) 1 capsule orally 6-hourly; OR
ii) 2 capsules 12-hourly 1 hour a.c. or 2
hours p.c.

Note

— 1 capsule contains tetracycline
250 mg and nystatin 250 000 units

DOXYCYCLINE

i) 100 mg orally 12-hourly first day,
then 100 mg as single daily dose or
50 mg 12-hourly; OR
ii) 200 mg orally stat and 100 mg nocte
first day, then 100 mg 12-hourly for 3
days (gonococcal infection); OR
iii) 150 mg orally 12-hourly for 10 days
(syphilis)

Note

— the 50 mg capsule is NOT a
paediatric formulation

MINOCYCLINE

i) 200 mg orally initially, then 100 mg
12-hourly; OR
ii) 200 mg IV initially, then 100 mg IV
12-hourly
Reconstitute powder with 5 ml
sterile water then dilute with
500–1000 ml of compatible solution
and infuse over $\frac{1}{2}$ to 1 hour (see
manufacturer's literature)

METHACYCLINE

i) 150 mg orally 6-hourly; OR
ii) 300 mg orally 12-hourly

OXYTETRACYCLINE

250–500 mg orally 6-hourly

ROLITETRACYCLINE

i) 350 mg IM daily or b.d.; OR
ii) 275 mg IV daily or b.d.

Note

— select correct preparation for prescribed route
— reconstituted drug stable under refrigeration for 24 hours

DEMECLOCYCLINE

Action

— as for tetracyclines
— selectively inhibits renal concentrating function by interfering with action of antidiuretic hormone in distal renal tubule

Use

— as for tetracyclines
— chronic hyponatraemia associated with the syndrome of inappropriate secretion of antidiurectic hormone (SIADH)

Dose

i) 150 mg orally 6-hourly 1 hour a.c.; OR
ii) 300 mg orally 12-hourly 1 hour a.c.; OR
iii) 600 mg orally initially, then 300 mg 12-hourly 1 hour a.c. for 4 days to a total of 3 g (gonococcal infection); OR
iv) 900–1200 mg orally daily in 2–4 divided doses 1 hour a.c. initially, then 600–900 mg daily in 2–4 divided doses (chronic hyponatraemia due to SIADH)

Adverse effects of tetracyclines

— nausea, vomiting, diarrhoea

— superinfection
— retardation of bone growth and tooth and nail discolouration if given during pregnancy or to children under 8 years
— allergic reaction
— photosensitivity
— rare but often fatal hepatotoxicity
— rarely, blood dyscrasias
— thrombophlebitis if prolonged IV therapy

Interactions of tetracyclines

— absorption of some reduced by milk, sodium bicarbonate, oral iron, calcium, magnesium and aluminium salts
— reduces activity of some penicillins
— affects stability of oral anticoagulant control
— tetracycline blood levels reduced by anticonvulsants
— increases blood levels of carbamazepine and phenytoin
— increases toxic effects of lithium
— may cause failure of oral contraceptives

Nursing points for tetracyclines

— taken at least 2 hours before or after calcium containing products, sodium bicarbonate, oral iron, magnesium and aluminium salts
— taken 1 hour a.c. or 2 hours p.c. except minocycline and doxycycline which may be taken with food or milk

Note

— degraded tetracyclines cause Fanconi syndrome

SULPHONAMIDES

Action

— compete with para-aminobenzoic acid (PABA) for incorporation into folic acid by microorganisms
— bacteria deprived of folic acid because of incomplete synthesis so cease to multiply
— bacteriostatic, broad spectrum
— thiazide diuretics, sulphonylurea oral hypoglycaemics and carbonic anhydrase inhibitors are sulphonamide derivatives

Preparations and dose

SULPHADIAZINE

1–1.5 g 4-hourly by IV infusion or diluted in 50–100 ml of isotonic saline and infused over at least 10 minutes

SULPHADIMIDINE (sulphamethazine)

2–3 g orally initially then 1 g 6-hourly

SULPHAFURAZOLE

2–4 g orally initially then 1–2 g orally 4- to 6-hourly or 2 g orally 8-hourly

SULPHAMETHIZOLE

i) 0.5 g orally 6-hourly; OR
ii) 1 g orally 8-hourly

Note

— highly soluble, so crystalluria rare

PHTHALYLSULPHATHIAZOLE

Bacillary dysentery

i) 1 g orally 12-hourly (prophylaxis); OR
ii) 2 g orally 8-hourly (treatment)

Bowel sterilization

250 mg/kg orally stat, then 1.5 g 3-hourly for 4 days both before and after surgery

SULPHAMETHOXAZOLE

2 g orally initially then 1 g 12-hourly

TRIMETHOPRIM 80 mg WITH SULPHAMETHOXAZOLE 400 mg
(co-trimoxazole)

Adult dose

i) 2 tablets (1 DS or Forte) orally b.d. p.c.; OR
ii) trimethoprim 160 mg with sulphamethoxazole 800 mg IM b.d.; OR
iii) 2–3 standard 5 ml ampoules diluted as instructed and given by IV infusion b.d., the duration of infusion should not exceed $1\frac{1}{2}$ hours.
iv) trimethoprim 20 mg/kg and sulphamethoxazole 100 mg/kg per 24 hours orally or IV infusion in 4 divided doses (*Pneumocystis carinii* pneumonitis)

Paediatric dose

Oral (each 5 ml of suspension contains trimethoprim 40 mg and sulphamethoxazole 200 mg)

6 weeks–2 years: 2.5 ml suspension b.d.
2–5 years: 2.5–5 ml suspension b.d.
6–12 years: 5–10 ml suspension or $\frac{1}{2}$–1 tablet b.d.

IV infusion (each 5 ml ampoule contains trimethoprim 80 mg and sulphamethoxazole 400 mg)

6 weeks–5 months: 1.25 ml
6 months–5 years: 2.5 ml
over 6 years: 5 ml

Note

— this combination is bactericidal as it blocks 2 consecutive steps in bacterial folate metabolism resulting in inability to synthesize nucleic acids
— DS, Forte denote double strength
— select the correct preparation for IV infusion and IM injection
— the manufacturer's literature must be

consulted for the correct dilution preparation for IV infusion
— must be diluted for IV administration and mixed thoroughly
— stable in IV solution up to 6 hours, but if visual turbidity or crystallization appear during infusion, replace with freshly prepared solution
— IV lines flushed with isotonic saline before and after administration
— may cause failure of oral contraceptives

Adverse effects of sulphonamides

— nausea, vomiting, malaise, headache
— rash, urticaria, dermatitis
— fever, symptoms resembling serum sickness
— crystalluria, oliguria, anuria
— blood dyscrasias
— Stevens-Johnson syndrome (rare but possibly fatal)
— photosensitivity

Interactions

— sulphonamides affect the stability of anticoagulant control
— sulphamethizole increases blood levels of phenytoin, tolbutamide and warfarin
— sulphonamides may enhance the effect of sulphonylurea hypoglycaemic agents
— co-trimoxazole may cause failure of oral contraceptives

Nursing points

— advise patient to increase fluid intake
— urinary output is monitored and kept above 1500 ml/day to reduce crystalluria and stone formation
— note and report oliguria and increasing urinary acidity
— alkalinization may be necessary to increase solubility of some sulphonamides and reduce risk of crystalluria
— note and report rash, fever, sore throat, purpura jaundice as these indicate the need to terminate therapy
— note instability in diabetics taking

sulphonylurea hypoglycaemics
— advise patient to avoid skin exposure to direct sunlight
— protect stock from light

Note

— blood cell counts necessary if prolonged therapy
— sulphonamides never given to nursing mothers as they may cause jaundice in the infant leading to kernicterus

PEPTIDE ANTIBACTERIAL AGENTS

POLYMYXIN B

Action and use

— attaches to the bacterial cell
  membranes causing disruption and
  lysis
— bactericidal
— effective mainly against Gram-
  negative bacilli, particularly
  pseudomonas and coliform
  organisms

Dose

i) 1 000 000 units orally 4-hourly
   (gastrointestinal infections); OR
ii) 15 000–25 000 units/kg/24 hours
    deep IM in 5 or 6 divided doses; OR
iii) 15 000–25 000 units/kg/24 hours
     dissolved in 200–500 ml 5% glucose
     and given as single IV infusion over
     60–90 minutes or 2 divided doses
     8–12 hours apart

Adverse effects

— local reaction and pain after IM
  injection
— gastrointestinal disturbances
— visual and speech disturbances
— proteinuria, oliguria
— drug fever, urticaria
— rarely, paraesthesia, respiratory arrest

Nursing points

— urinary output is monitored and kept
  above 1500 ml/day
— note and report oliguria, proteinuria
— encourage fluid intake
— procaine 1% 0.5 ml may be ordered
  as diluent to reduce the pain of IM
  injection
— dilutions according to manufacturer's
  literature

Note

— 500 000 units is equivalent to 50 mg
— may also be given intrathecally or by
  subconjunctival injection
  mucous membranes and into the eye

— combined with neomycin and
  bacitracin as intermittent or
  continuous bladder irrigation as
  prophylaxis against infections
  associated with catheterization and
  treatment of established infections of
  genitourinary system

POLYMYXIN E (colistin)

— as for polymyxin B

Dose

i) 2.5–5 mg/kg/24 hours deep IM in
   2–4 divided doses; OR
ii) ½ above total daily dose slowly IV
    then 1–2 hours later, remainder by
    IV infusion at 5–6 mg/hr

OTHER ANTIBIOTICS

CHLORAMPHENICOL

Action

— potent inhibitor of protein synthesis
— bacteriostatic
— broad spectrum antibacterial and antirickettsial antibiotic

Dose

i) 0.5–1 g orally or IM 6-hourly; OR
ii) 0.5–1 g IV 6-hourly diluted as directed and given by injection over 1 minute or in a larger volume of fluid by IV infusion

Note

— incompatibility may occur in the presence of other IV additives

Adverse effects

— nausea, vomiting, diarrhoea, stomatitis
— superinfection
— dose-related reversible bone marrow depression
— severe irreversible aplastic anaemia (remote, often fatal)
— peripheral neuritis, optic neuritis (prolonged therapy)
— Stevens-Johnson syndrome
— 'grey-syndrome' in neonates: ashen colour, vomiting, hypothermia, irregular respiration, pallid cyanosis, shock (fatal)

Interactions

— increases blood levels and adverse effects of tricyclic antidepressants
— increases blood level and activity of phenytoin
— increases effect of oral anticoagulants
— reduces therapeutic effect of penicillins
— phenobarb decreases chloramphenicol blood levels in children
— phenytoin increases chloramphenicol blood levels in children
— increases activity of oral hypoglycaemic agents

Nursing points

— check temperature 4- to 6-hourly as the drug may be discontinued if temperature normal for 48 hours
— note and report immediately sore throat, fever, bleeding tendency (early signs bone marrow depression)
— note and report stomatitis, glossitis, diarrhoea (superinfection)
— note instability in diabetics on oral hypoglycaemics
— select correct preparation for oral, parenteral or topical use

Note

— regular blood examinations do not warn of aplastic anaemia
— nursing mothers taking chloramphenicol should not breast-feed their infants

CLINDAMYCIN

Action

— binds to bacterial ribosomes inhibiting protein synthesis
— penetrates bone well
— reserved for patients where inappropriate to use penicillin
— similar to lincomycin but more active

Dose

i) 150–300 mg orally 6-hourly; OR
ii) 600–2400 mg/24 hours IM in 2, 3, or 4 divided doses; OR
iii) 900–2700 mg/24 hours in 2, 3 or 4 equal divided doses infused IV over 20–30 minutes

Adverse effects

— nausea, vomiting, diarrhoea, abdominal discomfort
— pain, sterile abscess (IM site)
— occasionally, rash, urticaria
— superinfection
— acute colitis (rare but possibly fatal)

Nursing points

— note and report immediately, diarrhoea, or abdominal discomfort
— not more than 600 mg given at single IM site
— dilutions according to manufacturer's literature

Note

— diarrhoea may begin several weeks after ceasing therapy

DILOXANIDE

Action

— anti-amoebic agent

Dose

500 mg orally t.d.s. for 10 days

Adverse effects

— occasionally, flatulence, vomiting, rash, albuminuria

Note

— used in conjunction with chloroquine metronidazole, and tetracycline
— 10-day course may be repeated if necessary

ERYTHROMYCIN

Action

— binds to bacterial ribosomes inhibiting protein synthesis
— bacteriostatic in low concentrations
— bactericidal in high concentrations

Adult dose

i) 250–500 mg orally 6-hourly 1 hour a.c.; OR
ii) 100 mg IM 6-hourly; OR
iii) 300 mg 8-hourly or 1 g 6-hourly either slowly IV or continuous infusion

Paediatric dose

30–50 mg/kg/24 hours orally or IV in divided doses

Adverse effects

— rash, urticaria
— occasionally nausea, vomiting, abdominal discomfort

Interactions

— reduces therapeutic effect of penicillins.
— increases theophylline blood levels

Nursing points

— oral preparations are taken 1 hour a.c. or 3 hours after evening meal as activity decreased in the presence of acid and food
— avoid taking oral preparations with acidic fruit juices or liquids as these decrease activity
— select the correct preparation for IV infusion and IM injection
— dilutions according to manufacturer's literature
— initial reconstitution of IV solution is with Water for Injection

FURAZOLIDONE

Action

— antibacterial, antiparasitic

Use

— bacillary dysentery
— diarrhoea (non-specific)

Dose

100 mg orally q.i.d. for 2–5 days

Adverse effects

— occasionally, nausea, vomiting, headache, rash
— disulfiram-alcohol-like reaction

Interactions

— increases activity of oral hypoglycaemic agents
— reduces antihypertensive effects of bretylium, debrisoquine, guanethidine

— enhances CNS depressant effects of alcohol, narcotic analgesics and most hypnotics
— disulfiram-like reaction when taken with alcohol
— increases activity of anticholinergic agents
— the 'cheese reaction', a combination of cheese, levodopa, some sympathomimetics and furazolidone can result in severe hypertension and subarachnoid haemorrhage even up to 2 weeks following cessation of furazolidone
— results in excitation, sweating, rigidity, hypertension or hypotension and coma when combined with pethidine
— last 2 interactions not likely until furazolidone has been taken for about 5 days

FUSIDIC ACID (sodium fusidate)

Action

— bactericidal

Dose

i) 500 mg orally t.d.s. with meals (for 6 days); OR
ii) 500 mg IV infusion 8-hourly
Reconstitute drug with diluent provided, then dilute according to manufacturer's literature and infuse over 2–4 hours

Adverse effects

— anorexia, nausea (mild)
— diarrhoea
— venospasm, thrombophlebitis (IV infusion)
— rarely, jaundice

LINOMYCIN

— as for clindamycin but less active

Dose

i) 500 mg orally 6- to 8-hourly 1 hour a.c. or p.c.
ii) 600 mg IM daily or 12-hourly; OR
iii) 600 mg 8- to 12-hourly added to 100 ml or more of 5% glucose or isotonic saline and infused IV over at least 1 hour

Interactions

— cyclamate and kaolin-pectin reduce blood levels of lincomycin markedly so give 2 hours apart

Note

— may cause diarrhoea when taken on a full stomach or with food

METRONIDAZOLE

Action and use

— thought to penetrate protozoal wall and stop nucleic acid synthesis
— antitrichomonal, antiamoebic and anaerobic antibacterial agent
— prevention of anaerobic infection in gynaecological and colonic surgery

Dose

i) 200 mg orally t.d.s. for 7 days (trichomoniasis); OR
ii) 2 g as single oral dose (trichomoniasis); OR
iii) 400–800 mg orally t.d.s. for 5–10 days (amoebiasis); OR
iv) 2 g orally daily for 3 days (giardiasis); OR
v) 200 mg orally t.d.s. for 3 days (acute ulcerative gingivitis); OR
vi) 400 mg orally t.d.s. for 7 days (anaerobic infection); OR
vii) 1 rectal suppository (1 g) 8-hourly for 3 days, then 12-hourly (anaerobic infection); OR
viii) 500 mg IV 8-hourly infused over 30 minutes

Adverse effects

— gastrointestinal disturbances
— rash, urticaria, pruritus

— superinfection (candida species)
— metallic taste
— headache, dizziness
— transient leucopenia and paraesthesias

Interactions

— if taken in combination with alcohol, may produce nausea, vomiting, abdominal cramps, headaches and flushing (disulfiram-like reaction)
— enhances activity of coumarin anticoagulants
— cimetidine increases metronidazole blood levels
— effects of metronidazole reduced by phenobarbitone

Nursing points

— tablets taken with meals, swallowed whole, suspension 1 hour a.c.
— warn patient to avoid alcohol while taking metronidazole
— warn patient that the urine may become a harmless dark colour during treatment

Note

— treatment for trichomonas should include the sexual partner to reduce incidence or reinfection
— nursing mothers taking metronidazole should not breast-feed their infants.

ORNIDAZOLE

Action and use

— antiprotozoal agent used to treat acute and chronic trichomoniasis

Dose

i) 1.5 g as single oral dose after evening meal; OR
ii) 25 mg/kg as single oral dose after evening meal if under 50 kg

Adverse effects

— mild gastrointestinal disturbances
— headache, dizziness, drowsiness

— fatigue, muscle weakness, rash
— rarely, blood dyscrasias

Note

— treatment for trichomonas should include the sexual partner to reduce incidence of reinfection

NALIDIXIC ACID

Action and use

— thought to inhibit bacterial DNA synthesis
— bactericidal to most Gram-negative organisms causing urinary tract infections

Dose

1 g orally q.i.d. for 1–2 weeks then 0.5 g q.i.d.

Adverse effects

— gastrointestinal disturbances and bleeding
— drowsiness, weakness
— dizziness, visual disturbances
— urticaria
— photosensitivity (necessitates stopping therapy)
— rarely, convulsions, blood dyscrasias, jaundice

Interactions

— may enhance effects of oral anticoagulants
— antagonizes nitrofurantoin

Nursing points

— note and report vomiting, irritability, drowsiness, photosensitivity
— advise patient to avoid exposure to direct sunlight
— may give false positive reaction for urinary glucose with Clinitest® tablets

Note

— mothers taking nalidixic acid should not breast-feed their infants

NORFLOXACIN

Action

— inhibits bacterial DNA synthesis
— bactericidal

Use

— urinary tract infections
— shigellosis
— traveller's diarrhoea

Dose

i) 400 mg orally b.d. 7–10 days (urinary tract infection): OR
ii) 400 mg orally b.d. 4–12 weeks (suppression of chronic recurrent urinary tract infection): OR
iii) 400 mg orally b.d. 5 days (shigellosis, traveller's diarrhoea)

Adverse effects

— gastrointestinal disturbances, constipation
— dizziness, lightheadedness, headache, depression, somnolence, insomnia
— fatigue
— rash

Interactions

— absorption reduced by antacids
— probenecid reduces urinary excretion of norfloxacin
— antibacterial effect of norfloxacin antagonized by nitrofurantoin

Nursing points

— tablets taken 1 hour before or 2 hours after meals with a glass of water
— taken 2 hours apart from antacids
— caution patient against driving or working in situations requiring mental alertness and co-ordination
— advise patient to drink sufficient fluids to maintain adequate hydration and urinary output to avoid crystalluria

Note

— not used in children or pregnant women
— mothers taking norfloxacin should not breast-feed their infants

NITROFURANTOIN

Action and use

— thought to interfere with several bacterial enzyme systems
— bacteriostatic in low concentrations
— bactericidal in high concentrations
— highly soluble in urine thereby effective mainly in urinary tract infections both prophylactically and in long term suppressive therapy

Dose

i) 50–100 mg orally q.i.d. with or after food for at least a week (not to exceed 400 mg/day); OR
ii) 50 or 100 mg orally nocte with or after food (prophylaxis)

Adverse effects

— anorexia, nausea, vomiting
— diarrhoea (occasionally)
— headache, drowsiness, dizziness, nystagmus
— peripheral neuritis (necessitates stopping therapy)
— rash
— blood dyscrasias
— hepatitis
— rarely, asthma, pulmonary oedema

Interactions

— taken with food or milk to enhance absorption and reduce gastrointestinal irritation
— antagonizes nalidixic acid
— absorption of nitrofurantoin reduced by magnesium trisilicate

Nursing points

— macrocrystalline preparation (Macrodantin®) reduces nausea
— advise patient that urine becomes harmless dark brown

— note and report muscle weakness, numbness and tingling (peripheral neuritis) as this necessitates ceasing drug

SPECTINOMYCIN

Action and use

— inhibits bacterial protein synthesis
— used in acute gonorrhoea

Dose

i) single dose of 2 g deep IM (male) and
ii) single dose of 4 g deep IM (female), divided between 2 gluteal sites

Adverse effects

— dizziness, nausea
— chills, fever
— discomfort at injection site

Nursing points

— dilute according to manufacturer's literature
— use accompanying special diluent
— not more than 5 ml into a single site

TINIDAZOLE

Action

— antiprotozoal

Use

— trichomonal vaginitis
— amoebic dysentery, amoebic liver abscess
— giardiasis
— reduce anaerobe population prior to bowel or gynaecological surgery

Adult dose

Trichomoniasis

2 g orally stat.

Amoebic dysentery and amoebic liver abscess

2 g orally as single daily dose for 2–3 days

Giardiasis

2 g orally stat.

Prevention of post-operative infection

2 g as single oral dose 12 hours before surgery

Paediatric dose

Giardiasis

50 mg/kg orally stat up to a maximum of 2 g or daily for 3 days

Adverse effects

— gastrointestinal disturbances
— metallic taste, fatigue, headache, dizziness
— rash, pruritus
— blood dyscrasias
— intolerance to alcohol

Note

— taken with or immediately after food
— warn patient to avoid alcohol while taking tinidazole
— should not be given to nursing mothers

TRIMETHOPRIM

Action

— interferes with bacterial biosynthesis of nucleic acid and proteins by inhibiting the enzyme dihydrofolate reductase

Use

— acute urinary tract infection

Dose

300 mg orally daily nocte with food for 7 days

Adverse effects

— nausea, vomiting, epigastric distress, glossitis
— rash, pruritus, fever
— bone marrow depression (prolonged therapy)

Nursing point

— note and report immediately sore throat, fever, bleeding tendency (early signs of bone marrow depression)

Note

— combined with sulphamethoxazole as was found to enhance its activity (co-trimoxazole)

VANCOMYCIN

Action and use

— inhibits bacterial wall synthesis
— bactericidal against Gram-positive bacteria
— indicated in life-threatening infections which cannot be treated by a less toxic agent

Dose

i) 500 mg orally 6-hourly (staphylococcal enterocolitis); OR
ii) 500 mg IV 6-hourly; OR
iii) 1 g IV 12-hourly by *infusion* only; OR
iv) 125 mg orally 6-hourly 7–10 days (anti-biotic-associated diarrhoea)

Adverse effects

— nausea, chills, fever
— urticaria, rash
— superinfection
— anaphylactoid reactions
— ototoxic, nephrotoxic
— blood dyscrasias
— thrombophlebitis (IV)
— nausea, diarrhoea, vomiting (oral)

Interactions

— streptomycin synergistic with vancomycin in treating enterococcal endocarditis
— concurrent and sequential use of other ototoxic and/or nephrotoxic antibiotics should be avoided

Nursing points

— for IV infusion, reconstitute drug with 10 ml Water for Injection, then dilute according to manufacturer's literature
— reconstituted drug stable under refrigeration for 96 hours
— note and report tinnitus and oliguria

ANTIFUNGAL AGENTS

AMPHOTERICIN B
Dose

i) 100 mg orally b.d. p.c. 2 weeks
   (prophylaxis); OR
ii) 100–200 mg orally q.i.d. p.c.
    (treatment); OR
iii) 1 lozenge (10 mg) dissolved slowly in
     the mouth q.i.d. p.c.; OR
iv) 0.25–1 mg/kg/24 hours or up to
    1.5 mg/kg on alternate days by IV
    Infusion.

Adverse effects

— oral administration; occasional
  nausea, vomiting, diarrhoea
— IV administration; fever (sometimes
  with shaking chills), headache,
  anorexia, nausea, vomiting, diarrhoea,
  dyspepsia, cramping epigastric pain,
  muscle and joint pains, some renal
  damage, hypokalaemia, anaemia

Interactions

— risk of cardiac glycoside toxicity
  increased in presence of
  hypokalaemia

Nursing points

— patients should remove dentures
  while sucking the lozenge,
  thoroughly cleaning them each time
— drug for IV use reconstituted and
  diluted according to manufacturer's
  literature
— protect from light by wrapping
  prepared IV solution and lines
  immediately in aluminium foil, black
  plastic sheeting or some other
  opaque material
— keep in the dark and store at correct
  temperature in refrigerator
— note and report fever, tinnitus,
  dizziness, oliguria, haematuria, signs
  of hypokalaemia such as drowsiness,
  muscle weakness, paraesthesias and
  ECG changes

FLUCYTOSINE (5-fluorocytosine)
Dose

37.5–50 mg/kg orally or IV infusion 6-
hourly

Adverse effects

— nausea, vomiting, diarrhoea
— blood dyscrasias

Nursing point

— adhere strictly to manufacturer's
  instructions for storing infusion
  solutions

GRISEOFULVIN
Dose

i) 125 mg orally q.i.d. or 500 mg orally
   daily (fine particle); OR
ii) 330–660 mg orally daily
    (ultramicrosize crystals)

Adverse effects

— nausea, vomiting, 'black tongue'
— mental confusion, headache, vertigo
— paraesthesia
— rash, urticaria, photosensitivity
— blood dyscrasias

Interactions

— if combined with alcohol, may cause
  headache, dyspnoea, nausea,
  giddiness and flushing (disulfiram-like
  reaction)
— reduces activity of oral anticoagulants
— phenobarbitone causes reduced
  griseofulvin blood levels when latter
  taken orally
— high fat-content meal enhances drug
  absorption

Nursing points

— infected hair removed
— advise patient of the need for
  cleanliness and keeping skin dry
— advise patient to avoid skin exposure
  to direct sunlight

Note

— treatment may last for at least 4
weeks and extend to 12 months in
some nail infections

MICONAZOLE
Dose

i) 200–1200 mg diluted to 200 ml with
isotonic saline or 5% glucose and
given by IV infusion over 30–60
minutes 8-hourly; OR
ii) 50 mg gel q.i.d. kept in mouth as
long as possible

Adverse effects

— pruritus, rash, anaphylactoid reaction
(indicating cessation of therapy)
— nausea, vomiting, diarrhoea, anorexia
— flushes, hypotension, fever
— tachycardia, arrhythmias
— hyperlipidaemia, hyponatraemia
— blood dyscrasias
— oral, gastrointestinal disturbances,
malaise, difficulty in visual
accommodation

Interactions

— enhances effect of oral anticoagulants

Nursing points

— dilutions according to manufacturer's
literature
— 50 mg gel may be applied to
dentures and left overnight

Note

— may also be given IT and instilled
into urinary bladder
— also available as cream, powder,
lotion and tincture for topical use

KETOCONAZOLE
Dose

200 mg orally daily or b.d. with food

Adverse effects

— gastrointestinal disturbances,
— rash, pruritus
— headache, dizziness, drowsiness,
fatigue, photophobia
— fever, chills
— rarely, hepatitis

Interactions

— increases cyclosporin blood levels
significantly
— effectiveness reduced by rifampicin
and isoniazid
— reduces effectiveness of rifampicin

NYSTATIN
Dose

500 000–1 000 000 units (1–2 tablets)
orally t.d.s.; OR
100 000 units q.i.d. (oral drops) held in
mouth as long as possible

Adverse effects

— rarely, nausea, vomiting, diarrhoea

Nursing points

— advise patient of the need for
cleanliness and keeping skin dry
— shake suspension vigorously

ANTIVIRAL AGENTS

ACYCLOVIR

Use

— herpes simplex virus infections

Dose

i) 5 mg/kg 8-hourly by slow IV infusion over 1 hour (immune-compromised patient); OR
ii) 200 mg orally 4-hourly while awake i.e. 5 doses daily for 10 days (treatment of initial genital herpes); OR
iii) 200 mg orally 4-hourly while awake, i.e. 5 doses daily for 5 days (intermittent treatment of genital herpes); OR
iv) 200 mg orally b.d. or t.d.s. for 6 months (intermittent treatment of genital herpes)

Adverse effects

— lethargy, confusion, hallucinations, tremor, agitation, convulsions, coma
— rash, urticaria
— nephrotoxicity
— nausea, vomiting, headache
— long term suppressive therapy: diarrhoea, vertigo, arthralgia

Interaction

— probenecid increases acyclovir blood levels

Nursing points

— follow preparation instructions carefully from manufacturer's literature
— reconstituted and diluted solutions are NOT refrigerated as this causes precipitation of crystals

AMANTADINE

Use

— influenza A prophylaxis (Asian and Hong Kong strains)

Dose

100 mg orally after breakfast and at midday meal for 10 days

Note

— see in anti-Parkinson section (p. 140)

VIDARABINE (adenine arabinoside, Ara-A)

Use

— herpes simplex virus encephalitis
— chickenpox or herpes zoster in an immunosuppressed patient

Dose

i) 15 mg/kg/day for 10 days (herpes simplex viral encephalitis); OR
ii) 10 mg/kg/day for 5 days (others) given by continuous IV infusion

Adverse effects

— anorexia, nausea, vomiting, diarrhoea
— occasionally, tremor, dizziness, confusion, ataxia

Nursing point

— follow preparation instructions carefully from manufacturer's literature

Note

— nursing mothers being treated with vidarabine should not breast-feed their infants

ZIDOVUDINE

Action

— appears to inhibit in vitro replication of retroviruses by interfering with viral RNA-directed DNA polymerase

Use

— active against human immunodeficiency virus (HIV)
— appears to slow down the progress of HIV disease

Dose

i) 200 mg orally 4-hourly; OR

ii) 500 mg orally 12-hourly; OR
iii) 250 mg orally at 4 evenly spaced
     intervals during the waking day

Adverse effects

— bone marrow depression resulting in
  severe anaemia and/or
  granulocytopenia necessitating
  reduced dose or discontinuation of
  therapy
— headache, insomnia
— nausea
— myalgia
— weakness

Interactions

— toxicity of zidovudine may be
  increased by dapsone, pentamidine,
  amphotercin B, flucytosine,
  vincristine, adriamycin, interferon
— probenecid may reduce renal
  excretion of zidovudine
— toxicity of either drug may be
  potentiated if paracetamol, aspirin or
  indomethacin used concurrently with
  zidovudine

Note

— regular blood monitoring to detect
  reduced haemoglobin,
  granulocytopenia
— zidovudine was previously known as
  azidothymidine or AZT

ANTITUBERCULOTIC AGENTS

The National Tuberculosis Advisory
Council recommends:
1. At least two drugs effective against
   the patient's mycobacteria should be
   administered at the same time to
   reduce the rate of the development
   of bacterial resistance
2. Until the sensitivities of the patient's
   organisms are known or until sputum
   conversion, treatment should begin
   with triple chemotherapy, followed by
   two-drug chemotherapy
3. The drugs for initial treatment may
   be selected from isoniazid, rifampicin,
   streptomycin and ethambutol

ETHAMBUTOL

Use

— first-line drug in treatment of
  tuberculosis

Dose

15–25 mg/kg/day as single oral daily
dose

Adverse effects

— visual acuity and colour vision
  disturbances
— occasionally, rash, gastrointestinal
  disturbances

Interaction

— absorption delayed and reduced by
  aluminium hydroxide

Nursing point

— advise patient to report any visual
  symptoms immediately as these are
  reversible if drug stopped early

ISONIAZID

Use

— first-line drug in treatment of
  tuberculosis

Dose

300 mg orally as single daily dose

Adverse effects

— peripheral neuritis
— nausea, vomiting, epigastric distress
— visual disturbances
— hepatitis (sometimes fatal)
— fever, rash, lymphadenopathy
— pyridoxine deficiency
— hyperglycaemia
— optic neuritis (rare)

Interactions

— absorption reduced by aluminium hydroxide gel
— increases effect of phenytoin
— effect of isoniazid increased by para-aminosalicylic acid
— combination with alcohol may produce hyperpyrexia, tremor and death
— isoniazid and rifampicin reduce vitamin D blood levels
— results in severe hepatitis when combined with rifampicin
— increases effect of carbamazepine
— decreases blood level of theophylline

Nursing points

— taken $\frac{1}{2}$ hour before food for peak levels but may be taken with food in divided doses to minimize nausea
— advise patient to report any visual disturbances and any numbness or tingling in the extremities

Note

— excreted in breast milk, so observe breast-fed infant for adverse effects
— pyridoxine (vitamin B_6) is given concurrently to prevent isoniazid-induced peripheral neuropathy
— used alone for chemoprophylaxis if inactive disease

RIFAMPICIN

Use

— first-line drug in treatment of tuberculosis

Dose

8–12 mg/kg (450–600 mg) orally as single daily dose taken 30 minutes before breakfast

Adverse effects

— occasionally, gastrointestinal disturbances, disorder of liver function and influenza-like symptoms

Interactions

— rifampicin blood levels reduced by para-aminosalicylic acid, phenobarbitone and phenytoin
— rifampicin blood level increased by probenecid
— rifampicin decreases effectiveness of theophylline, verapamil, prednisolone, tolbutamide, clofibrate, coumarin anticoagulants, diazepam and oral contraceptives
— reduces blood levels of metoprolol, chloramphenicol, cyclosporin, ketoconazole, norethisterone and quinidine
— rifampicin and isoniazid reduce vitamin D blood levels
— results in severe hepatitis when combined with isoniazid
— causes methadone withdrawal symptoms when rifampicin given

Nursing points

— advise patient that urine, faeces, sweat, sputum and tears may become a harmless red-orange
— rifampicin is taken 8–12 hours apart from para-aminosalicylic acid

Note

— used in combination with antileprotics

— advise patients taking oral contraceptives to use other forms of contraception

STREPTOMYCIN

Use

— first-line drug in treatment of tuberculosis
— see aminoglycoside section (p. 206)

CAPREOMYCIN

Use

— second-line drug in treatment of tuberculosis

Dose

1 g deeply IM daily for 60–120 days then 1 g IM 2 or 3 times each week

Adverse effects

— ototoxicity, nephrotoxicity
— blood dyscrasias
— pain, bleeding and induration at injection site
— when combined with other antituberculotic agents, rash, urticaria and fever

Nursing points

— note and report tinnitus, vertigo, hearing loss
— note urinary output
— dilute preparation according to manufacturer's instructions

CYCLOSERINE

Use

— second-line drug in treatment of tuberculosis

Dose

250 mg orally 12-hourly for first 2 weeks then increase to maximum daily dose of 1 g

Adverse effects

— neurotoxicity: headache, drowsiness, confusion, behaviour change, convulsions
— rash
— intolerance to alcohol

Nursing points

— note and report signs of neurotoxicity
— blood levels monitored weekly

SODIUM AMINOSALICYLIC ACID
(sodium PAS)

Use

— second-line drug in treatment of tuberculosis

Dose

12 g orally daily in 2–4 divided doses

Adverse effects

— nausea, vomiting, diarrhoea
— fever, rash, jaundice
— crystalluria

Interactions

— increases isoniazid blood levels
— probenecid increases sodium PAS blood levels
— toxicity of aspirin and sodium PAS increased when used in high doses in combination
— rifampicin given 8–12 hours apart from sodium PAS because PAS reduces rifampicin blood levels

Nursing points

— taken with or following food to minimize nausea
— note and report fever, sore throat, joint pains, oliguria
— encourage increased fluid intake
— advise patient of the importance of continuing therapy (often 2 years)

PROTHIONAMIDE

Use

— second-line drug in treatment of tuberculosis

Dose

0.5–1 g orally as single daily dose or in divided doses with food

Adverse effects

— anorexia, nausea, vomiting, diarrhoea
— metallic taste, stomatitis, excessive salivation

PYRAZINAMIDE

Use

— second-line drug in treatment of tuberculosis

Dose

20–35 mg/kg/day orally in 3 or 4 divided doses

Adverse effects

— jaundice indicating liver damage (serious)
— anorexia, nausea, vomiting
— fever, urticaria, joint pains
— dysuria
— hyperuricaemia leading to gout

ANTILEPROTICS

CLOFAZIMINE

Dose

i) 50–100 mg orally daily p.c.; OR
ii) 100 mg orally 3 times each week (leprosy); OR
iii) 300 mg orally daily for 3 months (lepra reaction)

Adverse effects

— red-brownish black discolouration of skin lesions and skin at sites exposed to light in lighter skinned patients, also sweat, sputum, urine and faeces (may persist for several months after ceasing drug)
— rash, pruritus, photosensitivity
— transient nausea, giddiness
— mild diarrhoea, abdominal discomfort, headache

Note

— used in combination with dapsone or rifampicin

DAPSONE

Dose

i) 100–200 mg orally daily; OR
ii) 200–400 mg orally twice weekly; OR
iii) 300–600 mg orally weekly; OR
iv) 50–200 mg orally daily (dermatitis herpetiformis)

Adverse effects

— allergic dermatitis
— rarely, gastrointestinal disturbances, blood dyscrasias

Interaction

— dapsone blood level increased by probenecid

THALIDOMIDE

Use

— treat lepra reaction

Dose

50–400 mg orally daily

Adverse effects

— birth defects
— paraesthesias, peripheral neuropathy

ANTIMALARIAL AGENTS

CHLOROQUINE

Action

— inhibits synthesis of parasitic DNA
— preferentially accumulates in infected erythrocytes

Use

— effective against *P. vivax, P. malariae, P. ovale* and susceptible strains of *P. falciparum*
— extraintestinal amoebiasis
— rheumatoid arthritis
— lupus erythematosis
— light-sensitive skin eruptions

Adult dose

Malaria (treatment)

Dose refers to chloroquine base
Day 1: 600 mg orally initially, then
300 mg 6 hours later
Days 2 and 3: 300 mg daily

Malaria (suppression)

Dose refers to chloroquine base
300 mg orally as single weekly dose
commencing 2 weeks before exposure
and continuing for 4 weeks after leaving
a malarious area

Amoebic hepatitis and liver abscess

Dose refers to chloroquine base
i) 300 mg orally b.d. for 2 days then
daily for 2 or 3 weeks; OR
ii) 160–200 mg IM daily for 10–12 days

Rheumatoid arthritis

Dose refers to chloroquine base
200 mg orally daily

Lupus erythematosis ·

Dose refers to chloroquine base
200 mg orally daily until maximum
improvement then dose reduced

Light-sensitive eruption

Dose refers to chloroquine base
400 mg orally during period of maximum
light exposure

Paediatric dose

Malaria (treatment)

Dose refers to chloroquine base
10 mg/kg daily for 3 days; OR
Day 1: 50 mg for each year of age (up
to 11 years) initially, then half the initial
dose 6 hours later
Days 2 and 3: repeat second dose daily

Malaria (suppression: single weekly
dose)

Dose refers to chloroquine base 5 mg/kg
commencing 2 weeks before exposure
and continuing 4 weeks after leaving
malarious area

Amoebic hepatitis and liver abscess

Dose refers to chloroquine base
  i) 6 mg/kg orally b.d. for 2 days then
     6 mg/kg daily; OR
 ii) 6 mg/kg IM daily for 10–12 days

Adverse effects

— gastrointestinal disturbances
— headache, skin eruptions
— depigmentation and loss of hair
— blurred vision, difficulty in visual
  accommodation, photophobia, corneal
  opacities, retinal degeneration
  (reversible if detected early and drug
  ceased immediately)
— rarely, headache, dizziness, tinnitus,
  deafness, blood dyscrasias

Note

— combined with primaquine to treat
  P. vivax, P. malariae or *P. ovale*
  because it dose not affect the
  malarial parasite in human liver cells

HYDROXYCHLOROQUINE

Action

— similar to chloroquine

Use

— suppression and treatment of malaria
— acute and chronic rheumatoid
  arthritis
— mild systemic and discoid lupus
  erythematosus

Dose

Malaria (treatment)

Day 1: 800 mg orally initially, then
400 mg 6 hours later
Days 2 and 3: 400 mg daily; OR 800 mg
as single oral dose

Malaria (suppression)

400 mg orally as single weekly dose
commencing 2 weeks before exposure
and continuing for 4 weeks after
leaving a malarious area

Rheumatoid arthritis

200 mg orally b.d. or t.d.s. p.c. for 4–12
weeks, then 200 mg daily or b.d. p.c.

Lupus erythematosus

200–400 mg orally b.d. p.c. for several
weeks, then 200 mg daily or b.d. p.c.

Adverse effects

— as for chloroquine

Nursing point

— advise patient to keep follow-up
  appointments
— advise patient to wear sunglasses in
  strong sunlight

Note

— not effective against chloroquin-
  resistant strains of *P. falciparum*
— routine ophthalmological
  examinations and blood cell counts
  during therapy

PRIMAQUINE PHOSPHATE

Use

— radical cure of relapsing *P. vivax* malaria
— acute attack of *P. vivax* malaria
— in conjunction with chloroquine if *P. falciparum* is associated with *P. vivax* in an acute attack

Adult dose

Treatment

15 mg orally daily for 14 days

Suppression

30–60 mg orally as a single weekly dose with chloroquine 300 mg

Paediatric dose

Treatment

1–7.5 mg orally daily according to weight for 14 days

Adverse effects

— nausea, vomiting, abdominal cramps, epigastric distress
— blood dyscrasias, uriticaria

Interactions

— primaquine toxicity enhanced by mepacrine

Nursing points

— may be taken with food or antacids to minimize gastrointestinal disturbances
— advise patient to report any reddening or darkening of urine or cyanosis (suggestive of haemolytic reaction)

Note

— frequent blood cell counts and haemoglobin estimations should be done during therapy

PROGUANIL

Dose

100 mg orally daily after food

Note

— suppression begins 24 hours before arrival in a malarious area then a daily dose continued for 1 month after leaving the area

PYRIMETHAMINE

Use

— prophylactic and suppressive against *P. falciparum*
— suppressant against *P. vivax*
— toxoplasmosis

Adult dose

Malaria prophylaxis

25 mg orally as single weekly dose commenced on arrival in a malarious area and continued for 4 weeks after leaving

Toxoplasmosis

50 mg orally initially, then 25 mg daily for 3–6 weeks

Paediatric dose

Malaria prophylaxis (single weekly dose 1 tablet = 25 mg)
under 5 years $\frac{1}{4}$ tablet
5–10 years $\frac{1}{2}$ tablet
over 10 years 1 tablet

Toxoplasmosis

under 3 months: $\frac{1}{4}$ tablet alternate days
3–9 months: $\frac{1}{4}$ tablet daily
10 months–2 years: $\frac{1}{2}$ tablet daily
2–6 years: 1 tablet initially, then $\frac{1}{2}$ tablet daily
over 6 years: 2 tablets initially, then 1 tablet daily

Adverse effects

— nausea, vomiting, diarrhoea, colic
— rash
— bone marrow depression (prolonged therapy or high doses)

Interactions

— antifolate effect of methotrexate may be increased
— increases toxicity of quinine

Note

— pyrimethamine combined with sulphonamides and calcium folinate or folic acid in treating toxoplasmosis
— treatment for toxoplasmosis should continue for 3 to 6 weeks

PYRIMETHAMINE WITH SULFADOXINE

Use

— treatment of chloroquine-resistant falciparum malaria
— short term prophylaxis of chloroquine-resistant falciparum malaria

Adult dose

Treatment

i) 2 or 3 tablets as single dose; OR
ii) 5–7.5 ml deep IM as single dose

Prophylaxis

i) 2 or 3 tablets once every 4 weeks (semi-immune)
ii) 2 tablets once every 2 weeks (non-immune)

Paediatric dose

Treatment

	Oral	IM
under 4 years	½ tablet	1–1.5 ml
4–8 years	1 tablet	2.5 ml
9–14 years	2 tablets	5 ml

Prophylaxis (semi-immune)

under 4 years: ½ tablet
4–8 years: 1 tablet
9–14 years: 2 tablets
tablets taken once every 4 weeks

Prophylaxis (non-immune)

under 4 years: ½ tablet
4–8 years: 1 tablet
9–14 years: 1½ tablets
tablets taken once every 2 weeks

Adverse effects

— as for pyrimethamine (p. 228) and sulphonamides (p. 210)

Note

— 1 tablet and each 2.5 ml ampoule contains 25 mg pyrimethamine and 500 mg sulfadoxine
— drug therapy ceased immediately if any skin reactions
— travellers should take the first dose 1–2 weeks before entering a malarious area and continue for 4 weeks after leaving
— if it is essential to give this preparation to a nursing mother, the infant should not be breast-fed for the first 4 weeks of life
— maintain adequate fluid intake

PYRIMETHAMINE WITH DAPSONE

Use

— prophylaxis of chloroquine-resisant malaria

Adult dose

1 tablet weekly

Paediatric dose

5–10 years: ½ tablet weekly
over 10 years: 1 tablet weekly

Adverse effects

— gastrointestinal disturbances
— allergic dermatitis

Note

— 1 tablet contains 12.5 mg
pyrimethamine and 100 mg dapsone
— travellers should start drug 1–2
weeks before entering a malarious
area and continue for 4 weeks after
leaving
— infants of breast-feeding mothers
receiving the drug should not be
breast-fed for the first 4 weeks of
life
— drug therapy ceased immediately if
any skin reactions

QUININE

Action

— antimalarial
— increases tension response to a
single maximal stimulus, but
increases muscle refractory period so
that reponse to tetanic stimulation is
diminished
— decreases excitability of motor end-
plate so response to repetitive nerve
stimulation and acetylcholine reduced
— salicylate-like analgesic effects on
joint and muscle pain and some
antipyretic effect

Use

— effective against *P. falciparum*
malaria resistant to other antimalarial
drugs
— radical cure of relapsing vivax malaria
— symptomatic relief of nocturnal leg
muscle cramps (elderly)

Dose

i) 300 mg orally daily or b.d. p.c.
(malaria)
ii) 300 mg orally nocte with food
(nocturnal cramps)

Adverse effects

— (cinchonism) tinnitus, hearing and
visual impairment, dizziness,
headache, fever, nausea, vomiting,
diarrhoea, abdominal pain
— rash, urticaria, pruritus
— blood dyscrasias

Interactions

— increases digoxin blood levels
— toxicity of quinine increased by
pyrimethamine
— may enhance effects of
anticoagulants

Note

— not to be confused with the anti-
arrhythmic, quinidine
— not used during pregnancy or if
patient has tinnitus or optic neuritis
— sulphate and bisulphate salts used
interchangeably

MEFLOQUINE

Action

— structurally related to quinine
— destroys asexual erythrocytic form of
malarial pathogens

Use

— acute attack of *P. falciparum* malaria
resistant to conventional antimalarial
drugs
— prophylaxis of multi-drug resistant
P. falciparum

Dose (adults and children more than 45 kg)

Treatment (non-immune)

750 mg orally followed by 500 mg 6–8
hours later. If more than 60 kg, a further
dose of 250 mg should be taken after
6–8 hours

Treatment (semi-immune)

750 mg orally as a single dose. If more
than 60 kg, a further dose of 250 mg
should be taken after 6–8 hours

Malaria prophylaxis

250 mg orally as single weekly dose
commencing 1 week before exposure
and continuing for 3 weeks after leaving
a malarious area

Adverse effects

— gastrointestinal disturbances
— dizziness, malaise
— uncommonly, headache, bradycardia, rash, muscle pain, tremors, sleep disturbances

Interactions

— must not be administered concurrently with quinine although may follow initial treatment of severe cases with IV quinine

Note

— tablet snould be swallowed whole with plenty of liquid
— avoid use in patients with cardiac disease
— women of childbearing potential should use an effective contraceptive throughout therapy and for at least 3 months after taking mefloquine
— should not be used in nursing mothers unless no alternative arrangements can be made for feeding the infant

9 Agents acting on the immune system

ANTIHISTAMINES

Action

— block the main actions of histamine except those stimulating secretion of gastric acid
— probably compete with histamine for the occupation of receptor sites
— reduces capillary permeability
— anticholinergic and antiserotonin effects
— most have local anaesthetic properties
— CNS stimulant in high doses, especially in children
— effective within 1 hour of oral administration
— conventional antihistamines are histamine H_1-receptor antagonists

Use

— respiratory allergies such as asthma, hay fever, sinusitis, vasomotor rhinitis
— urticaria
— pruritus
— angioneurotic oedema
— anaphylaxis, serum sickness, blood transfusion reaction
— insect bites and stings
— prevention and treatment of nausea, vomiting and motion sickness
— sedation in young and elderly
— premedication
— Ménière's disease

Preparations and dose

ASTEMIZOLE

Adult dose

10 mg orally daily

Paediatric dose

under 6 years: 2 mg/10 kg/24 hours
6–12 years: 5 mg orally daily

Note

— take 1 hour before or 2 hours after meals for better absorption
— does not cause sedation, presumably because does not cross blood brain barrier

AZATADINE MALEATE

Adult dose

1 mg orally b.d.

Paediatric dose

6–12 years: 0.5 mg orally b.d.

BROMPHENIRAMINE

i) 4–8 mg orally t.d.s. or q.i.d.; OR
ii) 12 mg orally (SR) b.d.

BUCLIZINE

25–50 mg orally 1–3 times daily

CHLORPHENIRAMINE

Adult dose

4 mg orally t.d.s. or q.i.d.

Paediatric dose

0.35 mg/kg/day orally in divided doses

CLEMASTINE

i) 1–3 mg orally b.d. a.c.; OR
ii) 2–4 mg IM or slow IV

CYPROHEPTADINE

Adult dose

i) 4–8 mg orally t.d.s. p.c.; OR

ii) 4 mg orally initially, repeated in ½ hour if necessary, then 4 mg 4- to 6-hourly (prophylaxis and treatment of migraine and histamine cephalalgia)

Paediatric dose

2–6 years: 2 mg t.d.s. (tablets or syrup)
6–14 years: 4 mg t.d.s. (tablets or syrup)

DEXCHLORPHENIRAMINE

Adult dose

i) 2 mg 4- to 6-hourly (tablet or syrup); OR

ii) 6 mg (Repetab) b.d.

Paediatric dose

0.15 mg/kg/day in divided doses

DIMENHYDRINATE

Adult dose

50 mg orally 4-hourly

Paediatric dose

Based on 5 mg/kg orally in 4 divided doses
2–6 years: 12.5–25 mg orally 6- to 8-hourly
6–12 years: 25–50 mg orally 6- to 8-hourly

DIPHENHYDRAMINE

Adult dose

25–50 mg orally t.d.s. p.c. and nocte

Paediatric dose

5 mg/kg/day orally in divided doses

DIPHENYLPYRALINE

i) 2.5–5 mg 3–4 times daily (tablet); OR

ii) 5 mg 3–4 times daily (syrup); OR

iii) 5 mg (SR) b.d.

DOXYLAMINE

25 mg orally up to 4 times a day

HYDROXYZINE

25–100 mg orally 3–4 times daily

MEBHYDROLIN

50–100 mg orally t.d.s. (tablet or syrup)

MECLOZINE

i) 25 mg orally b.d.; OR

ii) 50 mg orally nocte

iii) 25–50 mg orally b.d. (Ménière's disease)

METHDILAZINE

8–16 mg orally b.d.

PHENIRAMINE

Adult dose

i) 15–30 mg b.d. or t.d.s. (syrup); OR

ii) 20–30 mg t.d.s. (10 mg tablet); OR

iii) 25–50 mg b.d. or t.d.s. (50 mg tablet); OR

iv) 75 mg (SR) nocte

Paediatric dose

1–5 years: 7.5–15 mg orally b.d. or t.d.s.
6–14 years: 15–30 mg orally t.d.s.

PROMETHAZINE HYDROCHLORIDE

Adult dose

i) 10–20 mg orally b.d. or t.d.s. OR

ii) 25–50 mg orally or IM; OR

iii) 50–100 mg IM or diluted and given slowly IV (oculogyric crisis)

Paediatric dose

Based on 2 mg/kg/day orally or deep IM in divided doses
under 6 months: 5 mg b.d.
6–12 months: 5–10 mg b.d.
1–5 years: 10 mg b.d. or t.d.s.
over 5 years: up to 25 mg b.d.

Note

— compatible with morphine, pethidine or papaveretum when mixed in the same syringe as long as the resultant solution is used within 15 minutes and there is no precipitation

PROMETHAZINE THEOCLATE

Motion sickness

i) 25 mg orally nocte each night commencing night before starting long journey (prophylaxis); OR
ii) 25 mg orally 1–2 hours before starting short journey (prophylaxis); OR
iii) 25 mg orally stat, repeat same evening and again following evening (treatment)

TERFENADINE

60 mg orally b.d.

Note

— does not cause sedation, presumably because does not cross blood brain barrier

TRIMEPRAZINE

Adult dose

10 mg orally t.d.s. or q.i.d.

Paediatric dose

i) 0.5–1 mg/kg/day orally in divided doses; OR
ii) 2–4 mg/kg/dose orally (premedication); OR
iii) 0.6–0.9 mg/kg/dose IM (premedication)

TRIPROLIDINE

2.5–5 mg orally t.d.s.

Adverse effects of antihistamines

— sedation (may diminish after a few days) except astemizole, terfenadine
— lassitude, muscle weakness, incoordination
— hypotension, dizziness
— gastrointestinal disturbances
— CNS stimulation (large doses)
— allergic reaction (occasionally)
— (children), convulsions, hyperpyrexia

Interactions

— enchance the CNS depressant effects of alcohol, hypnotics, sedatives, tranquillizers and narcotic analgesics except astemizole, terfenadine
— some anticholinergics and tricyclic antidepressants may have enhanced effects

Nursing points for antihistamines

— usually taken after food to avoid gastric irritation
— sustained release (SR) preparations are swallowed whole, not crushed or chewed
— be aware that cotsides may be required if patient becomes drowsy or dizzy
— warn patient, about reduced tolerance to alcohol
— warn patient against driving a vehicle or operating machinery if drowsy
— advise patient to consult pharmacist before buying any OTC preparations especially 'common cold' preparations, many of which contain antihistamines
— take 1 or 2 hours before exposure to conditions that may precipitate motion sickness

Note

— nursing mothers should avoid taking antihistamines as lactation may be inhibited by the anticholinergic effect

VACCINES

Action

— antigenic materials which induce a specific active artificial immunity to infection by the corresponding infecting agent
— subsequent doses of vaccine (booster doses) provide protection by increasing declining antibody levels
— the effect of diphtheria and tetanus vaccines is enhanced when administered with pertussis vaccine

Use

— specific vaccine affords prophylaxis against some infectious diseases by providing complete or partial protection for months or years
— primary immunization schedule is undertaken early in life

Preparations (see literature for dose)

Bacterial vaccines (inactivated)

Cholera, Coryza, Diphtheria (adsorbed), Pertussis, Plague, Tetanus (adsorbed) (formerly Tetanus Toxoid), Typhoid, Meningococcal, Pneumococcal, Staphylococcus

Bacterial vaccines (live attenuated)

Bacillus Calmette-Guérin (BCG)

— indicated for tuberculin-negative contacts of known tuberculosis cases, medical and nursing personnel, mortuary attendants, bacteriology laboratory staff and other ancillary health workers, also aboriginal infants and children and high risk ethnic groups

Rickettsial vaccine (inactivated)

Typhus

Viral vaccine (inactivated)

Hepatitis B, Influenza, Rabies, Salk

Viral vaccine (live attenuated)

Measles, Mumps, Rubella, Sabin, Smallpox Varicella-zoster and Yellow Fever

Note

Triple antigen DTP contains Diphtheria, Tetanus and Pertussis vaccines. CDT is Combined Diphtheria and Tetanus vaccines. ADT vaccine contains Diphtheria and Tetanus vaccines diluted for use in individuals older than 8 years. Triple antigen is omitted and CDT given at 4, 6 and 18 months if child or family has a history of neurological disease

Adverse effects

— redness or sterile abscess at injection site
— fever, headache, myalgia and malaise for up to 1 to 2 days
— vaccines made from viruses or rickettsiae grown in eggs, e.g. Influenza, Measles, Typhus and Yellow Fever, may cause allergic reactions in hypersensitive persons
— vaccines containing animal serum or antibiotics, e.g. Rubella and Smallpox, may cause allergic reactions in hypersensitive persons
— pertussis vaccine, fever above 40.5°C, convulsions (uncommon), and very rarely, shock, anaphylaxis, thrombocytopenia, encephalopathy

Precautions

— enquire about previous hypersensitivity to immunizing agents
— vaccines containing live organisms are contraindicated during acute illness
— response may be diminished in patients receiving corticosteroids
— some vaccines containing live organisms are contraindicated during corticosteroid or immunosuppressive therapy including radiation
— hypersensitivity to diphtheria vaccine reduced by giving a low concentration preparation to persons over 8 years

PRIMARY IMMUNIZATION SCHEME*

Age	Disease	Agent	Route
2 months	Diphtheria-tetanus-pertussis	Triple antigen	IM
	Poliomyelitis	Sabin vaccine	Oral
4 months	Diphtheria-tetanus-pertussis	Triple antigen	IM
	Poliomyelitis	Sabin vaccine	Oral
6 months	Diphtheria-tetanus-pertussis	Triple antigen	IM
	Poliomyelitis	Sabin vaccine	Oral
15 months	Measles-mumps-rubella	Measles-mumps-rubella vaccine	SC
18 months	Diphtheria-tetanus-pertussis	Triple antigen	IM
5 years or prior to school entry	Poliomyelitis	Sabin vaccine	Oral
	Diphtheria-tetanus	CDT	IM
10–16 years (females)	Rubella	Rubella vaccine	SC
15 years or prior to leaving school	Diphtheria-tetanus	ADT	IM

* As recommended by the National Health and Medical Research Council, Australia
Consult current booklet, *Immunization Procedures.*

— there should be an interval of at least a month between the administration of any 2 live vaccines, however if it is necessary to administer 2 live vaccines within a month, the injections should be given in different arms
— pregnancy is an absolute contraindication to rubella vaccination and should be avoided for at least two full menstrual cycles following vaccination
— check manufacturer's information leaflet on specific contraindications for each vaccine

Nursing points

— primary immunization schedule, giving minimum time intervals may be followed easily
— medical officer will discuss benefits, possible adverse effects and take a careful history with special regard to previous reactions or allergies in patient or family
— products are kept at required temperature, not exposed to direct sunlight or high humidity according to the manufacturers' instructions to retain potency, activity and antigenicity

— live vaccines are not to be exposed to heat or sunlight
— killed vaccines are never allowed to freeze
— freeze-dried preparations stored in dried state at 2–8°C
— all vaccines are shaken well to ensure even dispersion before withdrawal
— outdated material is not used
— ensure recipient seated comfortably
— strict aseptic technique used
— a fresh needle is used for injecting aluminium carrier vaccines e.g. Hepatitis B Vaccine, Diphtheria Vaccine, Adsorbed, Tetanus Vaccine, Adsorbed, CDT and ADT, to prevent any vaccine being deposited superficially along the needle track
— ensure correct siting and route of administration
— avoid intravascular infection by withdrawing syringe plunger
— advise patient to avoid vigorous exercise and excessive alcohol consumption for several hours after vaccination

Note

— toxins which have been detoxified without loss of antigenicity are now classified as vaccines, e.g., Tetanus Toxoid is now Tetanus Vaccine, Adsorbed
— it is for the individual medical officer to decide on the type, dosage and timing of the vaccine given
— since smallpox has been eradicated world-wide, only laboratory workers directly involved with smallpox are vaccinated

ANTISERA

Action

— injectable serum containing the appropriate antibody provides transient passive immunity, or protection, against the specific invading microorganisms or toxins
— protection, although immediate, lasts only 2–3 weeks
— heterologous antiserum contains antibodies produced in horses or other animals by artificial active immunization
— homologous antiserum is the globulin fraction of human serum which contains antibodies

Use

— immediate protection against a particular infectious disease
— protection of contacts

Preparations (see literature for dose)

Antitoxins

Diphtheria Antitoxin (Equine Origin): used to treat all forms of diphtheria

Gas-Gangrene Antitoxin (Equine Origin): obtainable as monovalent antitoxin to treat a specific invading organism or polyvalent antitoxin which contains antitoxin to all 3 types of invading gas-gangrene organisms

Antivenoms (heterologous)

Red back spider, sea snake, stone fish, tick, box jellyfish, black snake, brown snake, death adder, taipan and tiger snake
Snake venom antiserum available for individual snakes if positively identified or for all five as polyvalent antivenom if snake species unknown

Immunoglobulins (human)

Normal Immunoglobulin (Human): given by deep IM injection, fractionally at different sites where more than 5 ml.

Indicated in agammaglobulinaemia, hypogammaglobulinaemia, hepatitis A, measles (morbilli), poliomyelitis, chicken pox (varicella), herpes zoster and overwhelming bacterial infections.

Normal Immunoglobulin (Human, For IV Use): used to treat patients with antibody deficiency and overwhelming bacterial infections. Observe for constitutional reaction by monitoring pulse, blood pressure and respiratory rate ¼ hourly and temperature hourly.

Diphtheria Immunoglobulin (Human): for passive immunization of unimmunized contacts

Hepatitis B Immunoglobulin (Human): for prophylaxis in persons accidentally exposed to material known to contain hepatitis B surface antigen (HBsAg)

Rabies Immune Globulin (Human): used in conjunction with Rabies Vaccine for prophylaxis in persons who have suffered bites from a suspected rabid animal. Half the single dose is infiltrated around the wound and the remainder given IM, but if no bite, total dose given IM. (Australia is free from rabies, but is used with vaccine in post-exposure prophylaxis).

Rh(D) Immunoglobulin (Human): given to an Rh-negative mother within 72 hours of delivery of an Rh-positive infant, stillbirth or abortion to protect against sensitization by the D antigen, so preventing subsequent formation of anti-D antibodies

Tetanus Immunoglobulin (Human) (TIG): for passive immunization of non-immune patients who sustain tetanus-prone wounds and who are known to be sensitive to tetanus antitoxin obtained from animals

Tetanus Immunoglobulin (Human, For IV Use): used in treatment of tetanus

Vaccinia Immunoglobulin (Human): for prevention and treatment of complications of smallpox vaccination

Zoster Immunoglobulin (Human): prevents onset of chicken pox (varicella) or herpes zoster in high-risk patients such as those with immune deficiency

disease or receiving immunosuppressive therapy

Adverse effects

(likely to occur after the injection of serum of animal origin)
— serum anaphylaxis within a few minutes of injection occurring as a condition of severe shock (dangerous but rare)
— serum sickness occurring 4–12 days later consisting of a syndrome of urticaria, fever and joint pains
— convalescent or adult serum carries the risk of transmitting viral hepatitis B

Precautions

— enquire about any previous injections of antisera or any allergies in patient or family especially asthma, hay fever and infantile eczema
— trial dose of 0.2 ml of 1 in 10 dilution in isotonic saline SC of Diphtheria Antitoxin or Gas-Gangrene Antitoxin will test for general sensitivity to horse serum (Gas-Gangrene Antitoxin test result may be unpredictable)
— if no general reaction such as pallor, tachycardia, urticaria, swelling of tongue or lips, bronchospasm, abdominal pain, unconsciousness or convulsions has occurred in 30 minutes, the full dose of antitoxin is administered and the patient observed for a further 30 minutes
— antivenom is diluted in isotonic saline or preferably Hartman's solution 1 in 10 and given by slow IV infusion without testing for sensitivity to horse serum
— have available adrenaline 1 in 1000 (drawn up), aminophylline, antihistamines, IV corticosteroid, oxygen, suction and resuscitation equipment whenever foreign serum is administered

Nursing points

— store antisera between 2 and 8°C, **NOT TO BE FROZEN**
— protect from light
— outdated material not used
— allow preparation to reach room

temperature before injection
— ensure patient seated comfortably or recumbent
— trial dose given where indicated (see precautions)
— avoid intravascular injection (where not intended) by withdrawing syringe plunger
— if horse serum-sensitive patient, observe airway and vital signs closely
— keep patient warm and recumbent until recovery

Tetanus-prone wound

The growth of *Cl. tetani* is favoured in compound fractures, penetrating wounds, wounds complicated by extensive tissue damage including burns, pyogenic infection or wood splinters or superficial wounds contaminated with soil, dust or horse manure which have remained untreated for 4 hours. Immunoprophylaxis depends on the patient's immunization status and ranges from a booster dose to a full course of Tetanus Vaccine (Adsorbed) with or without Tetanus Immunoglobulin (TIG). A complete active immunization course comprises 3 doses of Tetanus Vaccine (Adsorbed) with 6–12 weeks between the first and second doses and 6–12 months between the second and third. When Tetanus Vaccine and Tetanus Immunoglobulin are administered at the same time, each is given into a different limb and a separate syringe is used.
A booster dose of Tetanus Vaccine should be given if 2 or more years have elapsed since the previous dose

Note

— where a patient is known or likely to be sensitive to horse serum, it may be given in divided doses under cover of an antihistamine, adrenaline and corticosteroid
— follow passive immunity as soon as practicable with a course of suitable active immunity
— see current edition of National Health and Medical Research Council *Immunization Procedures* for availability of immunoglobulins

DIAGNOSTIC PRODUCTS

TUBERCULIN PURIFIED PROTEIN DERIVATIVE (PPD)

OLD TUBERCULIN, DILUTED 'C' STRENGTH

Use

— diagnosis of tuberculosis (Mantoux or Heaf test)

Result

— Mantoux positive recorded at 72 hours if an area of oedema 5 mm or more in diameter present
— Heaf positive recorded from 72 hours to 7 days and is graded according to degree of induration and oedema
— 0.1 ml PPD = 10 I.U.

Note

— measles virus inhibits the response to tuberculin
— a positive test may be an indication of previous or present natural infection, BCG vaccination, or some partial immunity to tuberculosis

SCHICK TEST TOXIN AND TEST CONTROL

Use

— to detect susceptibility to diphtheria in older children and young adults

Result

— read between 24 and 48 hours and between 5 and 7 days, a positive result is a red raised area on the left forearm into which the toxin was given and indicates susceptibility to diphtheria and the person requires active immunization with diphtheria vaccine

Note

— although many Australians are Schick-positive, very few adult cases of diphtheria seen

IMMUNOSUPPRESSIVE AGENTS

AZATHIOPRINE

Action

— suppresses the immune response
— converts to mercaptopurine in the body
— effect appears in several weeks

Use

— prolong survival of organ and tissue transplants
— autoimmune diseases such as lupus erythematosus, rheumatoid arthritis, renal, hepatic and skin disorders

Dose

Transplantation

1–5 mg/kg/day orally or IV

Autoimmune disorders

1–2.5 mg/kg/day orally or IV

Adverse effects

— generally reversible bone marrow depression especially leucopenia and thromboxytopenia
— anorexia, nausea, diarrhoea
— pancreatitis
— cholestatic hepatotoxicity
— serum sickness
— mouth ulcers
— infection
— abnormal bleeding

Interactions

— effects enhanced by allopurinol
— reverses effects of tubocurarine
— enhances effects of succinylcholine
— allows reduction of corticosteroid dose when used together

Nursing points

— tablets taken with food to reduce gastric irritation
— IV injection prepared immediately before use by dissolving vial

contents in 5 ml sterile water
— injection given slowly into tubing of running IV infusion of isotonic saline or glucose and saline
— any remaining solution discarded
— note and report any signs of infection, abnormal bleeding, jaundice, dark urine or clay-coloured stools
— record fluid intake and output carefully
— explain to patient and family about the need for reverse isolation in hospital and the need to keep a high standard of personal hygiene
— advise patient about the need to keep appointments for blood cell counts and to avoid contact with persons with infections and to report early signs and symptoms of infections

Note

— patient to have complete blood cell count regularly during therapy
— drug is discontinued if WCC falls to 3000/mm^3
— drug discontinued or reduced if signs of infection

ANTITHYMOCYTE IMMUNOGLOBULIN

Action

— produced by immunizing horses with human thymus lymphocytes
— reduces peripheral T-lymphocyte function

Use

— prolong the survival of organ and tissue transplants

Dose

i) 15 mg/kg/day for 14 days commencing 24 hours before or after transplant, then alternate days for 14 days (delay onset of rejection); OR
ii) 10–15 mg/kg/day for 14 days with optional additional treatment (treatment of rejection)

Prepared according to manufacturer's literature and given IV after a skin test

Adverse effects

— anaphylaxis
— haemolysis, thrombocytopenia, leucopenia
— fever, chills, pruritus, erythema
— phlebitis at IV site

Nursing points

— obseve patient closely during infusion for possible allergic reaction
— store between 2–8°C and do not freeze

CYCLOSPORIN

Action

— suppresses the immune response

Use

— prevention of graft rejection following renal transplantation

Dose

i) 14 to 17.5 mg/kg orally 4–12 hours prior to transplantation then daily, reducing gradually over several months to a maintenance dose of 6–8 mg/kg/day as a single dose or 2 divided doses (see nursing points)
ii) 3–5 mg/kg/day IV initially (if unable to take drug orally), the concentrate being diluted 1:20 to 1:100 with isotonic saline or 5% glucose and given by slow IV infusion over 2–6 hours commencing 4–12 hours prior to transplantation. A post-operative loading dose is prepared by diluting the concentrate to 500 ml and infusing over 24 hours.

Adverse effects

— impaired renal function
— impaired hepatic function
— hyperkalaemia, fluid retention,
— hypertension
— hirsutism
— tremor
— anorexia, nausea, vomiting, diarrhoea
— gingival hypertrophy
— rash
— burning sensation in hands and feet (may occur in first week of oral administration)
— anaphylactoid reaction (IV infusion) necessitating discontinuation

Interactions

— nephrotoxicity of cyclosporin increased when taken in combination with amphotericin B, aminoglycosides, cefotaxime, co-trimoxazole, frusemide, melphalan
— blood cyclosporin levels increased by ketoconazole, miconazole, erythromycin, verapamil, diltiazem, methyltestosterone
— blood cyclosporin levels decreased by phenytoin, rifampicin, isoniazid, IV sulphadimidine

Nursing points

— oral solution to be taken in fixed relation to food for consistent absorption
— dilute with milk or chocolate milk in a glass or cup (not plastic) immediately before being taken
— ensure that cup rinsings are also taken
— after use, the measuring pipette is not washed but is dried with a clean tissue and replaced in its protective cover
— oral solution should *not* be refrigerated and should be used within 2 months of opening
— any diluted infusion solution is discarded after 48 hours
— if blood to be sampled for cyclosporin levels, patient instructed not to take morning dose until after blood taken
— may be increased incidence of infection and delayed healing, so patient advised that dental work should be undertaken with caution and dental floss and toothpicks used carefully
— observe patient continuously for first

30 minutes of IV infusion, then at frequent intervals to detect anaphylactoid reaction (IV infusion concentrate contains polyoxyethylated castor oil which has been reported to cause anaphylactoid reactions
— have available adrenaline and resuscitation equipment

Note

— blood levels monitored to minimize toxicity and rejection episodes
— liver function monitored when oral contraceptives given concomitantly
— may need less cyclosporin if given with corticosteroid therapy
— mothers receiving cyclosporin should not breast-feed their infants

MUROMONAB-CD3

Action

— suppresses the immune response
— reverses graft rejection, most probably by blocking the function of all T cells which play a role in acute renal rejection

Use

— treat acute graft rejection following renal transplantation

Dose

5 mg IV daily for 10–14 days

Adverse effects

— first 2 days, pyrexia, chills, dyspnoea, wheezing, chest pain, nausea, vomiting, diarrhoea, tremor
— 'first dose effect' potentially fatal, severe pulmonary oedema (if fluid overload present before treatment)

Nursing points

— observe patient closely during first 6 hours of infusion
— note and report significant fever, chills, dyspnoea, malaise

— have available adrenaline and resuscitation equipment

Note

— evaluate patient for fluid overload by chest X-ray or weight gain if greater than 3%
— fever greater than 37.8°C should be reduced by antipyretics prior to commencing treatment
— patient should be informed of the expected first dose effects

10 Drugs acting on the blood

IRON PREPARATIONS

Action

— necessary for haemoglobin formation

Use

— iron deficiency anaemia resulting from severe or chronic blood loss
— dietary insufficiency
— increased demand e.g. pregnancy

Preparations and dose

FERROUS SULPHATE

Adult dose

320–350 mg orally 1–2 times daily

Paediatric dose

Prophylaxis

10 mg/kg/day (mixture or tablet)

Therapeutic

30 mg/kg/day (mixture or tablet)

FERROUS GLUCONATE

Adult dose

600 mg orally 1–3 times daily

Paediatric dose

Prophylaxis

18 mg/kg/day (elixir or tablet)

Therapeutic

54 mg/kg/day (elixir or tablet)

IRON-DEXTRAN COMPLEX

Dose

2–5 ml (50 mg Fe/ml) IM, IV or by single continous IV infusion (Total Dose Infusion)

IRON POLYMALTOSE COMPLEX

Dose

i) 1–2 tablets 1–3 times daily OR
ii) 4 ml (200 mg of iron) IM daily OR
iii) total dose infusion, calculated from a dosage table (up to 2500 mg may be given in 500 ml isotonic saline)

Note

— tablets (40 mg of iron per tablet) may be chewed or swallowed whole and may be taken with or without food
— total dose by IM injection is 2 ml alternate days until total dose attained or 4 ml at longer intervals
— first 50 ml of total dose infusion given slowly at 5–10 drops/min and if tolerated increased to 30 drops/min
— treatment monitoried by regular determination of haemoglobin

Adverse effects of iron preparations

— gastrointestinal irritation
— skin staining and/or abscess formation (IM)
— anaphylactoid reaction (IV)

Overdose of oral iron preparations

— very serious in small children as the gut lining may be destroyed

— treated urgently by stomach washout
and the iron chelating agent,
desferrioxamine (p. 289)

Interactions or iron preparations

— absorption of oral iron compounds
reduced by antacids and
tetracyclines, cereals, milk and eggs
— absorption of oral tetracyclines
reduced by oral iron compounds
— absorption of oral iron compounds
increased by ascorbic acid

Nursing points for iron preparations

— gastrointestinal irritation reduced if
oral iron preparations taken with or
• immediately after food although iron
is absorbed better between meals
— oral iron, tetracyclines and aluminium
salts are each given at least 2 hours
apart to allow adequate absorption
— iron mixtures are taken in milk or
through a straw to avoid temporary
staining of teeth
— warn patient that faeces become
darker during treatment
— give IM injection deeply into buttock
by drawing subcutaneous tissue to
one side before inserting the needle
(Z track technique) to promote
absorption and prevent skin staining
and pain
— observe patient carefully during the
initial stages of IV injection or
infusion in case of anaphylactoid
reaction
— have available adrenaline,
aminophylline, antihistamines,
hydrocortisone and resuscitation
equipment
— advise patient to keep iron
preparations out of the reach of
children

Note for iron preparations

— folic acid, liver extract and vitamins,
mainly B group and C have been
added to some oral iron preparations

HAEMATINICS

HYDROXOCOBALAMIN (Vitamin B_{12})

Action

— necessary for maturation of red
blood cells
— required for normal function of
nervous system and the formation of
epithelial cells in the mouth and gut

Use

— prevent or treat pernicious anaemia
— treat certain other megaloblastic
anaemias
— treat optic neuropathies

Dose

i) 250–1000 micrograms IM alternate
days for 1–2 weeks, then 250
micrograms IM weekly until blood
count normal, then 1000 micrograms
every 2–3 months for life (macrocytic
anaemia); OR
ii) 1000 micrograms IM alternate days
for 1–2 weeks, then 1000
micrograms every 2 months for life
(macrocytic anaemia with
neurological involvement); OR
iii) 1000 micrograms IM daily for 2
weeks, then twice weekly for 4
weeks, then monthly for life (optic
neuropathies)

Note

— iron and folic acid supplements may
also be necessary if severe anaemia

CYANOCOBALAMIN (Vitamin B_{12})

— as for hydroxocobalamin but not as
effective in optic neuropathies

Dose

i) 250–1000 micrograms IM alternate
days for 1–2 weeks, then 250
micrograms IM weekly until blood
count normal, then 1000 micrograms
monthly for life (macrocytic
anaemia); OR

ii) 1000 micrograms IM alternate days until improvement, then 1000 micrograms monthly for life (if neurological involvement); OR

iii) 50 micrograms orally 1–3 times daily 1 hour a.c. (tablets); OR

iv) 35–70 micrograms orally t.d.s. 1 hour a.c. (syrup)

Note

— patients sensitized to cyanocobalamin by injection are often able to take it orally

FOLIC ACID

Action

— required for the maturation of red blood cells
— necessary for DNA synthesis and mitosis hence for growth
— member of the vitamin-B group

Use

— prevent or treat megaloblastic anaemia caused by folic acid deficiency, e.g. in pregnancy

Dose

i) 0.5–15 mg orally daily; OR
ii) 15 mg IM daily

Interactions

— absorption of oral folic acid reduced by phenytoin
— folic acid blood levels reduced by phenobarbitone, phenytoin and primidone

Note

— folic acid may obscure the diagnosis of pernicious anaemia by improving the anaemia but allowing progression of irreversible neurological degeneration, therefore contraindicated in undiagnosed megaloblastic anaemia
— iron and/or liver extract and vitamins have been added to some folic acid preparations

OXYMETHOLONE

Action and use

— anabolic steroid used to treat aplastic anaemia by stimulating haemopoiesis

Dose

50–100 mg orally t.d.s.

Adverse effects

— see androgens (p. 163)

PARENTERAL ANTICOAGULANTS

HEPARIN (Heparin sodium)

Action

— direct anticoagulant which potentiates the naturally occurring inhibitors of coagulation, antifactor Xa and antithrombin III which then slows conversion of prothrombin to thrombin and fibrinogen to fibrin
— acts for 4–6 hours and trebles blood clotting time to 15–30 minutes

Use

— prophylaxis and treatment of thrombosis and embolism
— disseminated intravascular coagulation
— anticoagulant in blood collected for transfusion or laboratory tests
— extracorporeal circulation (heart/lung and renal dialysis machines)
— in locks giving access to veins

Dose

Prophylaxis (no laboratory control)

i) 5000 units SC 2 hours before surgery then 8- to 12-hourly until patient mobile
ii) 5000 units/ml made up to 5 ml with isotonic saline and injected up to 3 times/day into capped cannula in situ giving access to vein (heparin lock flush)

Therapeutic (laboratory control required)

i) 2000–5000 units IV bolus followed by 20 000–60 000 units in 24 hours by IV infusion; OR
ii) 5000–10 000 units IV 4- to 6-hourly; OR
iii) 10 000–20 000 units SC initially then 5000–15 000 units 8- to 12-hourly

Other

50 units made up to 5 ml with isotonic saline and injected 6-hourly into the cannula of a running IV infusion to maintain patency of the cannula (heparinized saline)

Treatment of heparin overdose

Protamine sulphate, a small basic protein, counteracts the anticoagulant effect of heparin by neutralizing its acidic charge (see p. 251)

Adverse effects

— bleeding, therefore contraindicated in gastric ulcer
— febrile or allergic reaction (rare)
— slight epistaxis, bruising, slight haematuria (overdose)

Interactions

— dipyridamole and salicylates enhance the activity of heparin by interfering with platelet aggregation so increasing the risk of haemorrhage
— effects enhanced by oral anticoagulants and phenylbutazone
— effects reduced by protamine sulphate
— as heparin is incompatible with many other drugs in aqueous solution it should only be mixed with another drug if prescribed by the medical officer or pharmacist

Nursing points

General

— heparin sodium given IV but heparin sodium or calcium may be used by SC injection (see below)
— avoid giving heparin IM to prevent painful haematoma formation
— be alert to the early signs of overdose by looking for bruising and testing the urine for blood daily (therapeutic dose only)
— monitor IV infusion rate closely by using a burette or infusion pump
— any IV solutions containing heparin and having any drug added should be screened carefully for signs of incompatibility
— protect heparin from light and heat
— have protamine sulphate available

Subcutaneous injection technique

— careful SC injection technique to

avoid local haematoma formation and ensure uniform absorption
— use a tuberculin syringe and a short 25 or 26 gauge needle
— the injection site is the subcutaneous fat of the anterior abdominal wall
— the needle is introduced perpendicularly to the skin surface into a pinched-up fold of skin and subcutaneous tissue until the tip enters the subcutaneous fat
— avoid intravascular injection by withdrawing the plunger
— inject slowly at the rate of 1 ml per minute
— withdraw the needle and exert firm palm pressure with an alcohol swab over the site for 5 minutes, the patient usually assisting with this
— rotate the injection sites regularly

Note

— ineffective if given orally
— prevents further clotting
— coagulation tests performed midway between injections
— test dose of 1000 units may be given if history of allergy
— heparin dose adjusted to keep the activated partial thromboplastin time (APTT) or the whole blood clotting time (WBCT) at $1\frac{1}{2}$–$2\frac{1}{2}$ times the control value
— oral anticoagulants may be commenced 3–5 days before gradually reducing then discontinuing heparin

CALCIUM HEPARIN

— prevent or treat thrombo-embolic disorders in the short term, otherwise as for heparin
— given by deep SC injection

INDIRECT (ORAL) ANTICOAGULANTS
(vitamin K antagonists)

Action

— reduce the formation of vitamin K-dependent clotting factors in the liver such as factor II (prothrombin) and factors VII, IX and X
— effective in 12–18 hours, peaks at 36–48 hours and persists for 5–6 days

Use

— prevent and treat venous thrombosis and pulmonary embolism
— cardiac valve prosthesis
— rheumatic valvular disease
— atrial fibrillation
— transient ischaemic attacks

Preparations and dose
WARFARIN
Dose

10–15 mg orally initially, then maintained on 3–10 mg daily

Note

— a long acting coumarin derivative

NICOUMALONE
Dose

20–28 mg orally initially, then maintained on 2–12 mg daily

Note

— a coumarin derivative of intermediate duration

PHENINDIONE
Dose

100 mg orally 12-hourly first day, 50 mg 12-hourly second day, then maintained on 12–50 mg 12-hourly

Note

— an indanedione derivative of intermediate duration

Adverse effects of oral anticoagulants

— bleeding
— nausea, vomiting, diarrhoea
— hypersensitivity reaction
— bleeding from the gums and haematuria (overdose)

Treatment of oral anticoagulant overdose

— phytomenadione (synthetic vitamin K)

Interactions of oral anticoagulants

— activity enhanced by salicylates, indomethacin, oxyphenbutazone, chloral hydrate, clofibrate, thyroid hormones, diflunisal, disulfiram, mefenamic acid, quinidine, antibiotics, phenylbutazone, phenytoin, tolbutamide, anabolic steroids, cimetidine, ranitidine and many other agents, hence leads to bleeding episodes
— activity reduced by cholestyramine, rifampicin, griseofulvin, carbamazepine, chlorthalidone, some hypnotics, vitamin K and many other agents, hence leads to loss of control of thrombo-embolic episodes

Nursing points for oral anticoagulants

— observe for early signs of overdose such as bleeding, especially from the gums
— urine not routinely tested daily for blood
— a metabolite of phenindione often causes red coloured urine, but this disappears when urine is acidified, distinguishing it from haematuria
— advise the patient to carry the anticoagulant handbook or booklet at all times in which is recorded laboratory test results and daily anticoagulant dose, or obtain 'Identicare' bracelet or pendant and enter the relevant information

— advise the patient to report melaena, excessive bleeding or bruising immediately to the medical officer
— advise the patient to notify his or her dentist of the anticoagulant therapy
— warn the patient that aspirin enhances the effects of anticoagulants and check OTC medications
— advise the patient that drug therapy is best withdrawn over 3–4 weeks unless urgent need to stop abruptly

Note for oral anticoagulants

— warfarin can be used safely by nursing mothers
— oral anticoagulants usually commenced at the same time as heparin, the heparin being stopped gradually once effect of oral anticoagulant apparent, usually in 36–48 hours
— dose adjusted by monitoring the prothrombin activity of the blood which is maintained at between 2–2½ times normal
— when heparin and warfarin are given together, blood for prothrombin activity taken 5 hours after last IV dose of heparin
— oral anticoagulants withdrawn gradually over 3–4 weeks

ANTITHROMBOTIC AGENT

DIPYRIDAMOLE

Action

— anti-thrombotic agent which reduces platelet aggregation mainly in arteries
— coronary vasodilator

Use

— as adjunct to anticoagulant therapy
— arterial thrombosis
— renal transplantation
— cardiac valve prosthesis

Dose

i) 100 mg orally q.i.d. 1 hr a.c.; OR
ii) 10 mg IM or slowly IV t.d.s.

Adverse effects

— headache (sometimes severe)
— gastrointestinal disturbances
— facial flushing
— dizziness, rash

Interactions

— when used with heparin, increases risk of haemorrhage

ASPIRIN (low dose)

Action

— blocks synthesis of thromboxane A_2 in platelets, so inhibits platelet aggregation

Use

— prophylaxis and treatment of transient ischaemic attacks
— secondary prevention of myocardial infarct
— prophylaxis against stroke, vascular occlusion and deep vein thrombosis

Dose

50–100 mg orally daily

Adverse effects

— as for aspirin (see p. 99) but minimized in low dose

Note

— high doses of aspirin cause platelet aggregation by blocking the synthesis of prostacyclin which normally inhibits platelet aggregation

CLOTTING AGENTS AND HAEMOSTATICS

AMINOCAPROIC ACID

Action

— causes haemostasis by inhibiting fibrinolysis

Use

— severe haemorrhage associated with excessive fibrinolysis, e.g. in haemophilia and following surgery
— subarachnoid haemorrhage

Dose

5 g initially orally or slow IV infusion then 1 g/hour for 8 hours or until bleeding controlled

Adverse effects

— nausea, abdominal cramps, diarrhoea
— nasal stuffiness, rash
— headache, dizziness, diuresis
— hypotension, bradycardia (if rapid IV injection)

Nursing points

— monitor vital signs, noting and recording response to therapy
— ensure IV needle remains firmly fixed in position to prevent thrombophlebitis

TRANEXAMIC ACID

Action

— inhibits fibrinolysis by reducing the conversion of plasminogen to plasmin

Use

— hereditary angioedema
— decreases risk of bleeding after tooth extraction in haemophiliacs

Dose

1–1.5 g orally 2–3 times daily

Adverse effects

— nausea, vomiting, diarrhoea
— giddiness

Note

— should be discontinued if patient develops a colour vision or other vision defect

CONJUGATED OESTROGENS

Action

— strengthens capillary walls and increases resistance to bleeding

Use

— haemostasis at the capillary level during and after surgery, epistaxis, hyphaema, dysfunctional uterine bleeding
— oestrogen replacement therapy

Dose

i) 25 mg slowly IV or IM, repeated in 1 hour as required (rapid control of spontaneous bleeding); OR
ii) 25 mg slowly IV or IM the evening before or a least 1 hour pre-operatively and may be repeated during and after surgery (control post-operative capillary bleeding); OR
iii) 25 mg slowly IV or IM, repeated in 6–12 hours as required plus oral preparation on designated days (dysfunctional uterine bleeding) (see p. 165)

Adverse effects

— too rapid IV, nausea, vomiting, flushing

Note

— shake vial gently when reconstituting with supplied diluent

PHYTOMENADIONE (Vitamin K₁)

Action

— similar to naturally occurring vitamin
  K which promotes the hepatic
  biosynthesis of prothrombin and
  coagulation factors VII, IX and X
— antagonizes the effects of indirect,
  orally-acting anticoagulants

Use

— prothrombin deficiency
— prophylaxis and therapy of
  haemorrhagic disease of the
  newborn (neonatal
  hypoprothrombinaemia)
— hypovitaminosis K
— reverses the effects of oral
  anticoagulants

Adult dose

5–20 mg orally IM or IV depending on
the severity of the condition. Repeat
doses determined by prothrombin time
estimations

Paediatric dose

Neonatal hypoprothrombinaemia

0.5–1 mg IM (prophylaxis)
1–2.5 mg IM (therapeutic) and if
necessary, further doses of 1 mg may
be given 8-hourly

Adverse effects

— hypersensitivity reaction (rare)
— hyperbilirubinaemia in newborn infant
  (rare)

Nursing point

— tablets chewed thoroughly and
  allowed to dissolve in the mouth

Note

— ineffective in heparin overdose

MENAPHTHONE

— as for phytomenadione but with less
  rapid and shorter duration of action

Dose

i) 1–2 mg SC or IM daily; OR
ii) 10 mg orally t.d.s. with food

PROTAMINE SULPHATE

Action

— basic protein which combines with
  acidic heparin to form a stable,
  inactive complex

Use

— neutralizes the anticoagulant action
  of heparin

Dose

based on 1 mg neutralizing
approximately 100 units of heparin;
given slowly by IV injection over 10
minutes and repeated depending on the
whole blood clotting time or plasma
activated partial thromboplastin time
(APTT)

Adverse effects

— hypotension, bradycardia
— dyspnoea

Nursing point

— vital signs monitored closely

Note

— no more than 50 mg given in any 10
  minute period
— if used in excess, has an
  anticoagulant action
— ineffective in overdose of oral
  anticoagulants

THROMBIN

Action and use

— a bovine plasma product used topically to control capillary bleeding during surgery

Dose

1000–2000 units topically

Adverse effects

— allergic reaction

FIBRINOLYTIC AGENTS (thrombolytics)

STREPTOKINASE

Action

— rapidly activates endogenous fibrinolytic system by converting plasminogen into the fibrinolytic enzyme plasmin

Use

— dissolves intravascular blood clots

Dose

50 000–750 000 units by IV infusion according to manufacturer's literature and medical officer

Adverse effects

— mild fever
— hypersensitivity reaction (common)
— haemorrhage (rare)

Nursing points

— monitor vital signs closely especially if given rapidly
— reconstituted streptokinase can be refrigerated at 4°C to 6°C for 5–6 hours
— any unused solution is discarded

Note

— best stability achieved when mixed with the gelatin plasma substitute Haemaccel®, but if unavailable, isotonic saline, 5% glucose or Ringer's lactate solution may be used
— allergic reaction reduced if initial dose given with hydrocortisone
— when combined with streptodornase, may be applied topically or instilled in body cavities to remove fibrinous or purulent accumulations (streptokinase-streptodornase)

RECOMBINANT TISSUE PLASMINOGEN ACTIVATOR (rt-PA)

Action

— fibrinolytic glycoprotein which binds fibrin in the thrombus and converts entrapped plasminogen to plasmin which results in clot dissolution with minimal systemic effects
— produced by recombinant DNA technology

Use

— lysis of suspected occlusive artery thrombi associated with myocardial infarction

Dose

100 mg infused over 3 hours via dedicated IV line with an infusion pump:
1st hour: 60 mg of which 6–10 mg is given as IV bolus over first 1–2 minutes and remainder by continuous infusion
2nd and 3rd hours: 20 mg during each hour by continuous infusion

Adverse effectrs

— internal bleeding involving gastro-intestinal or genitourinary tracts, retroperitoneal or intracranial sites
— superficial or surface bleeding from arterial and venous puncture sites or surgical incisions
— epistaxis, bleeding gums, bruising
— nausea, vomiting, hypotension, fever which are also frequent sequelae of myocardial infarction

Nursing points

— reconstitute to concentration of 1 mg/ml by adding to the 50 mg vial of powder 50ml of accompanying sterile Water for Injection according to the manufacturer's instructions
— do not use vial if vacuum not present
— powder is reconstituted immediately before use and can be kept for up to 8 hours at 25°C or for up to 24 hours at 2–8°C

— any unused solution is discarded
— avoid excessive or vigorous shaking
— IM injections and non-essential handling of patient avoided during therapy
— if arterial puncture is necessary during therapy, an upper extremity vessel is used which is accessible to manual compression which is applied for 30 minutes, followed by a pressure dressing
— puncture sites checked frequently for evidence of bleeding, especially if heparin is being used concomitantly
— if serious bleeding (not controllable by local pressure), cease rt-PA infusion and heparin
— heparin effects can be reversed by protamine sulphate
— have available anti-arrhythmic therapy for bradycardia and/or ventricular irritability when infusion administered

Note

— heparin 1000 units/hour is usually commenced prior to termination of rt-PA infusion through a separate IV line to maintain an activated partial thromboplastin time (APTT) $1\frac{1}{2}$ to 2 times the control

HYPOLIPIDAEMIC AGENTS

CLOFIBRATE

Action

— reduces elevated blood triglyceride and cholesterol levels
— reduces platelet stickiness and prolongs platelet survival time

Use

— hypercholesterolaemia
— some types of hyperlipoproteinaemia
— diabetic retinopathy
— adjunctive in treatment of angina pectoris
— xanthoma

Dose

20–30 mg/kg orally daily in 2 or 3 divided doses after meals

Adverse effects

— nausea and abdominal discomfort

Interactions

— enhances effect of oral anticoagulants and possibly oral hypoglycaemic agents
— effect reduced by rifampicin

Nursing points

— note instability in diabetes in patients receiving oral hypoglycaemics

CHOLESTYRAMINE

Action

— anion-exchange resin which forms an insoluble non-absorbable complex with intestinal bile salts, so reduces blood cholesterol level

Use

— reduce blood cholesterol level
— relieve pruritus associated with partial biliary obstruction

— diarrhoea following ileal resection or disease

Adult dose

i) 1–3 level scoops t.d.s. a.c.; OR
ii) ½–1 sachet t.d.s. a.c.
(1 scoop provides 4 g and 1 sachet 9 g)

Paediatric dose

6–12 years determined by Clark's rule

Adverse effects

— constipation, faecal impaction, haemorrhoids
— mild transient nausea, diarrhoea
— reduced absorption of fat-soluble vitamins
— steatorrhoea

Interactions

— reduces absorption of thyroid hormones, warfarin and hydrochlorothiazide

Nursing points

— place scoop or sachet contents on the surface of 120–180 ml of water, fruit juice, apple sauce or crushed pineapple in a large glass
— allow to stand for 1–2 minutes to hydrate then stir to uniform suspension
— ensure that glass rinsings are also taken
— other oral drugs given either 1 hour before or 4–6 hours after resin for better absorption

Note

— should not be taken in dry form
— if prolonged therapy, may require supplementary vitamins A and D

COLESTIPOL

As for cholestyramine

Dose

15–30 g daily 2–4 divided doses
(1 sachet supplies 5 g)

PROBUCOL

Action

— reduces blood cholesterol level

Use

— familial hypercholesterolaemia
unresponsive to other treatment

Dose

500 mg orally b.d. with food

Adverse effects

— nausea, abdominal pain, diarrhoea
— paraesthesia

11 Vitamins and mineral supplements

VITAMINS

VITAMIN A (retinol)

Action

— fat-soluble vitamin necessary for normal formation and function of epithelial and mucosal cells
— necessary for formation and regeneration of rhodopsin (visual purple)

Deficiency

— night blindness, later xerophthalmia
— dry rough skin
— infection

Use

— deficiency states, some skin diseases, night blindness
— chronic infection, sunburn
— supplement in pregnancy and lactation
— replacement in decreased intestinal absorption conditions, e.g. steatorrhoea, biliary obstruction, coeliac disease

Adult dose

Optimal daily requirements

750 micrograms (2500 units) (increase required during pregnancy and lactation)

Prophylactic

1.5–2.4 mg (5000–8000 units) orally once daily

Therapeutic

3–150 mg (10 000–500 000 units) orally once daily

Paediatric dose

Prophylactic

up to 1 year: 450 micrograms (1500 units)
1–3 years: 600 micrograms (2000 units)
3–6 years: 750 micrograms (2500 units)
6–10 years: 1.05 mg (3500 units)
10–12 years: 1.35 mg (4500 units)

Therapeutic

3.6 mg (12 000 units) orally once daily

Adverse effects

— fatigue, anorexia, vomiting, abdominal discomfort, weight loss, fever
— irritability, headache
— dry lips, yellow skin pigmentation, desquamation, pruritus
— hepatosplenomegaly
— premature closure of epiphyses

Interaction

— excess amounts of liquid paraffin reduces absorption

THIAMINE (vitamin B_1, aneurine)

Action

— water-soluble member of the vitamin B group necessary for carbohydrate metabolism and nutrition of nerve cells

Deficiency

— dietary deficiency, e.g. chronic
  alcoholism
— neuritis
— beri beri

Use

— neuritis, polyneuritis
— anorexia
— faulty carbohydrate metabolism
— constipation
— beri beri
— Wernicke's encephalopathy

Adult dose

Optimal daily requirements

200 micrograms per 4200 kj (1000 kcal)
of carbohydrate intake

Prophylactic

2–5 mg daily

Therapeutic

i) 50–100 mg orally daily as single dose
   or 2 divided doses; OR
ii) 100 mg IM daily

Paediatric dose

1–5 mg orally daily in a vitamin B group
or multivitamin preparation

Adverse effects

— anaphylactic shock following rapid IV
  injection

Note

— thiamine requirements increase as
  carbohydrate intake increases

RIBOFLAVINE (vitamin B₂)

Action

— water soluble member of the vitamin
  B group necessary for carbohydrate
  and protein metabolism and red
  blood cell production

Deficiency

— angular stomatitis, glossitis, ano-
  genital dermatitis
— 'burning feet'
— photophobia

Use

— ariboflavinosis
— neurological symptoms of pellagra

Adult dose

Optimal daily requirements

1.3–1.8 mg daily (increase required
during pregnancy and lactation)

Therapeutic

2–10 mg orally daily

Paediatric dose

1–2.5 mg orally daily in a vitamin B
group or multivitamin preparation

Adverse effects

— none known

Note

— urine becomes a harmless intense
  yellow

NICOTINIC ACID (niacin)

Action

— water soluble member of the vitamin
  B group
— peripheral vasodilator
— hypolipidaemic, hypotriglyceridaemic
  and hypocholesterolaemic
— form co-enzymes important in tissue
  respiration

Deficiency

— pellagra

Use

— pellagra

— hypercholesterolaemia
— hypertriglyceridaemia
— peripheral vascular disorders
— Ménière's disease

Adult dose

Optimal daily requirements

15–20 mg depending on the protein intake

Pellagra

i) 15–50 mg orally daily (prophylaxis); OR
ii) 250 mg orally b.d. p.c. (therapeutic)

Hypercholesterolaemia and hypertriglyceridaemia

250 mg orally t.d.s. p.c. increasing to 1.5 g t.d.s. p.c.

Peripheral vascular disorders and Ménière's disease

50 mg orally t.d.s.

Adverse effects

— flushing, strong sensation of warmth, pounding in head
— pruritus, urticaria, dry skin, exfoliation
— nausea, vomiting, diarrhoea, activation of peptic ulcer
— nervousness
— hepatotoxicity

Nursing point

— warn patient of the occurrence of flushing of the face and chest 30 minutes after taking nicotinic acid

Note

— see peripheral vasodilators

PYRIDOXINE (vitamin B$_6$)
Action

— water soluble member of the vitamin B group important in carbohydrate, lipid and protein metabolism
— assists in formation of haem

Deficiency

— irritability, convulsions
— hypochromic anaemia
— peripheral neuritis
— angular stomatitis, glossitis

Use

— prophylactically to avoid isoniazid-induced peripheral neuritis
— some types of anaemia
— premenstrual tension

Adult dose

Optimal daily requirements

2 mg

Prophylactic

50 mg orally t.d.s. (isoniazid-induced peripheral neuritis)

Therapeutic

25–50 mg orally t.d.s. (anaemia)
25–50 mg orally b.d. or t.d.s. 1–3 days before expected onset of symptoms until onset of menstruation (premenstrual tension)

Paediatric dose

25–50 mg orally daily (prevention of isoniazid-induced neuropathy)
50 mg IV (pyridoxine-dependent convulsions infants)

Adverse effects

rarely, slight flushing, paraesthesia

Interactions

— reduces effects of levodopa
— reduces blood levels of phenobarbitone and phenytoin

CYANOCOBALAMIN (vitamin B$_{12}$)

— see haematinics

HYDROXOCOBALAMIN (vitamin B_{12})

— see haematinics

FOLIC ACID (vitamin B group)

— see haematinics

FOLINIC ACID (calcium folinate)

Action

— member of vitamin B group neutralizes folic acid antagonists
— administered a few hours after methotrexate to 'rescue' the normal cells of the host preferentially after the drug has been bound within tumor cells

Use

— antidote to folic acid antagonists, e.g. methotrexate
— megaloblastic anaemia (not vitamin B_{12} deficient)
— pyrimethamine overdose

Dose

'Folinic acid rescue'

Depends on dose of methotrexate so following is an example only
 i) 75 mg IV infusion within 12 hours, then 12 mg IM 6-hourly for 4 doses; OR
 ii) 6–12 mg IM 6-hourly for 4 doses; OR
 iii) 15 mg orally 6-hourly for 48–72 hours

Megaloblastic anaemia

1 mg IM daily

Pyrimethamine overdose

3–9 mg/day IM for 3 days

Adverse effects

— fever, rash, pruritus
— nausea, vomiting

ASCORBIC ACID (vitamin C)

Action

— water soluble agent necessary for development of collagen and intercellular material
— necessary for wound healing
— necessary for the conversion of folic acid to folinic acid
— necessary for red blood cell production

Deficiency

— scurvy

Use

— supplement when on restricted diet
— treatment of scurvy
— promotion of healing of wounds and fractures
— some types of anaemia
— urinary acidification

Adult dose

Optimal daily requirements

30 mg (increase required in adolescence, pregnancy, lactation, infections, thyrotoxicosis and after surgery

Prophylactic

25–75 mg orally daily

Therapeutic

200–600 mg orally daily
0.5–1 g orally b.d. or t.d.s. (scurvy)

Paediatric dose

 i) 25–50 mg orally daily (prophylaxis); OR
 ii) 100 mg orally t.d.s. for 7–10 days (scurvy treatment)

Adverse effects

— large doses may cause diarrhoea and renal calculi

Interactions

— chronic administration of aspirin reduces ascorbic acid blood levels
— increases absorption of oral iron in anaemic partial gastrectomy patients
— increases activity of co-trimoxazole against pseudomonas organisms

Note

— infants fed on cow's milk alone require ascorbic acid supplement
— ascorbic acid mixture available 25 mg/ml, kept in refrigerator

CALCIFEROL (vitamin D$_2$)

Action

— fat soluble vitamin necessary for the absorption of calcium, an essential requirement in bone formation

Deficiency

— rickets (in children)
— osteomalacia (in adults)

Use

— rickets
— osteomalacia
— hypoparathyroidism
— tuberculous bone disease
— chilblains

Adult dose

Optimal daily requirements

2.5 micrograms (100 units) (increase required in infancy, pregnancy and lactation)

Prophylactic

20 micrograms (800 units)

Therapeutic

1.25–5 mg (50 000–200 000 units) orally daily depending on the condition
15 mg (600 000 units) orally weekly for 3 weeks (chilblains)

Paediatric dose

10–20 micrograms (400–800 units) for rickets prophylaxis
75–2500 micrograms (3000–100 000 units) orally daily depending on the condition

Adverse effects

— prolonged administration of 2.5–3.75 mg (100 000–150 000 units) daily in adults or 750 micrograms (30 000 units) in children causes anorexia, lassitude, nausea, vomiting, diarrhoea, profuse sweating, polyuria, excessive thirst, weight loss, headache, dizziness, hypertension, renal failure
— hypercalcaemia

Interactions

— phenobarbitone, phenytoin and primidone reduce the effects of vitamin D resulting in hypocalcaemia
— combined rifampicin and isoniazid therapy causes reduced vitamin D blood levels

Note

— liquid paraffin reduces absorption of vitamin D
— vitamin D is synthesized from steroids in the skin by the action of sunlight

CALCITRIOL

(1,25-dihydroxycholecalciferol)

Action

— a potent metabolite of vitamin D
— as for calciferol

Use

— renal osteodystrophy conditions including osteitis fibrosa cystica, osteomalacia and osteoporosis

Dose

0.25 micrograms orally daily increasing by 0.25 micrograms at 2–4 week intervals as required up to 0.5–1 microgram daily

Adverse effects

— as for calciferol

Interactions

— magnesium preparations reduce calcium absorption in gut
— concurrent cardiac glycoside therapy may precipitate cardiac arrhythmias
— cholestyramine reduces absorption of calcitriol

Note

— an adequate daily intake of 400–800 mg of calcium is necessary

TOCOPHEROLS (vitamin E)

Action

— function as antioxidants
— fat soluble
— deficiency may cause anaemia in infants

Use

— may be used in treating haemolytic anaemia in premature infants

Adult dose

Optimal daily requirements

10–30 mg depending on intake of polyunsaturated fatty acids

Therapeutic

10–800 mg orally daily depending on the response

Paediatric dose

5–100 mg orally daily depending on the response

Adverse effects

— high doses may cause nausea, fatigue and weakness

PHYTOMENADIONE (vitamin K)

— see clotting agents

MULTIVITAMIN PREPARATIONS

Many mixed vitamin preparations containing vitamins A, B group, C, D and E are available, some also containing minerals. Prolonged courses of high doses are of little value if a well-balanced diet is also being taken, and can lead to serious results in the case of excessive intake of the fat-soluble vitamins A and D. Deficiency states are rare in people living in communities where an adequate diet can be taken. However, vitamin and mineral supplements are necessary in cases of restricted diet, malabsorption syndrome, and where there are increased requirements such as in pregnancy, lactation, fever, hyperthyroidism and wasting diseases.

MINERAL SUPPLEMENTS

CALCIUM CARBONATE

Use

— antacid
— calcium supplement in prophylaxis and treatment of calcium deficiency
— supplement in pregnancy
— phosphate binder in chronic renal failure

Dose

1–3 g orally 1–3 times daily with meals

Adverse effects

— constipation, nausea, flatulence
— prolonged high doses, hypercalcaemia, hypophosphataemia, renal calculi

Interactions

— reduces absorption of oral iron
— phenobarbitone, phenytoin and primidone reduce calcium absorption
— reduces blood level of tetracyclines
— reduces absorption of phosphate from food

Nursing points

— give calcium salts at least 2 hours apart from oral iron compounds and oral tetracyclines
— note nausea, constipation, confusion, weakness, as these are early signs of hypercalcaemia
— give with food if using as phosphate binder

Note

— see antacids

CALCIUM CHLORIDE

Use

— given IV to initiate cardiac rhythm in asystole if patient fails to respond to other measures
— potassium overdose
— magnesium overdose

Dose

5–10 ml of solution IV bolus slowly over 2–3 minutes

Adverse effects

— peripheral vasodilatation, bradycardia, hypotension
— can cause asystole if injected too quickly

Note

— 10% solution contains 6.8 mmol Ca^{++}/10 ml
— continuous auscultation or ECG monitoring during IV injection
— not added to sodium bicarbonate as forms precipitate

CALCIUM GLUCONATE

Use and adverse effects

— as for calcium chloride

Adult dose

10 ml of 10% solution IV bolus slowly over 2–3 minutes

Paediatric dose

0.1 ml/kg IV

Note

— solution 1 g/10 ml (2.2 mmol Ca^{++}/10 ml)
— continuous auscultation or ECG monitoring during IV injection
— also given orally as calcium supplement
— not added to sodium bicarbonate as forms precipitate
— not as potent as calcium chloride
— should not be given to patients taking digoxin

FLUORIDE

Use

— help in formation of healthy teeth and help prevent tooth decay

Dose (non-fluoridated areas)

Consult dentist or medical officer if in fluoridated area
under 12 months: 0.55 mg daily
12–24 months: 1.1 mg daily
24 months and over: 2.2 mg daily
pregnancy: 3.3 mg daily

Adverse effects

— large doses cause weakness, convulsions and cardiopulmonary failure

Nursing points

— tablets to be crushed or chewed for maximum benefit
— dentist may prescribe an external preparation which is made into a solution and applied to the teeth

Note

— optimal level in fluoridated water supply in 1 mg/l (1 ppm) in temperate regions
— at higher concentrations, teeth develop brownish mottling

POTASSIUM CHLORIDE

Use

— as potassium replacement therapy after long term use or high doses of potassium-depleting diuretics especially if patient also receiving digoxin
— long term corticosteroid therapy especially if patient also receiving digoxin
— digoxin toxicity precipitated by loss of potassium
— poor absorption or loss from gastrointestinal tract after excessive vomiting or diarrhoea, or use of laxatives
— diabetic ketoacidosis
— metabolic alkalosis
— hyperaldosteronism

Dose

Slow Release Tablets

i) 1 or 2 tablets daily (prophylaxis); OR
ii) 1 or 2 tablets 2–3 times daily (therapeutic)
(1 tablet contains 312 mg or 8 mmol potassium)
Tablets are swallowed *whole* with a little water or fruit juice preferably after meals

Effervescent Tablets

i) 1 tablet daily (prophylaxis); OR
ii) 2 tablets b.d. (therapeutic) (1 tablet contains 548 mg or 14 mmol potassium)
(Tablets are dissolved in ½ glass of water and taken orally)

Oral liquids

15 ml b.d.
(15 ml contains 786 mg or 20 mmol potassium)
Dilute in one glass of water or fruit juice after breakfast and after the evening meal

Intravenous preparations

80–400 mmol/24 hours as a *dilute* solution
N.B. IV potassium must be given as a thoroughly mixed dilute solution of uniform concentration of not more than 80 mmol/1 and run slowly at a rate not exceeding 30 mmol/hour. This avoids a sudden increase in plasma potassium concentration which may lead to cardiac arrest and death.
If potassium chloride is to be added to a hanging IV solution, ensure there is sufficient solution to make the correct dilution, then after adding the medication, invert the container several times to guarantee complete mixing.

Adverse effects

— effervescent tablets and liquids; nausea, vomiting, bad taste, diarrhoea, abdominal pain and heartburn

— slow release tablets; nausea,
vomiting, diarrhoea, abdominal pain,
and rarely, stricture, ulceration or
perforation of bowel
— parenteral; pain and phlebitis at IV
site, nausea, vomiting, abdominal
pain
  Overdose: lethargy, confusion,
weakness, flaccid paralysis, paraesthesia
of extremities, hypotension, cardiac
arrhythmias, cardiac arrest

Interactions

— hyperkalaemia may occur if
potassium supplements given in
conjunction with the potassium-
sparing diuretics amiloride,
spironolactone and triamterene

Nursing points

— advise patient to swallow slow
release (SR) tablets whole with a
little water and do not allow to
dissolve in the mouth
— advise patient to dissolve
effervescent preparation, 1 tablet to ½
glass of water
— advise patient to report to the
medical officer any gastrointestinal
symptoms
— ensure all IV solutions containing
potassium are mixed thoroughly and
labelled carefully
— monitor IV infusion rate by using a
burette or infusion pump
— potassium *must not* be added to a
burette or into an injection port
— have available calcium gluconate (if
patient not receiving cardiac
glycosides), 5% or 10% glucose,
soluble insulin and sodium
bicarbonate

Note

— IV potassium chloride is *not*
compatible with adrenaline,
phenytoin, thiopentone, mannitol,
diazepam, amphotericin B and
streptomycin
— a 1 g ampoule contains 13 millimoles
of potassium ion

SODIUM BICARBONATE

Use

— alkalinizing agent given IV to correct
acidosis in cardiopulmonary arrest

Adult dose

1 mmol/kg IV over 1–3 minutes, repeat
½ dose every 10 minutes as required,
but avoid exceeding 50 mmol/hr

Paediatric dose

Dilute 8.4% solution 1 in 10 before
administration
2 mmol/kg IV initially then 1 mmol/kg
incremental doses if necessary (about
every 10 minutes) to a maximum rate
of 0.1 mmol/kg/min

Adverse effects

— alkalosis with skeletal muscle and
cardiac irritability, apathy and mental
confusion

Note

— 8.4% solution (1 mEq/ml)
— 1 mEq is equivalent to 1 mmol of
sodium bicarbonate
— sodium overload may provoke
pulmonary oedema

SODIUM CHLORIDE

Use

— prevention and correction of fluid and
electrolyte deficits or imbalance
— prevention or treatment of sodium
chloride loss in sweat when heavy
work is being done in a hot
atmosphere
— replacement of urinary sodium
chloride loss in Addison's disease
(adrenocortical atrophy)
— dialysis fluid
— eye lotion, mouth wash and irrigating
solution

Dose

i) mainly given by IV infusion as

sodium chloride injection 0.9%
(isotonic saline); OR
ii) 10–12 g orally daily in 3–4 divided
doses; OR
iii) 0.45% sodium chloride solution
administered rectally; OR
iv) as basis of fluid for peritoneal
dialysis or haemodialysis

Adverse effects

— restlessness, weakness, dizziness,
headache
— thirst, swollen tongue
— flushing
— oliguria
— hypotension, tachycardia
— cerebral oedema, peripheral oedema
— delirium
— respiratory arrest

Interaction

— high sodium intake reduces effect of
lithium

Nursing points

— select the correct preparation for
administration
— select the correct concentration of
saline, isotonic (0.9%), hypotonic
(less concentrated), or hypertonic
(more concentrated) noting also that
sodium chloride is often combined
with glucose
— monitor heart rate, blood pressure,
fluid intake and output
— note and report any dependant
oedema or pulmonary oedema

Note

— IV solutions incompatible with
amphotericin B, noradrenaline or
mannitol
— avoid giving saline emetics as many
tragedies have resulted especially in
children

12 Antineoplastic agents

Used alone or in combination with glucocorticoids, sex hormones, azathioprine, B.C.G. vaccine, radiopharmaceuticals, radiotherapy and/or surgery against malignant disease to provide palliation with regression of the neoplasm. Very toxic agents are used to inhibit the growth of malignant cells by attacking them at different stages in the cell cycle. However, all rapidly dividing cells are affected, malignant and normal, so limiting the use of these agents. Generally, malignant cells surviving treatment recover less readily than do normal cells surviving treatment.

Adverse effects result from attack on the rapidly dividing cells in tissues such as hair follicles, bone marrow, gut and lymphatic tissues (see adverse effects). Cancer cells, taking longer to recover, can be attacked by multiple therapy (protocols) in different ways, the courses being repeated over a long period.

These drugs, often called cytotoxics, may be given orally, intravenously or by regional perfusion, often in a specialized unit, the maximum tolerated doses are administered, the dose being controlled by the patient's blood picture, tumour size and general health. Combinations of high doses of cytotoxic drugs are often given intermittently, to allow normal cells to recover.

Use

— most leukaemias
— multiple myeloma
— Hodgkin's disease
— lymphosarcoma
— lymphoma
— Burkitt's lymphoma
— osteogenic sarcoma
— reticulum cell sarcoma
— carcinoma breast, lung, prostate, testis, ovary, uterus
— carcinoma gastrointestinal tract
— choriocarcinoma
— neuroblastoma
— Ewing's tumour
— Wilms' tumour
— polycythaemia vera
— carcinoid syndrome
— retinoblastoma
— rhabdomyosarcoma

ALKYLATING AGENTS

Action

— arrest cell division by damaging DNA during all phases of cell cycle
— cell cycle non-specific agents

Preparations and usual route of administration

BUSULPHAN (oral)

CARMUSTINE (IV)

CHLORAMBUCIL (orally a.c.)

CYCLOPHOSPHAMIDE (oral, IV)

Note

— encourage high fluid intake to reduce risk of cystitis

LOMUSTINE (orally a.c.)

MELPHALAN (oral, IV)

MUSTINE (IV, intracavity)

Note

— strong vesicant and nasal irritant, therefore wash any spillage from skin immediately and avoid leaking from injection site

THIOTEPA (IM, IV, IA, intracavity, local)

ANTIMETABOLITES

Action

— competes with essential substances required by cell so prevents synthesis of bases or their incorporation into nucleic acids
— cell cycle specific agents

Preparations and usual route of administration

CYTARABINE (Cytosine arabinoside) (SC, IV)

Note

— also has antiviral properties

FLUOROURACIL (IV, IA, local)

MERCAPTOPURINE (oral)

Note

— allopurinol enhances effects of mercaptopurine

METHOTREXATE (Amethopterin) (oral, IM, IV, IT)

Note

— severe haematological effects reversed by folinic acid within 12 hours of infusion then at 6-hourly intervals ('folinic acid rescue' (p. 259))
— excretion of methotrexate enhanced by sodium bicarbonate
— blood levels increased by probenecid

THIOGUANINE (oral)

ANTIBIOTICS

Action

— inhibits RNA synthesis by binding with DNA
— cell cycle non-specific agents

Preparations and usual route of administration

ACTINOMYCIN D (Dactinomycin) (IV)

BLEOMYCIN (SC, IM, IV, IA)

Note

— note and report fever, dyspnoea and cough as it is pulmonary toxic

DAUNORUBICIN (Rubidomycin) (IV)
Note

— cardiotoxic therefore requires cardiac monitoring
— transient red coloured urine

DOXORUBICIN (Adriamycin) (IV)

Note

— cardiotoxic therefore requires cardiac monitoring
— urine may be coloured red

EPIRUBICIN (IV)

Note

— careful monitoring to minimize risk of cardiac failure
— urine may be coloured red

MITHRAMYCIN (IV)

Note

— early sign of bleeding syndrome, epistaxis

MITOMYCIN (IV, IA)

Note

— also used as bladder instillation

VINCA ALKALOIDS

Action

— cell division is arrested in metaphase because of the inhibition of spindle formation
— cell cycle stage-specific

Preparations and usual route of administration

VINBLASTINE (IV)

VINCRISTINE (IV)

Note

— severe constipation and faecal impaction likely

VINDESINE (IV)

HORMONES

CYPROTERONE (oral)

Note

— an anti-androgen with progestogenic activity used in prostatic carcinoma
— see (p. 164)

DROSTANOLONE (IM)

Note

— anabolic steroid with weak androgenic activity, promotes regression of breast cancer

FOSFESTROL (Stilboestrol diphosphate) (oral, IV)

Note

— controls androgen-dependent prostatic carcinoma

MEDROXYPROGESTERONE (oral, IV)

MEGESTROL (oral)

NORETHISTERONE ACETATE (oral)

Note

— progestogenic, oestrogenic and androgenic agent used in breast cancer

POLYESTRADIOL (IM)

Note

— an oestrogen used in prostatic carcinoma

TAMOXIFEN (oral)

Note

— anti-oestrogen, causes regression in oestrogen-dependent breast tumours
— activity enhanced by concurrent administration of bromocriptine to decrease prolactin levels

MISCELLANEOUS AGENTS

AMINOGLUTETHIMIDE (oral)

Note

— inhibits production of adrenal steroids producing a 'medical' adrenalectomy

AMSACRINE (central vein infusion)

Note

— cardiotoxic therefore requires cardiac monitoring

CARBOPLATIN (IV)

Note

— not compatible with IV needles, syringes or sets containing aluminium

CIS-PLATINUM (IV)

Note

— action similar to alkylating agent
— note tinnitus, hearing loss
— IV hydration prior to administration to try to reduce nephrotoxicity
— protect from light by wrapping prepared IV solution and lines immediately in aluminium foil, black plastic sheeting or some other opaque material

COLASPASE (L-asparaginase) (IV)

Note

— acts by decreasing blood levels of L-asparagine, on which certain tumour cells are metabolically dependent
— after a test dose (SC), the patient is observed for about 3 hours for signs of hypersensitivity

DACARBAZINE (IV)

Note

— restriction of food for 4–6 hours prior to treatment may reduce severity of nausea and vomiting
— avoid contact with skin and eyes
— must be protected from light

ETHOGLUCID (local)

Note

— use glass syringe to prepare
— used as bladder instillation

ETOPOSIDE (oral, IV)

HYDROXYUREA (oral)

Note

— inhibits ribonucleotide reductase

LEUPRORELIN (SC)

MITOZANTRONE (IV)

Note

— urine may be blue-green
— cardiotoxic therefore requires cardiac monitoring

PROCARBAZINE (oral)

Note

— is a weak monoamine oxidase inhibitor, so alcohol, cheese etc. should be avoided, as for phenelzine (p. 130)

TENIPOSIDE (VM 26) (IV)

Adverse effects of cytotoxic agents

— anorexia, nausea, vomiting, diarrhoea
— bone marrow depression resulting in immunosuppression, infection and bleeding
— hyperuricaemia
— oesophagitis
— stomatitis
— gastrointestinal ulceration
— alopecia
— rash, dermatitis
— fever, malaise
— pulmonary toxicity
— nephrotoxicity
— cardiotoxicity
— hepatotoxicity
— neurotoxicity
— ototoxicity
— sterility, mutations, teratogenesis, and abortion
— tissue sloughing (local)
— impaired wound healing

Nursing points for cytotoxic agents

— assure patient that nausea, vomiting are transient and that drugs are available to counteract these adverse effects
— prevent extravasation of cytotoxic drugs by ensuring IV cannula remains securely in position, thereby avoiding severe pain and tissue damage
— observe closely for and report extravasation immediately
— protect patient from infection by maintaining strict asepsis and high standard of hygiene and nursing in reverse isolation if practicable
— observe closely for signs of infection, bleeding tendencies, paraesthesia, loss of reflexes, ataxia, mouth ulcers and alopecia
— advise the patient that hair will regrow and that a wig may be worn in the meantime
— when handling any cytotoxic agents, avoid inhaling, and any contact with skin or eyes
— staff handling cytotoxics will have clear guidelines regarding preparation, administration, dealing with spillage, extravasation and disposal of used equipment and patients' body wastes

Note for cytotoxic agents

— cytotoxic agents cause the lysis of a massive number of cells resulting in the production of large amounts of uric acid from the breakdown of the nucleoproteins but the resulting hyperuricaemia is reduced by allopurinol
— treatment with cytotoxics is commonly referred to as 'chemotherapy'

ANTITUMOUR AGENT

INTERFERON

Action

— naturally occurring small protein molecule produced and secreted by cells in response to viral infections or to various synthetic and biological inducers
— produced by recombinant DNA technology
— inhibits replication in virus-infected cells by binding to cell surface receptors and inducing production of intracellular enzymes
— suppression of immunomodulating activity

Use

— treatment of hairy cell leukaemia in patients over 18 years
— condylomata accuminata (genital warts)

Dose

Hairy cell leukaemia

i) 2 million IU/m^2 SC 3 times a week (interferon alpha-2b); OR
ii) 3 million IU SC or IM 3 times a week (interferon alpha-2a)

Condylomata accuminata

1 million IU into lesion 3 times a week on alternate days for 3 weeks (interferon alpha-2b)

Adverse effects (systemic use)

— fever, fatigue, chills, headache, myalgia, arthralgia
— nausea
— thrombocytopenia, transient granulocytopenia
— transient mild skin rash

Note

— at the discretion of the medical officer, patient may self-administer medication SC before retiring
— patient advised not to change brands without consulting the medical officer
— paracetamol 0.5–1 g is taken 30 minutes before administration of interferon to alleviate symptoms of fever and headache, then up to 1 g q.i.d.
— patient should be well hydrated especially during initial stages of treatment
— reconstituted solution stable at room temperature for 2 hours or 24 hours at 2–8°C as it contains no preservative
— do not freeze
— blood cell counts and liver function monitored before therapy and then at monthly or appropriate intervals during treatment

13 Drugs acting on the skin and mucous membranes

Applications to the skin and mucous membranes contain active ingredients (see lists) which may be formulated, depending on the desired effect, in preparations such as lotions, solutions, paints, creams, ointments, pastes, soaps, shampoos, powders and aerosols.

Nursing points for application of preparations

— use powders and lotions sparingly to prevent excessive drying and cracking
— apply ointment as a thin smear
— avoid applying ointments to hairy areas or to discharging lesions as exudate drainage is inhibited
— creams absorb exudate, do not inhibit drainage and are applied as a thin smear
— creams are not substituted for ointments
— creams are not suitable for chronic scaling
— dried out creams are not used because of the increased concentration of medicament
— ointments and creams do not have to be washed off prior to reapplication
— excessive use of soaps, being caustic (alkaline) may damage the protective horny epidermal layer
— replace container caps and lids to reduce escape or contamination of contents and dehydration
— protect clothing where possible

TOPICAL SOOTHING AND PROTECTIVE AGENTS

Action and use

— prevent skin from drying, softens crusts
— lubricate surface to prevent chafing
— protect skin from excoriation

Ingredients

acrylic resin transparent wound dressing, aluminium acetate solution, calamine, calamine with lignocaine, carmellose with gelatin and pectin, coal tar, dimethicone (silicone), glycerine, ichthammol, lanoline, magnesium silicate, methylsalicilate liniment, methylsalycilate liniment with menthol, methylsalicylate liniment with eucalyptus, peppermint ointment, mineral oil, petroleum jelly (white soft paraffin), Pinetarsol, starch, talc, titianium dioxide, triethanolamine with pine tar, urea 10%, vitamin A, vitamin A and D, zinc oxide

Nursing points

— open wet dressings used when a cooling effect desired
— talcum powder used sparingly to prevent any absorption which may result in an undesirable systemic effect
— solutions used to treat generalized itch are added to a half full bath in which the patient soaks for 10–15 minutes, then is patted dry with a soft towel

KERATOLYTICS AND CLEANSERS

Action and use

— remove accumulation of kertinized cells which cause flaking and scaling
— soften horny layer and reduce epidermal thickening (psoriasis)

Ingredients

allantoin, benzalkonium, benzoyl peroxide, cetalkonium, cetrimide, chlorhexidine, chloroxylenol, coal tar, dithranol, gentian violet 0.5%, 1%, hydrogen peroxide, iodine 2%, iodine tincture, mercurochrome, methylated spirit, nitromersol, plasmin (fibrinolysin), podophyllum, potassium permanganate, resorcinol, salicylic acid, selenium sulphide, silver nitrate 0.5%, soaps, sodium hypochlorite, streptokinase-streptodornase, sulphur, tretinoin

Nursing points

— resorcinol may darken fair hair, so ensure that hair is free of soap before applying resorcinol
— skin around a wart being treated with podophyllum is protected with adhesive strapping or petroleum jelly
— apply medicaments gently and sparingly
— avoid contact with eyes and mucous membranes

TOPICAL ANTIBACTERIALS

Use

— impetigo, folliculitis, pyoderma
— prophylactically against infection in burns and ulcers

Ingredients

bacitracin, benzoic acid, cetrimide, chloramphenicol, chlorhexidine, chloroxylenol, chlorquinaldol, chlortetracycline, clioquinol, clotrimazole, colistin, dequalinium, dibromopropamidine, framycetin, fusidic acid, gentamicin, gentian violet, gramicidin, hexachlorophene, hydroxyquinoline, iodine, mafenide, mupirocin, neomycin, nitrofurazone, oxytetracycline, polymyxin B, polynoxylin, povidine-iodine, propamidine, resorcinol, salicylic acid, silver nitrate, silver sulphadiazine, triclosan, tyrocidin

Nursing points

— recurrent inflammation, despite prescribed treatment may indicate sensitivity to an ingredient
— ototoxicity may result from prolonged neomycin irrigation therapy on a large infected wound

Treatment of burns

— 1 jar or tube of silver sulphadiazine cream is reserved for 1 patient, any remaining cream being discarded after completion of treatment
— silver sulphadiazine is applied in a layer 3–5 mm thick using a sterile spatula or a hand covered with a sterile glove

Note

— neomycin, bacitracin and polymyxin B are combined in ointment form and used for impetigo

TOPICAL ANTIFUNGAL AGENTS

Use

— topical mycoses such as tinea, ringworm, moniliasis

Ingredients

amphotericin B, benzoic acid, chlorphenesin, chlorquinaldol, clotrimazole, dithranol, econazole, gentian violet, isoconazole, miconozole, nystatin, polynoxylin, povidine-iodine, salicylic acid, sodium thiosulphate, tolnaftate, triacetin, undecylenic acid, zinc undecanoate

Note

— dithranol may change the colour of fair hair and skin and requires a sensitivity test prior to use

TOPICAL ANTIPARASITICS

Use

— kill lice and scabies

Ingredients

benzyl benzoate, crotamiton, gamma benzene hexachloride, monosulfiram

Nursing points

— see manufacturer's directions for use
— sources of lice infestation are cleared by boiling, ironing or dusting with dicophane powder
— other household members are checked for lice and treated if necessary
— sources of infestation with scabies are soon reduced if clean clothing and bedding are used after treatment and personal hygiene improved
— keep agents away from the eyes

TOPICAL CORTICOSTEROIDS

Action

— penetrate through skin and hair follicles
— suppress inflammation and allergic reactions

Use

— dermatitis, eczema, pruritus, psoriasis

Ingredients

beclomethasone, betamethasone, clobetasone, fluocortin butyl, dexamethasone, fluoclorolone, flucortolone, fludrocortisone, flumethasone, fluocinolone, flurandrenolone, halcinonide, hydrocortisone, triamcinolone

Nursing points

— corticosteroid creams and ointments are applied thinly and not rubbed in
— frequently an occlusive dressing of impermeable polythene is used to maintain a high local concentration
— topical corticosteroids are applied with an applicator, gauze or gloved hand to protect against cutaneous absorption

Note

— topical corticosteroids are used alone or in combination with one or more other preparations such as soothing, cleansing, antibacterial or cell growth stimulant
— topical corticosteroids provide a way of delivering large doses locally without serious systemic effects
— topical corticosteroids increase the risk of infection due to the immunosuppressant action
— lower strength preparations should be used on the face
— topical steroids should not be used on infected areas as they will mask the infection

TOPICAL ANTIHISTAMINES

Use

— allergic dermatoses

Ingredients

mepyramine, promethazine

Adverse effects

— hypersensitivity reactions

TOPICAL HEPARINOID AGENTS

Action

— anticoagulant
— anti-inflammatory
— promote fibrinolysis

Use

— sprains
— haematoma
— superficial thrombosis
— varicose ulcers
— soften scar tissue

Agents

heparinoid, hyaluronidase, nicotinic acid

Nursing points

— not applied to bleeding or infected areas or broken skin
— cream massaged into skin

TOPICAL ANAESTHETICS

Use

— ano-genital pruritus
— painful haemorrhoids
— prior to bronchoscopy, catheterization, cystoscopy

Agents

amylocaine, benzocaine, butyl aminobenzoate, butyl aminobenzoate with nitromersol, cinchocaine, dimethisoquin, fluorochloromethanes, orthocaine and lignocaine which maybe formulated as a solution, spray, jelly or ointment

Note

— repeated topical use of local anaesthetic agents often leads to hypersensitivity reactions, e.g. dermatitis, asthma, anaphylaxis
— see alimentary system for rectal preparations
— topical anaesthetic agent may be used alone or combined with vitamins A, D and E or ephedrine or allantoin

SUNSCREEN AGENTS

Use

- prevent or reduce drug-induced photosensitivity and solar herpes
- reduce sensitivity of certain skin diseases to UV light
- erythropoietic protoporphyria

Agents

β-carotene (oral)
mexenone, padimate,
p-methoxycinnamate

MISCELLANEOUS TOPICAL AGENTS

acriflavine	— disinfectant
allantoin	— stimulates tissue formation
aluminium chloride	— antiperspirant
aminacrine	— disinfectant
boric acid	— weak disinfectant
crotamiton	— antipruritic
dextroanomer	— absorbent for cleansing discharging wounds
dihydroxyacetone	— increases skin pigmentation
diphemanil	— antiperspirant (amputation stump)
ephedrine	— vasoconstrictor
hydroquinone	— reduces skin pigmentation
idoxuridine	— antiviral
magnesium sulphate	— osmotic anti-inflammatory
mequinol	— reduces skin pigmentation
methotrexate	— folic acid antagonist (psoriasis)
methoxsalen	— increases skin pigmentation
monobenzone	— reduces skin pigmentation
panthenol	— promotes healing
phenol	— disinfectant
propantheline	— antiperspirant
pyrithione zinc	— antidandruff
selenium sulphide	— antidandruff
triclosan	— antiperspirant, bacteriostatic
trioxsalen	— increases skin pigmentation
zinc and castor oil	— 'nappy' rash

ORAL DERMATOLOGICAL AGENT

ETRETINATE

Action

— derivative of tretinoin, a metabolite of vitamin A, but less likely to cause hypervitaminosis A
— reverses epidermal proliferation and increased keratinization

Use

— severe psoriasis
— keratinization skin disorders

Dose

0.75–1 mg/kg orally daily in 2–3 divided doses until response, then 0.3–0.6 mg/kg/day

Adverse effects

— dryness of mucous membranes
— hair loss
— paronychia
— transient increase in blood levels of bilirubin, transaminase, alkaline phosphatase and triglyceride

Interactions

— concomitant oral vitamin A could lead to hypervitaminosis A
— increases phenytoin blood levels

Nursing points

— advise patient to avoid taking vitamin A supplements
— advise patient to use a lip salve frequently
— warn patient about the increased susceptibility to sunburn

Note

— etretinate is a potent teratogen , so pregnancy must be avoided during, and for 12 months following cessation of, treatment

14 Drugs acting on the eye

MIOTIC DROPS

Action and use

— constrict pupil and decrease intraocular pressure
— antagonize effects of short acting mydriatic

Parasympathomimetic drugs

acetylcholine, carbachol, pilocarpine

Anticholinesterase drugs

neostigmine, physostigmine (eserine), demecarium, dyflos, ecothiopate, pyrophos

Adverse effects

— blurred vision
— headache

Nursing points

— see at end of chapter

Other agents used to reduce intraocular pressure

Topical

adrenaline, dipivefrin (prodrug of adrenaline), timolol

Note

— adrenaline drops used in simple glaucoma to reduce production of aqueous humour and when instilled 2–3 minutes after a miotic, produce mild mydriasis, so reducing the visual handicap of miosis and ciliary spasm caused by miotics

— absorption of timolol eye drops has resulted in the patient experiencing systemic effects of beta-adrenoceptor blocking agents

Systemic

carbonic anhydrase inhibitors (acetazolamide, dichlorphenamide, methazolamide) (pp. 280, 281) osmotic agents (mannitol, glycerine, urea)

CARBONIC ANHYDRASE INHIBITORS

ACETAZOLAMIDE

Action

Sulphonamide derivative which inhibits the action of carbonic anhydrase resulting in:
— inhibition of secretion of aqueous humour so reduces intraocular pressure
— apparent retardation of abnormal paroxysmal excessive discharge from CNS neurones
— increase in bicarbonate excretion in the renal tubules and consequently sodium, potassium and water excretion resulting in an alkaline diuresis

Use

— adjunctive treatment in chronic simple (open angle) glaucoma, secondary glaucoma and pre-operatively in acute closed angle glaucoma
— some types of epilepsy
— cardiac and drug-induced oedema

Dose

Glaucoma

  i) 250 mg orally 1–4 times/day; OR
 ii) 500 mg orally initially, then 125 or 250 mg 4-hourly; OR
iii) 500 mg orally b.d. (SR); OR
 iv) 500 mg slowly IV over 1 minute (rapid reduction of intraocular pressure)

Epilepsy

250–1000 mg orally daily

Diuretic

250–375 mg orally daily or alternate days

Adverse effects

— drowsiness, paraesthesias, confusion, excitement, hyperpnoea, fatigue, ataxia, headache, dizziness, tinnitus, deafness
— thirst, anorexia
— allergic reactions
— crystalluria, renal calculi
— transient myopia
— rare, but occasionally fatal blood dyscrasias
— prolonged therapy, hypokalaemic acidosis

Interactions

— risk of digoxin toxicity increased by acetazolamide-induced hypokalaemia
— reduces effect of hexamine
— reduces blood doxycycline levels

Note

— parenteral solution prepared by reconstituting with 5 ml Water for Injection
— given IV as IM injection too painful
— effectiveness as a diuretic diminishes with continuous use
— hypokalaemic acidosis corrected by administering bicarbonate

DICHLORPHENAMIDE

Action

— partially suppresses secretion of aqueous humour so reduces intraocular pressure

Use

— adjunctive treatment in chronic simple (open angle) glaucoma, secondary glaucoma and pre-operatively in acute closed angle glaucoma

Dose

100–200 mg orally initially, then 100 mg 12-hourly until response, then maintenance of 25–50 mg 1–3 times/day

Adverse effects

— as for acetazolamide

Interaction

— reduces effect of hexamine

METHAZOLAMIDE

Action

Sulphonamide derivative which is a
potent inhibitor of carbonic anhydrase
secretion resulting in:
— inhibition of secretion of aqueous
  humour so reduces intraocular
  pressure
— increase in bicarbonate excretion in
  renal tubules and consequently
  sodium, potassium, chloride and
  water excretion resulting in a mild
  alkaline diuresis

Use

— chronic simple (open angle)
  glaucoma, secondary glaucoma and
  pre-operatively in acute closed angle
  glaucoma

Dose

50–100 mg orally 2–3 time daily

Adverse effects

— anorexia, nausea, vomiting
— malaise, fatigue or drowsiness,
  headache, vertigo, confusion,
  depression, paraesthesias

MYDRIATIC DROPS

Action

— dilate pupil by stimulating dilator
  muscles of iris

Use

— retinoscopy
— break posterior synechiae

Drugs

adrenaline, cocaine, ephedrine,
phenylephrine

Nursing points

— see at end of chapter (p. 284)

CYCLOPLEGIC MYDRIATIC DROPS

Action

— antimuscarinic drugs, act by blocking the actions of acetylcholine which normally causes miosis and allows accommodation, hence these drugs cause mydriasis and flattening of the lens, hence focussing for distant vision

Use

— retinoscopy in children
— treat uveitis

Drugs

atropine sulphate, cyclopentolate, homatropine, hyoscine, lachesine, tropicamide

Adverse effects

— dilatation of the pupil with loss of accommodation and photophobia
— atropine-like drugs can increase intraocular pressure in patients predisposed to glaucoma
— systemic absorption of atropine-like drugs can result in toxicity (see atropine) (p. 13)

Nursing points

— atropine is *never* put into an eye without a medical officer's order as its effects cannot be reversed quickly and it would cause an increase in intraocular pressure in susceptible patients
— see nursing points at end of chapter (p. 284)

TOPICAL CORTICOSTEROIDS

Agents

betamethasone, dexamethasone, fluorometholone, hydrocortisone, medrysone, methylprednisolone, prednisolone

Nursing points

— topical corticosteroids are *never* put into an eye without a medical officer's order, as healing is impaired, the herpes simplex virus is potentiated resulting in a dendritic ulcer, cataract may start to form in the lens and intraocular pressure may be increased in some patients
— see nursing points at end of chapter (p. 284)

Note

— topical corticosteroids are used alone or in combination with other active ingredients including antibacterial and antifungal agents to treat underlying disease as well as reduce the risk of infection

LOCAL ANAESTHETICS

Agents

amethocaine, cocaine, lignocaine, oxybuprocaine, proxymetacaine (proparacaine)

Nursing points

— local anaesthetics are *never* put into an eye without a medical officer's order, as healing is impaired and secondary bacterial infection is possible

TOPICAL ANTI-INFECTIVE AGENTS

Antibacterials

bacitracin, chloramphenicol, dibromopropamide, framycetin, gentamicin, mafenide propionate, mercuric oxide, neomycin, oxytetracycline, polymyxin B, propamidine, sulphacetamide, sulphafurazole, tetracycline, tobramycin

Antifungal

amphotericin B

Antivirals

acyclovir, idoxuridine, vidarabine

Note

— corticosteroids may be used topically against herpes zoster, but they exacerbate corneal herpes simplex infection
— use only topical ophthalmic preparation of idoxuridine in the eye

Antiseptics

aminacrine, boric acid

TOPICAL NON-STEROIDAL ANTI-INFLAMMATORY AGENTS

Antihistamine

antazoline

Astringents

zinc sulphate with adrenaline, zinc sulphate with phenylephrine

Vasoconstrictors, decongestants

adrenaline, naphazoline, phenylephrine, tetrahydrozaline, xylometazoline

OTHER AGENTS USED IN THE EYE

Diagnostic stains

fluorescein strips and drops, Rose Bengal

Useful for dry eyes

hypromellose, methylcellulose, polyvinyl alcohol

Toxoplasmosis

clindamycin (systemic), pyrimethamine (systemic)

Trachoma and related inclusion conjunctivitis (TRIC)

co-trimoxazole (systemic), sulphacetamide (topical), tetracycline (topical and systemic)

Miscellaneous

chymotrypsin (for cataract extraction)
ethylene diamine tetramine acetate (EDTA, chelating agent used to remove calcium deposits from the cornea)
sodium cromoglycate (optical hay fever)
contact lens preparations
thiotepa (prevents recurrence of pterygium and prevents corneal vascularization after graft)

Nursing points for the treatment of eye conditions

General

— drops or ointment are only put into the eye if ordered by a medical officer, especially drops containing local anaesthetics, atropine-like drugs and corticosteroids
— try to prevent contamination of the container contents
— the presence of pus and other exudates can decrease the effectiveness of anti-infective agents

Instillation of eye drops

— have the patient sitting or lying comfortably
— advise the patient if the drops cause smarting or visual disturbances
— select the correct drug preparation and check which eye is to be treated
— evert the lower lid and ask the patient to look up
— instil the correct number of drops into the lower conjunctival sac midway between the inner and outer canthus avoiding contact of the container with the skin or lashes
— ask the patient to close the eye gently and not squeeze the lids
— systemic absorption may be reduced by compressing the lacrimal sac after instilling the drops
— when separate solutions of a miotic and adrenaline are to be instilled, the adrenaline is instilled 2–10 minutes after the miotic
— check expiry date before use

Insertion of eye ointment

— have the patient sitting or lying comfortably
— advise the patient that the ointment will cause blurred vision

— select the correct drug preparation and check which eye is to be treated
— the first centimetre of ointment from the tube is discarded onto a sterile swab
— evert the lower lid and ask the patient to look up
— commencing at the inner canthus, squeeze the tube and insert the ointment along the lower fornix, ending at the outer canthus avoiding contact of the container with the skin or lashes
— ask the patient to close the eye gently

Application of ointment to lid margins

— crust or exudate is cleaned from lid margins
— ointment is applied directly onto the closed lid and spread gently over the lid margins using a swab

Contact lens preparations

— ensure that the correct solution is used with the particular lens type i.e. either hard lens or soft lens

15 Drugs administered topically to the ear, nose and oropharynx

EAR

Agents are introduced into the ear to treat inflammation, infection and to remove wax.

Analgesics and anaesthetic agents

benzocaine, bismuth iodoform paraffin paste (BIPP), phenazone

Anti-inflammatory agents (non-steroid)

acetic acid, glycerine ichthammol

Anti-infective agents

bacitracin, benzethonium, boric acid, chloramphenicol, chlorhexidine, clioquinol, colistin, dequalinium, framycetin, gramicidin, hydrogen peroxide, hydroxyquinolone, isopropyl alcohol, neomycin, nystatin, oxyquinoline, oxytetracycline, polymyxin B, salicylic acid, sodium propionate

Corticosteroids

betamethasone, dexamethasone, flumethasone, hydrocortisone, prednisolone, triamcinolone

Wax softeners

dichlorobenzene with chlorbutol and turpentine oil (Cerumol), glycerine

Other

ephedrine (decongestant)
isopropyl alcohol (drying)

Note

— agents are often combined, administered as drops, solutions, ointments, creams,

Nursing points

Instillation of ear drops

— patient sits or lies comfortably
— select the correct preparation and check which ear is to be treated
— ensure drops at room temperature
— with the affected ear uppermost, pull the auricle upward and backward to straighten the external auditory canal (if a child, pull the auricle downward)
— instill the required amount of solution into the canal without touching ear with dropper and return dropper to bottle without washing
— press the tragus over the meatus
— position maintained for 2–3 minutes so drops reach ear drum

Insertion of ear ointment

— patient sits or lies comfortably
— select the correct preparation and check which ear is to be treated
— a syringe plunger is removed, the ointment squeezed into the barrel and the plunger replaced
— a special wide bore blunt cannula is attached *firmly* to the syringe
— with the affected ear uppermost, pull the auricle upward and backward to straighten the external auditory canal (if a child, pull the auricle downward)
— the cannula is introduced just inside the canal and the canal filled until ointment appears at the meatus
— alternatively, applied directly from tube supplied with cannula tip

NOSE

Agents are introduced into the nose to treat infection, sinusitis and various types of rhinitis.

Anaesthetics

cocaine 10% with adrenaline 1 in 2000

Anti-infective agents

chlorhexidine, framycetin, gramicidin, neomycin, polymyxin B, silver vitellin

Corticosteroids

beclomethasone, dexamethasone, flunisolide

Sympathomimetic nasal decongestants

ephedrine, methoxamine, naphazoline, oxymetazoline, phenylephrine, phenylpropanolamine, propylhexedrine, tetrahydrozaline, tramazoline, xylometazoline

Other

antazoline, triprolidine (antihistamines), camphor, menthol (nasal decongestants) pseudoephedrine (oral decongestant), sodium cromoglycate (allergic rhinitis prophylaxis)
bismuth iodoform paraffin paste

Note

— two or more types of agents are often combined, administered as drops, creams, jellies, sprays, metered aerosols, etc.
— topical use of sympathomimetic nasal decongestants may cause drug-induced rhinitis
— rebound rhinitis may also be a problem

Nursing points
Instillation of nasal drops

— have the patient recumbent but with a pillow under the shoulders so that the neck is hyperextended to prevent entry of drops into the throat
— select the correct preparation
— ask the patient to breathe through the mouth
— instil the prescribed volume of drops into each nostril, turning the head to the same side as the nostril being dealt with
— maintain the position for several seconds to enable wide coverage of the nasal mucosa

OROPHARYNX

Agents are introduced into the mouth
and throat to treat mouth ulcers,
infections and inflammation.

Analgesics and anaesthetic agents

benzocaine, choline salicylate,
dihydrocodeine, lignocaine solution and
spray (topical), salicylic acid
cocaine mouth wash

Anti-infective agents

amphotericin B, amylmetacresol,
bacitracin, benzalkonium, cetalkonium,
cetylpyridinium, chlorhexidine,
dequalinium, dichlorobenzyl alcohol,
hydrogen peroxide, neomycin,
nitromersol, nystatin, sodium perborate

Corticosteroids

hydrocortisone, triamcinolone

Other

anthraquinone, benzydamine, (anti-
inflammatory)
carbenoxolone, panthenol, carmellose
with gelatin and pectin (mouth ulcers)
clove oil (tooth ache)
idoxuridine, povidone-iodine (herpes
simplex)
thymol (mouth wash)

Note

— two or more types of agent are
  often combined
— these agents are intended for topical
  application and may be formulated as
  sprays, metered aerosols, ointments,
  mouth washes, lozenges, tablets,
  paints, drops, pastes, suspensions,
  gels, lotions, and dental cones

Nursing points

— ensure that analgesic or anaesthetic
  agents are given to patients with
  painful mouth ulcers a few minutes
  before eating
— do not give anything to drink if
  patient has had pharynx
  anaesthetized until at least 1 hour
  after application to prevent aspiration
  of fluid
— if idoxuridine has been prescribed,
  use as early as possible at hourly
  intervals for 24 hours then 4-hourly
— idoxuridine not used during
  pregnancy
— mouth washes are beneficial before
  as well as after meals
— remove dentures where necessary
  to allow access to ulcers

16 Miscellaneous agents

DESFERRIOXAMINE

Action

— chelating agent which forms a non-toxic stable complex (chelate) with iron
— parenteral desferrioxamine removes iron from various iron-containing proteins but not from haemoglobin or iron-containing enzymes, and the chelate is excreted rapidly in the urine and some in bile
— oral desferrioxamine binds iron in the gastrointestinal tract, preventing its absorption in cases of acute iron poisoning

Use

— iron storage disease (haemochromatosis)
— transfusion haemosiderosis in thalassaemia and haemolytic anaemia
— acute iron poisoning

Adult and paediatric dose

i) 1.5–4 g over 12 hours by continuous IV or SC infusion at a maximum rate of 15 mg/kg/hour up to 80 mg/kg/24 hours; OR
ii) 0.5–1 g deeply IM daily as single dose or 2 divided doses, then maintenance dose according to response
iii) in acute poisoning, 5–10 g dissolved in water and given orally or by intragastric tube; AND
iv) 1–2 g deeply IM 3- to 12-hourly; OR
v) 1.5–4 g over 12 hours by continuous IV or SC infusion if severe shock

Adverse effects

— pain and induration at IM site
— pruritus, erythema, swelling (prolonged SC infusion)
— abdominal discomfort, diarrhoea, dysuria
— blurred vision, dizziness, convulsions
— rash, urticaria, fever
— rarely, cataract (prolonged therapy)
— circulatory collapse if too rapid IV

Nursing points

— reconstitute by adding 5 ml sterile water making 10% solution (see manufacturer's literature)
— slight opalescence of reconstituted solution precludes IV use but not IM or SC
— any unused solution discarded after 24 hours
— monitor IV infusion rate closely by using a burette or infusion pump
— continuous SC infusion controlled by battery-operated syringe pump and can be given over 12 hours 6 nights/week
— a reddish discoloration in the urine indicates the presence of excreted iron complex

Note

— in thalassaemia 500 mg desferrioxamine is given IV SC or IM per unit of blood transfused, to minimize iron deposition during blood transfusion
— urinary iron is measured at specified intervals
— also used as diagnostic test for iron-storage disease

DIMERCAPROL (BAL)

Action

— a chelating agent which combines in

the body with arsenic, mercury, and other heavy metals to form stable compounds which are excreted rapidly by the kidneys

Use

— acute poisoning by arsenic, gold, mercury, bismuth, thallium and antimony
— lead poisoning (with sodium calciumedetate)
— hydroxychloroquine overdose

Adult dose

Arsenic or gold poisoning

3–4 mg/kg IM 4-hourly for 48 hours, 6-hourly for 24 hours, then 12-hourly for 10 days or until recovery complete

Mercurial poisoning

5 mg/kg IM initially, then 2.5 mg/kg IM daily or 12-hourly for 10 days

Lead poisoning

3–4 mg/kg IM 4-hourly in combination with sodium calciumedetate for 2–7 days

Hydroxychloroquine overdose

2.4–3 mg/kg 4- to 6-hourly for 3 days then 12-hourly for 10 days

Paediatric dose

3–5 mg/kg IM 4-hourly for 2 days, 2.5–3 mg/kg IM 6-hourly for next 2 days, then 12-hourly for next 7 days; OR 4 mg/kg IM 4-hourly in combination with sodium calciumedetate for 3–7 days (lead poisoning)

Adverse effects

— hypertension, tachycardia
— nausea, vomiting, headache, restlessness
— burning sensation of lips, mouth, throat, eyes
— salivation, lachrymation, rhinorrhoea, sweating
— tingling of extremities
— sensation of constriction of throat and chest
— muscle pain and spasm, abdominal pain
— pain at IM injection site, sterile abscess
— fever, especially in children

Nursing points

— drug stock may become cloudy in cold weather, but will clear if warmed slightly before use
— rotate injection sites, only given IM
— monitor temperature, heart rate and blood pressure noting pyrexia, tachycardia, hypertension
— monitor urinary output, noting oliguria
— urine tested daily for pH and protein

Note

— not used in iron, cadmium or selenium poisoning or if impaired hepatic function
— some adverse effects may be reduced if ephedrine or an antihistamine given ½ hour beforehand
— urine alkalinized to maintain stable complex and so reduce renal damage during elimination
— irritating to skin and mucous membranes and imparts strong garlic-like odour to breath

DISULFIRAM

Action

— interferes with alcohol metabolism by inhibition of aldehyde dehydrogenase, causing an accumulation of acetaldehyde, resulting in the 'aldehyde reaction'
— inhibits hepatic microsomal (drug-metabolizing) enzymes

Use

— deterrent to alcohol consumption in the management of chronic alcoholism under strict medical supervision

Dose

500 mg orally daily initially on waking (nocte if sedative effect) for 1–2 weeks, then 125–500 mg daily

Adverse effects of disulfiram

— drowsiness, lassitude
— psychotic reactions
— peripheral neuropathy

Interactions

— enhances effects of chlordiazepoxide, diazepam, phenytoin, isoniazid and oral anticoagulants

Disulfiram-alcohol reaction

— intense flushing of face and neck accompanied by heat and sweating
— tachycardia, palpitation, dyspnoea
— dizziness, headache
— hypertension initially then hypotension
— nausea, vomiting, abdominal cramps
— exhaustion, then sleep
— severe reactions may result in convulsions and cardiopulmonary arrest

Management of reaction

— ascorbic acid 1 g IV
— chlorpromazine 50–100 mg IM
— resuscitation measures

Nursing points

— patient and relatives or responsible household member must understand the basis of treatment and be informed of the disulfiram-alcohol reaction and its consequences
— the patient is cautioned against taking alcohol or alcohol-containing preparations such as certain cough syrups, sauces, vinegar and food prepared in wine
— alcoholic back-rubs and after-shave lotions should be avoided

Note

— disulfiram should not be given to patients receiving paraldehyde or metronidazole
— therapy commences only after abstinence from alcohol for 24 hours

METHYLENE BLUE

Action

— reduces methaemoglobin in red blood cells to haemoglobin

Use

— treatment of drug-induced methaemoglobinaemia

Dose

1–2 mg/kg by slow IV infusion

Adverse effect (large dose)

— nausea, abdominal and chest pain
— headache, dizziness, mental confusion
— profuse sweating
— formation of methaemoglobin and cyanosis

Note

— also used for the delineation of body structures, e.g. parathyroid glands, fistulae

METYRAPONE

Action

— reduces production of hydrocortisone, corticosterone and aldosterone by the adrenal cortex
— if pituitary feedback control system is intact, also causes a compensatory increase in ACTH resulting in increased hydrocortisone precursor production

Use

— diagnostic agent for assessing anterior pituitary function and adrenocortical function
— antagonize aldosterone production to reduce severe oedema associated with excess aldosterone secretion

Dose

Short single dose text

1–2 g (based on 30 mg/kg) orally at
about midnight with yogurt or milk
8 hours later, blood taken for estimation
of ACTH and/or 11-desoxycortisol and
cortisone acetate 50 mg given
prophylactically

Multiple dose test

Control values of urinary steroid
excretion obtained in 24 hours prior to
test
500–750 mg orally 4-hourly for 6 doses
p.c. or with milk
All urine collected for next 24 hours and
stored at −10°C until analysis

Therapeutic

2.5–4.5 g orally daily in divided doses
usually with a corticosteroid
250 mg–6 g orally daily (Cushing's
syndrome)

Adverse effects

— occasionally, nausea, vomiting,
dizziness, headache, hypotension,
allergic skin reactions

Note

— drugs affecting pituitary or
adrenocortical function must be
withdrawn before the test, e.g.
anticonvulsants, psychoactive drugs,
hormone preparations, anti-thyroid
drugs

PENICILLAMINE

Action

— forms stable complex (chelate) with
heavy metals such as copper, lead,
gold and mercury
— combines with cystine in a more
soluble, readily excretable complex

— beneficial effect on rheumatoid
arthritis

Use

— severe active rheumatoid arthritis
— Wilson's disease (deficiency of
copper-binding protein)
— treatment of heavy metal poisoning
— treatment of cystinuria

Dose

250–2000 mg orally daily depending on
the condition treated taken in divided
doses if dose more than 500 mg/day

Adverse effects

— allergic reaction with rash, fever, joint
pains
— diminution in taste perception
— blood dycrasias including neutropenia
— renal damage including
glomerulonephritis and nephrotic
syndrome especially if taking iron
concomitantly and iron withdrawn
— prolonged use can lead to iron-
deficiency anaemia

Interactions

— enhances urinary excretion of copper,
lead, gold, mercury and other heavy
metals
— oral iron reduces effects of
penicillamine

Nursing points

— check temperature, skin, urine each
day prior to giving drug and note
fever, bruising, rash, sore throat,
proteinuria, or haematuria which
must be reported immediately to the
medical officer as it indicates the
need to stop the drug
— advise patient against abrupt
withdrawal of therapy
— taken with water 1 hour a.c. and 1
hour apart from milk or other drugs

Appendix 1: Drugs in lactation

Most drugs taken by the nursing mother will be excreted to some extent in her milk, the amount ingested by the infant generally being extremely small and harmless. Clinical side effects in the infant are rare and thus the actual presence of a drug in the infant need not be a contraindication to breast-feeding.

Some drugs are concentrated in breast milk relative to the maternal plasma concentration and may be toxic to infants because of the immaturity of hepatic and renal detoxification systems. Also the neonate may be more sensitive than the mother to the drug. The infant may needlessly be exposed to the risk of subsequent allergy if the mother receives allergenic antibiotics, e.g. penicillin.

Administration of the drug at or immediately after the infant nurses will result in the lowest amount of drug in the milk at subsequent feedings. Most drugs probably will not exert a harmful effect on the infant. However, if a potent drug is essential for the mother but of uncertain effect on the infant, it may be necessary to change to artificial feeding.

The infant should always be closely observed for any side effects which, if they occur, should be reported. The following drugs, if prescribed for the mother, may cause adverse effects in the baby.

Drug	Possible effect in infant
alprenolol	observe for signs of beta-blockade, especially bradycardia, hypoglycaemia
ampicillin	diarrhoea, candidiasis
antibiotics	see individual drug
anticonvulsants	see individual drug
antihistamines	no known harmful effects, but single-case report of drowsiness and irritability and refusal to feed; when clemastine used by mother may inhibit lactation due to anticholinergic effects
antipsychotic agents	not contraindicated, but drowsiness or other CNS effects may occur with high dosage or parenteral use
antithyroid drugs	monitor thyroid function in infant

Drug	Possible effect in infant
aspirin	bleeding tendency, possibly rash, acidosis, poor growth, neonatal jaundice which may lead to kernicterus (G6PD deficiency)
atenolol	observe for signs of beta-blockade especially bradycardia, hypoglycaemia
atropine	inhibits lactation and may cause atropine toxicity in infant
barbiturates	high doses, monitor infant for sedation, poor feeding, drowsiness, induces hepatic drug metabolizing enzymes
benzodiazepines	see individual drugs
benzylpenicillin	rash, fever (caution with high injectable dose)
beta-receptor blocking agents	see individual drugs observe for signs of beta-blockade with high dosage
bethanecol	abdominal pain, diarrhoea
bromocriptine	used to suppress lactation, monitor infant growth
caffeine	infant wakefulness and hyperactivity with high doses; suggest taken 4–6 hours before feeding
cascara	diarrhoea
chloral hydrate	drowsiness (high dose) monitor for sedation, poor feeding
chloramphenicol	neonatal jaundice which may lead to kernicterus (G6PD deficiency)
chloroquine	neonatal jaundice which may lead to kernicterus (G6PD deficiency)
chlorpromazine	may cause drowsiness in infant, galactorrhoea in mother
clindamycin	bloody diarrhoea (high dosage)
co-trimoxazole	slight risk from sulpha component neonatal jaundice which may lead to kernicterus (G6PD deficiency)

Drug	Possible effect in infant
dapsone	neonatal jaundice which may lead to kernicterus (G6PD deficiency)
dextropropoxyphene	drowsiness, difficulty with feeding
diazepam	avoid if possible as metabolized slowly in young infants and causes lethargy, difficulty with feeding, weight loss and possibly hyperbilirubinaemia
diphenoxylate	effects may appear in infant
ergot preparations	mutliple doses may suppress lactation, contraindicated in large doses (migraine treatment) vomiting, diarrhoea, unstable blood pressure, convulsions
fluphenazine	not contraindicated, but caution with high dose or parenteral use; potential for drowsiness and other CNS effects
hydroxychloroquine	neonatal jaundice which may lead to kernicterus (G6PD deficiency)
indomethacin	convulsions (high dose)
isoniazid	neonatal jaundice which may lead to kernicterus (G6PD deficiency); theoretical risk of convulsions — prophylactic pyridoxine advisable for mother and infant
labetalol	observe for signs of beta-blockade especially bradycardia, hypoglycaemia
laxatives	docusate could cause diarrhoea in infant
lithium	lithium toxicity syndrome — hypotonia, difficulty in feeding, may inhibit sucking reflex; not recommended
metoprolol	observe for signs of beta-blockade especially bradycardia, hypoglycaemia
metronidazole	loss of appetite, vomiting, diarrhoea rarely, blood dyscrasia; may be given as a single dose and breast-feeding discontinued for 24 hours to allow excretion and so expose infant to minimum amount of drug
nalidixic acid	neonatal jaundice which may lead to kernicterus (G6PD deficiency)

Drug	Possible effect in infant
nicotine	may decrease milk supply and cause nausea and vomiting in infants
nitrazepam	avoid repeated doses; may cause lethargy and weight loss
nitrofurantoin	neonatal jaundice which may lead to kernicterus (G6PD deficiency)
opiates	may cause withdrawal symptoms in infant
oral contraceptives	avoid oestrogen-containing preparations which may suppress lactation
oxprenolol	observe for signs of beta-blockade especially bradycardia, hypoglycaemia
penicillins	possibility of hypersensitivity in infant
phenobarbitone	drowsiness, decreased weight gain, may inhibit sucking reflex methaemoglobinaemia
phenytoin	drowsiness, poor feeding, methaemoglobinaemia
pimozide	monitor infant for excessive drowsiness, normal growth and development
pindolol	observe for signs of beta-blockade especially bradycardia, hypoglycaemia
probenecid	neonatal jaundice which may lead to kernicterus (G6PD deficiency)
procainamide	neonatal jaundice which may lead to kernicterus (G6PD deficiency)
propranolol	observe for signs of beta-blockade especially bradycardia, hypoglycaemia
pyridoxine	avoid dosage above 200 mg/day; may suppress lactation in high dosage; monitor infant growth
quinidine	neonatal jaundice which may lead to kernicterus (G6PD deficiency)
quinine	neonatal jaundice which may lead to kernicterus (G6PD deficiency)

Drug	Possible effect in infant
salicylates (high dose)	metabolic acidosis, rash, may affect platelet function
sotalol	observe for signs of beta-blockade especially bradycardia, hypoglycaemia
streptomycin	diarrhoea, superinfection
tetracycline	possible mottling of teeth
theophylline	irritability, restlessness
thiazides	may cause jaundice, thrombocytopenia
timolol	observe for signs of beta-blockade especially bradycardia, hypoglycaemia
vitamin D	hypercalcaemia

Appendix 2: Poisoning and its treatment

AIM

— assess severity of poisoning
— detect poison or poisons
— remove or neutralize the poison before absorption or corrosion occurs

ACTION

Hospital

— take history, if possible, to ascertain substance ingested and the likely amount
— observe level of consciousness, colour, heart rate, blood pressure and respiratory rate and character
— collect evidence and samples of gastric contents, urine and blood, if required

Home

— take history, if possible, to ascertain substance ingested and the likely amount
— observe level of consciousness, colour, heart rate, peripheral perfusion and respiratory rate and character
— contact Poisons Information Centre, as listed on pages 300–1, for advice as soon as possible
— collect evidence such as drug container and samples of vomitus and urine, if possible

TREATMENT

— *induce vomiting* with ipecacuanha syrup (see table for dose) EXCEPT if patient very drowsy or unconscious, if the poison ingested is an acid, an alkali, a petroleum distillate, a convulsant or drug overdose
— after emesis has occurred, activated charcoal is given, if indicated

Ipecacuanha syrup dose

under 2 years: 15 ml
2–3 years: 20 ml
3–4 years: 25 ml
over 4 years: 30 ml
Follow with large glass of water, lemonade or cordial. Repeat once in 20 minutes if vomiting has not occurred

Activated charcoal

Adsorbs most inorganic and organic compounds in the alimentary tract so reduces or prevents systemic absorption. Given preferably after emptying stomach contents by emesis or wash-out

Adult dose

i) 1 sachet (5 g) suspended in 100 ml water is taken orally as soon as possible after ingestion or suspected ingestion of the potential poison or after induced emesis or stomach washout. Dose repeated at about 20-minute intervals up to a maximum of 50 g if required; or
ii) 30–50 g per $\frac{1}{2}$–1 litre of irrigation water used in stomach washout

Paediatric dose

suspension 100 mg/ml
1–2 g/kg orally or via nasogastric tube,
then 0.5–1 g/kg orally 4-hourly for
12 hours

Note

— reduces emetic activity of
   ipecacuanha so not used
   simultaneously
— concurrent medication should
   preferably be given parenterally
— colours faeces black

Very drowsy or unconscious patient

— maintain clear airway and remove
   patient to hospital

Acid ingestion (includes acids and zinc chloride)

— give large quantities of milk or water,
   milk of magnesia or aluminium
   hydroxide mixture, and olive oil or
   beaten egg whites
— hospital check essential

Alkali ingestion (includes ammonia, drain and oven cleaners and floor strippers)

— give large quantities of milk or water,
   and lemon juice or vinegar and olive
   oil or beaten egg whites
— hospital check essential

Paracetamol ingestion

Acetylcysteine (Parvolex®)

Patients presenting within 15 hours of
ingestion
— obtain urgent blood paracetamol
   levels
— if overdose within last 4 hours
   administer ipecacuanha
— decision to give acetylcysteine made
   on basis of the amount of
   paracetamol ingested and should not
   be delayed pending laboratory results

Dose 150 mg/kg IV in 200 ml 5%
glucose over 15 minutes followed by
continuous infusion of 50 mg/kg in
500 ml in 4 hours, followed by
100 mg/kg in 1 litre over 16 hours. Total
dose 300 mg/kg in 20 hours.
   Note Acetylcysteine ineffective if
given 15 hours after paracetamol
ingestion

Petroleum distillate ingestion (includes petrol, kerosene, lighter fluid, turpentine, paint thinners and dry cleaning fluid)

— give milk
— observe for signs of bronchial
   aspiration of poison

Drug overdose ingestion (aspirin, phenobarbitone, tricyclic antidepressants

— give activated charcoal to adsorb
   poison (see p. 298)

Convulsant ingestion (camphor, strychnine and nicotine)

— give activated charcoal to adsorb
   poison (see p. 298)

Inhaled poison

— move patient into fresh air or admit
   fresh air to area
— hospital check, if required

Poison in contact with skin

— drench contacted area with water for
   at least 15 minutes
— if organophosphorus, will need
   hospital check

Poison in contact with eyes

— wash eyes thoroughly with water for
   at least 15 minutes
— evert the lids to ensure adequate
   removal of agent

Appendix 3: Poisons Information Centres

New South Wales	Poisons Information Centre Royal Alexandra Hospital for Children Pyrmont Bridge Road Camperdown NSW 2050	Sydney (02) 5190466 (008)251525
Victoria	Poisons Information Centre Royal Childrens Hospital Flemington Road Parkville VIC 3052	Melbourne (03) 3455678 (008)133890
Queensland	Brisbane Royal Childrens Hospital Herston Road Herston QLD 4006	Brisbane (07) 2538233 (008)17733
South Australia	Adelaide Childrens Hospital King William Road North Adelaide SA 5006	Adelaide (08) 2677000 (008)182111
Western Australia	Princess Margaret Hospital for Children Thomas Street Subiaco WA 6008	Perth (09) 3811177 (008)119244
Tasmania	Royal Hobart Hospital Liverpool Street Hobart TAS 7000	Hobart (002) 388485 (008)001400
Northern Territory	Royal Darwin Hospital Darwin N.T. 0800	Darwin (089) 274777 (008)251525
Australian Capital Territory	Royal Canberra Hospital Canberra A.C.T. 2601	Canberra (062) 432154
New Zealand	National Poisons and Hazardous Chemicals Information Centre PO Box 913 Dunedin	Dunedin (024) 740999

Hong Kong	Drug and Poisons Information Unit Department of Clinical Pharmacology 9/F, Clinical Sciences Building Prince of Wales Hospital Shatin, New Territories	Hong Kong (852) 0–6363130
United Kingdom	Royal Victoria Hospital Grosvenor Road Belfast BT12 6BA	Belfast (0232) 240503
	West Midlands Poisons Unit Dudley Road Hospital Birmingham B18 7QH	Birmingham (021) 554 3801
	Ambulance Headquarters St Fagans Raod Fairwater Cardiff	Cardiff (0222) 569200
	Royal Infirmary Lauriston Place Edinburgh EH3 9YW	Edinburgh (031) 229 2477
	General Infirmary Great George Street Leeds LS1 3EX	Leeds (0532) 430715
	New Cross Hostpital Avonley Road London SE14 5ER	London (01) 635 9191
	Royal Victoria Infirmary Queen Victoria Road Newcastle upon Tyne NE1 4LP	Newcastle (091) 232 1525
Ireland	Jervis Street Hospital Dublin	Dublin (0001) 745588

Bibliography

Analgesic guidelines 1988 Analgesic Guidelines Sub-Committee, Victoria Drug Usage
Advisory Committee
Antibiotic Guidelines 1987 5th edn. Antibiotic Guidelines Sub-Committee, Standing
Committee on Infection Control, Health Commission of Victoria
Australian Pharmaceutical Formulary and Handbook 1988 14th edn. Pharmaceutical
Association of Australia and New Zealand, South Australia
Batagol R (ed) 1980 The 3AW reference guide on drugs and pregnancy. Royal
Women's Hospital, Melbourne
Bennett V R, Brown L K (eds) 1989 Myles textbook for midwives, 11th edn. Churchill
Livingstone, Edinburgh
Clark J B, Queener S F, Karb V B 1982 Pharmacological basis of nursing practice.
Mosby, St Louis
Cohen M 1984 Diabetes A pocket book of management, 2nd edn. Commonwealth
Serum Laboratories, Parkville
Commonwealth Department of Health 1977 Treatment of tuberculosis with particular
reference to chemotherapy. Recommendations of the National Tuberculosis
Advisory Council, 4th edn.
Goodman L S, Gilman A (eds) 1985 The pharmacological basis of therapeutics, 7th
edn. Macmillan, New York
Govoni L E, Hayes J E 1982 Drugs and nursing implications, 4th edn. Appleton-
Century-Crofts, New York
Hipwell C E, Mashford M L, Robertson M B 1984 Guide to parenteral administration
of drugs. ADIS Health Science Press, Sydney
Immunization procedures 1986 National Health and Medical Research Council, 3rd
edn. Commonwealth Department of Health
Langslow A 1981 A macabre landmark case. The Australian Nurses' Journal
11(1): 23–26
Laurence D R, Bennett P N 1987 Clinical pharmacology, 6th edn. Churchill
Livingstone, Edinburgh
Lowe R F, Wong E E S 1987 Lectures in diseases of the eye, 2nd edn revised.
Royal Victorian Eye and Ear Hospital, Melbourne
Macleod J, Edwards C, Bouchier I (eds) 1988 Davidson's principles and practice of
medicine, 15th edn. Churchill Livingstone, Edinburgh
Miller E A (ed) 1987 A study of the ear, nose and throat for nurses. Royal Victorian
Eye and Ear Hospital, Melbourne
O'Sullivan J 1983 Law for nurses, 3rd edn. Law Book Co, Sydney
Rao J M, Arulappu R G 1984 Drugs and breast feeding Avoiding complications.
Current Therapeutics January 55–58
Reynolds J (ed) 1989 Martindale the extra pharmacopoeia, 29th edn. Pharmaceutical
Press, London
Roberts R (ed) 1988 Mims annual 1988 Intercontinental Medical Statistics
(Australasia), Sydney
Royal Children's Hospital, Melbourne 1985 Paediatric pharmacopoeia, 2nd edn.
Melbourne

Saunders A, Fong L, Elliot P 1988 Mixing premedication drugs in the syringe. The Australian Nurses' Journal 17(9): 38

Society of Hospital Pharmacists of Australia 1985 Pharmacology and drug information for nurses, 2nd edn. W B Saunders Sydney

Speight T M (ed) 1987 Avery's drug treatment. Principles and practice of clinical pharmacology and therapeutics, 3rd edn. Churchill Livingstone, Edinburgh

Thomas J (ed) 1989 Prescription product guide, 18th edn. Australian Pharrnaceutical Publishing, Melbourne

Trinca J C (ed) 1979 CSL medical handbook, 5th edn. Commonwealth Serum Laboratories, Parkville

Warden-Flood J 1984 Handbook for patient medication counselling, 4th edn. Pharmaceutical Society of Australia.

Index and key to proprietary names